LOW FODMAP DIET GUIDE AND COOKBOOK

Alleviate IBS & Digestive Disorders, with Over 100 Science-Backed Recipes. Explore a 28-Day Gut-Healing Journey, Meal Plan and Get Expert Tips.

Emma Greenfield

3+1 EXTRA BONUS
INSIDE THE BOOK

PRACTICAL GUIDE TO LOW FODMAP DIET FOR KIDS
+
DINING OUT CARD for KIDS
and
DINING OUT CARD for ADULTS

2 BONUS IN 1:

PRACTICAL GUIDE to LOW FODMAP DIET for Kids
&
DINING OUT CARD for Adults and Kids

FODMAP GROCERY LIST

FODMAP GROCERY LIST

DAILY SYMPTOMS TRACKER

DAILY SYMPTOMS TRACKER

Scroll to page 18, and SCAN the QR CODE!

Table of Content

Introduction

Purpose of the book

The journey to better health often begins with understanding our bodies and the food we consume. The purpose of this book, "LOW FODMAP DIET GUIDE AND COOKBOOK" is to guide you through a transformative dietary approach known as the low FODMAP diet.

For those who suffer from digestive disorders or have family members who do, the path to relief can feel overwhelming and complex. The information available might be confusing and the dietary guidance can often be conflicting.

That's where this book comes into play. It's designed specifically for three core audiences:

- If you're dealing with IBS or other digestive issues, the principles in this book aim to alleviate your symptoms by offering a clear and scientifically backed dietary plan.
- Parents who are concerned about their family's digestive health will find this book to be a valuable resource. It provides kid-friendly recipes and guidance on creating meals that everyone can enjoy without triggering discomfort.
- If you're someone who values wellness and wants to explore a diet that promotes optimal digestive health, this book offers insights and recipes that align with a health-conscious lifestyle.

What You'll Find Inside

This book is more than just a cookbook; it's a comprehensive guide to the low FODMAP diet. Here's what you'll find:

- An overview of the low FODMAP diet, its principles and benefits.
- A detailed section on which foods to avoid and which to include, ensuring a variety of delicious options.
- Quick and easy-to-follow recipes for breakfast, meat, fish, vegetables, pasta and vegan and vegetarian options, drinks and desserts, including meals for work.
- A 28-day meal plan based on the recipes in the book.
- Tips for managing your diet sustainably, with step-by-step guidance to maximize effectiveness.
- Advice for when eating out or at restaurants, so you can enjoy social occasions without stress.

The "LOW FODMAP DIET GUIDE AND COOKBOOK" is a tool, a friend and a guide that accompanies you on a path to better digestive health. Its purpose is to demystify a complex subject and make it accessible and enjoyable for all who wish to explore this dietary approach.

Welcome to the journey. The path to a more comfortable and joy-filled life with food begins here.

Part I: Understanding the low FODMAP Diet

1. What is the low FODMAP Diet?

A. Definition and Origin

The low FODMAP diet is more than just a trendy dietary approach; it's a scientifically researched and supported pathway to improved digestive health. But what does "FODMAP" mean and where did this diet come from? In this chapter, we will explore the definition and origin of the low FODMAP diet.

What Are FODMAPs?

FODMAP is an acronym that stands for Fermentable Oligosaccharides, Disaccharides, Monosaccharides and Polyols. These are specific types of carbohydrates that are found naturally in a wide variety of foods, including fruits, vegetables, grains and dairy products.

While these carbohydrates are part of a regular diet for many people, some individuals find them difficult to digest. They may ferment in the large intestine, leading to symptoms like bloating, gas, abdominal pain, diarrhea and constipation.

Definition of the low FODMAP Diet

The low FODMAP diet focuses on reducing the intake of these fermentable carbohydrates to alleviate digestive symptoms. It's not about eliminating them completely but rather understanding which foods contain high levels of FODMAPs and moderating or substituting them with low FODMAP alternatives.

The diet typically involves three phases:

1. **Elimination Phase**: Temporarily removing high FODMAP foods.
2. **Reintroduction Phase**: Gradually reintroducing them to identify personal triggers.
3. **Personalization Phase**: Creating a long-term dietary plan based on individual tolerances.

Origin of the low FODMAP Diet

The low FODMAP diet was developed by researchers at Monash University in Australia in the early 2000s. The diet was created after recognizing that certain carbohydrates were common triggers for digestive discomfort, particularly for those with Irritable Bowel Syndrome (IBS).

Under the guidance of Dr. Sue Shepherd, the team conducted extensive research to identify which foods were high or low in FODMAPs. Their findings have since been validated by numerous scientific studies around the world.

Adoption and Global Reach

Since its inception, the low FODMAP diet has gained international recognition and adoption. Healthcare professionals, particularly dietitians and gastroenterologists, now often recommend this diet as a management strategy for IBS and other functional gastrointestinal disorders (FGIDs).

The adoption and global reach of the low FODMAP diet has been increasing over the last few years. As awareness of irritable bowel syndrome (IBS) and other digestive disorders grows, so does the interest in effective dietary interventions such as the low FODMAP diet.

Alongside awareness, accessibility to low FODMAP foods and resources has improved. Supermarkets, health food stores, and online platforms now offer products explicitly labelled as low FODMAP. Moreover, the availability of apps, books, and online guides has made it easier for individuals to embark on this dietary journey regardless of their geographical location.

B. Principles of the low FODMAP Diet

1. Understanding FODMAPs

It can be a challenge to determine which foods are safe to eat as part of a low FODMAP diet. The low FODMAP list in this book provides an easy-to-understand summary of high and low FODMAP foods that are safe to eat individually. What happens when you eat adequate amounts of foods from the low FODMAP list? If IBS symptoms begin, we look at the concept of FODMAP stacking.

FODMAP stacking occurs when low FODMAP foods are consumed with other low FODMAP foods that surpass an individual's threshold, known as "dose response", leading to IBS symptoms. As the threshold varies from person to person, it is essential to consult a dietician, maintain a food diary, and customize an individual low FODMAP food list by adjusting the food amount based on one's symptoms

Some foods have shown no detectable levels of FODMAPs in testing. Therefore, you can consume them more frequently. The list of **FODMAP-free foods** to mitigate FODMAP stacking is provided in the following chapters.

2. Phases of the Diet

The low FODMAP diet is typically implemented in three main phases: the **Elimination phase**, the **Reintroduction Phase** and the **Personalization Phase**. During the elimination phase, all high FODMAP foods are excluded from the diet for a set period, usually 4–6 weeks, to allow the gut to heal. This phase is usually followed by the more complex reintroduction phase, where individual FODMAPs are gradually reintroduced to identify personal triggers and individual tolerance levels. This step-by-step process is essential in identifying personal triggers and developing the personalization phase, a long-term eating plan that minimizes discomfort, considering individual sensitivities and preferences.

3. Individualized Approach and Balanced Nutrition

Every person's body is different and so an individualized approach is key to the success of the low FODMAP diet. What might be a trigger food for one person may be well-tolerated by another. Working with healthcare professionals, such as dietitians, to create a tailored plan allows for adjustments based on personal preferences, cultural considerations and specific nutritional needs, leading to a more sustainable and effective dietary regimen. While focusing on FODMAPs, it's essential not to overlook overall nutrition. Balanced nutrition involves including a variety of foods that provide essential nutrients, even while following dietary restrictions. This can be challenging on a low FODMAP diet, but with careful planning and perhaps supplementation as advised by a healthcare provider, it is possible to meet all nutritional needs without triggering gastrointestinal symptoms, also finding suitable low FODMAP alternatives for high FODMAP foods rather than merely excluding them.

4. Mindfulness and Patience

One of the key aspects of mindfulness in this diet involves keeping track of symptoms and dietary intake to understand personal triggers. A detailed food diary, documenting both food intake and any corresponding symptoms, can be invaluable in identifying the specific foods or ingredients that might be causing discomfort. By reflecting on this information, one can create a more personalized diet plan that suits individual needs and sensitivities. Understanding that results may take time is crucial to success. The process of eliminating and reintroducing foods requires careful observation and adaptation. During this time, it may be tempting to rush the process or become frustrated with the pace of progress. However, this journey towards digestive comfort is often gradual and patience enables a more thoughtful, intentional approach that considers the complexity of individual responses to different foods.

5. Holistic Approach

A holistic approach recognizes that the low FODMAP diet is just one part of a broader strategy for managing digestive health. This includes considering not only food but also lifestyle factors like stress management, exercise and sleep. Working with a healthcare team that includes specialists in various fields can provide comprehensive support that looks at the whole person and not just individual symptoms.

C. Benefits for Digestive Health

The low FODMAP diet has emerged as a valuable tool in the management and alleviation of various digestive symptoms. In this chapter, we will delve into the specific benefits for digestive health that this diet can offer.

1. Alleviation of IBS Symptoms

- **Reduction in Bloating**: By minimizing the intake of fermentable carbohydrates, the low FODMAP diet can lead to a noticeable decrease in abdominal bloating.
- **Relief from Constipation and Diarrhea**: By regulating the digestive tract's response to certain foods, this diet can help normalize bowel movements.

2. Improvement in Overall Digestive Comfort

- **Less Gas and Pain**: The reduced fermentation in the gut minimizes gas production, leading to less discomfort and cramping.
- **Enhanced Gut Motility**: The diet promotes smoother passage of food through the digestive system, easing sensations of fullness and pressure.

3. Identification of Personal Triggers

- **Tailored Approach**: The phased approach helps identify specific foods or food groups that might cause symptoms, allowing for a personalized dietary plan.
- **Increased Dietary Awareness**: Building a deeper understanding of how different foods affect your body can lead to more conscious and satisfying food choices.

4. Support for Other Digestive Disorders

- **Management of Inflammatory Bowel Disease (IBD)**: Though not a cure, the low FODMAP diet can support the management of conditions like Crohn's Disease and Ulcerative Colitis.
- **Help for Functional Dyspepsia**: The diet may alleviate symptoms like stomach pain and burning, particularly when used in conjunction with medical treatment.

5. Holistic Wellness and Lifestyle Alignment

- **Emphasis on Whole Foods**: Encouraging the consumption of natural, unprocessed foods supports overall health and well-being.
- **Alignment with Other Dietary Preferences**: The diet can be adapted to suit vegan, vegetarian, gluten-free, or other specific dietary needs.

6. Enhancement of Mental and Emotional Well-being

- **Reduction in Anxiety Related to Eating**: Knowing which foods to avoid and having a plan can reduce meal-related stress.
- **Improved Quality of Life**: Alleviating chronic digestive discomfort can lead to a more active and joyful life.

D. How it Alleviates Symptoms of IBS and Other Digestive Disorders

Irritable Bowel Syndrome (IBS) and other digestive disorders are multifaceted conditions that can significantly impact an individual's quality of life. Symptoms like bloating, gas, constipation, diarrhea and abdominal pain can be persistent and frustrating. The low FODMAP diet has become a renowned approach for alleviating these symptoms and this chapter will delve into how the diet works to provide relief for IBS sufferers and those with other digestive issues.

IBS is a chronic disorder characterized by recurring abdominal pain and changes in bowel habits, often without a known organic cause. Other disorders like Functional Dyspepsia, Crohn's Disease and Ulcerative Colitis also present with digestive discomfort. These conditions are complicated and may lead to significant daily challenges for those affected by them.

A major factor in the development of these symptoms is the role of FODMAPs. High FODMAP foods can cause increased fermentation in the gut, leading to gas and bloating. Additionally, these carbohydrates may draw water into the gut, causing diarrhea or contributing to constipation. Some individuals may have heightened gut sensitivity to FODMAPs, leading to abdominal pain and discomfort, further compounding the issue.

The low FODMAP diet addresses these challenges by reducing fermentable carbohydrates. By limiting foods that contain FODMAPs, the diet reduces the substrates for fermentation, thus decreasing gas production. The dietary approach also controls osmotic effects, helping to normalize bowel habits. Crucially, the phased approach of the diet allows for the identification of specific triggers, leading to a personalized and sustainable dietary plan that can make a real difference for many sufferers.

Evidence and research back up the diet's efficacy. Numerous clinical trials have supported the positive effects of the low FODMAP diet in reducing IBS symptoms and gastroenterologists and dietitians worldwide recommend this approach for suitable patients.

However, it's vital to recognize that the diet is not a cure for underlying conditions. It serves as a management tool and must be implemented with professional guidance. Working with a healthcare provider specialized in the low FODMAP diet ensures that it's suitable for the individual's condition and that essential nutrients are not lacking. The diet often works best in conjunction with other medical therapies and lifestyle modifications and an integrated approach may provide the most significant relief for those struggling with IBS and related disorders.

2. Foods to Include

A. List and explanation of safe ingredients

Navigating the low FODMAP diet requires careful attention to ingredients that can be enjoyed without triggering digestive discomfort. Below is a detailed list and explanation of safe ingredients within various food categories.

The underlined foods in the following list are identified as being free from FODMAPs. These foods are safe to eat because they do not contain FODMAPs, and the amounts can also be consumed without worry.

Fruits

- **Breadfruit**
- **Bananas (unripe)**: they contain less fermentable sugars than ripe ones.
- **Clementines, Lemon, Mandarins and Oranges (navel)**: citrus fruits that are low in FODMAPs.
- **Kiwi, Passion Fruit, Papaya, Coconut and Pineapple**: tropical choices that are FODMAP-friendly.
- **Papaya**
- **Strawberries, Raspberries and Blueberries**: sweet options for desserts or breakfast.

Vegetables

- **Alfalfa**
- **Bamboo shoots**
- **Beansprouts**
- **Ginger and Rhubarb**
- **Olives**
- **Carrots, Parsnips and Radish**: great for roasting or in soups.
- **Cucumbers, Red Bell Peppers, Eggplant and Zucchini**: ideal for grilling or stir-frying.
- **Broccoli, Cabbage, Lettuce (iceberg, red coral, butterhead, rocket), Kale and Spinach**: nutrient-rich leafy greens.
- **Potatoes, Pumpkin and Tomatoes**: versatile and filling, suitable for numerous dishes.

Proteins

- **Meat and Poultry**: most fresh, unprocessed meats are low in FODMAPs.
- **Canned fish**: (e.g. tuna, sardines)
- **Fish and Seafood**: fresh fish and shellfish are safe.
- **Eggs**: perfect for breakfast or adding protein to salads.
- **Firm Tofu**: unlike softer varieties, it's low in fermentable carbs.

Grains

- **Rice**: brown or white, a safe staple in many diets.
- **Oats**: ideal for breakfast, ensure they are gluten-free.
- **Quinoa**: a protein-rich grain that's versatile.
- **Sourdough Spelt Bread**: a low FODMAP bread option.

Dairy Alternatives

- **Lactose-free Milk and Yogurt**: created to remove or break down lactose.
- **Hard Cheeses**: such as Parmesan or Feta, which has less lactose.
- **Plant-based Alternatives**: almond or coconut milk without additives.

Nuts and Seeds

- **Walnuts, Almonds, Hazelnuts, Peanuts and Macadamia Nuts**: healthy fats and crunchy textures.
- **Chia, Pumpkin and Sunflower Seeds**: excellent in baking or as toppings.

Beverages

- **Water and Herbal Teas**: always safe and hydrating.
- **Coffee and Tea**: generally safe in moderate amounts, watch for additives.

Herbs and Spices

- **Fresh Herbs**: such as basil, chives, thyme, mint, parsley or rosemary.
- **Spices**: like ginger, saffron, cumin or turmeric to enhance flavors.

Condiments

- **Butter and Ghee**
- **Mustard, Vinegar and Soy Sauce (Gluten-Free)**: for added flavor.
- **Oils** (e.g. olive, coconut, sesame, sunflower)
- **Garlic-Infused Oil and Onion-Infused Oil**: FODMAPs are not soluble in oil, so infused oils are safe.
- **Seaweed (nori)**

Snacks

- **Popcorn and Rice Cakes**: light snacks that won't weigh you down.

– IN THE BONUSES YOU WILL FIND A COMPLETE LIST OF SAFE FOOD PRODUCTS TO HELP YOU WHEN YOU GO TO THE GROCERY STORE –

B. Importance of portion sizes

The understanding and management of portion sizes in a low FODMAP diet are central to success, balancing both physical well-being and satisfaction in eating. Some foods contain FODMAPs in quantities that are tolerable in smaller servings but may trigger symptoms in larger portions. This highlights the need to understand personal sensitivity. Everyone has a different threshold for FODMAPs and understanding portion sizes helps tailor the diet to individual sensitivities.

It may take some trial and error to find the right portion sizes that do not trigger symptoms. Recording reactions in a food diary can be a very effective way to track what works and what doesn't. Personalization is key and a dietitian can guide adjustments to portion sizes based on individual needs, preferences and reactions.

Practical Tips

Monash University has given some advice on how to avoid FODMAP stacking. Here's what you can do to avoid it:

- **Space out your meals by leaving 3 to 4 hours in between.** This helps reduce the additive effects of FODMAPs. If you feel hungry, try snacking on FODMAP-free foods.

- **Snack on FODMAP-free foods to avoid stacking issues.** These foods are free of FODMAPs and ideal for snacking between meals. Check the list below for examples of FODMAP-free foods.

- **Try to eat more foods that are naturally low in FODMAPs.** This way, you won't need to worry as much about combining them. Actually, many foods contain very few FODMAPs, even if you eat a lot of them. Some examples of foods that are naturally low in FODMAPs are rice, carrots, and meat, fish, or eggs.

- **Keep an eye on your fruit intake.** Eating too much fruit, especially at one time, may increase your risk of FODMAP-related bloating. Limit your total fruit intake to two servings per day and eat only one serving of low-FODMAP fruit per meal.

- **Eating a variety of foods is important.** Try to avoid eating the same meal or foods repeatedly to prevent FODMAPs stacking. Keep in mind that FODMAP-free protein sources include plain meat, chicken, fish, and eggs.

- **Relax, and don't stress out if you inadvertently exceed the recommended low FODMAPs servings.** It's not going to wipe out all your progress. If you do feel any symptoms, take care of yourself, do some self-care measures to alleviate discomfort, and start with a fresh mindset tomorrow.

- **Lactose is not involved in the stacking process.** Lactose only affects people with IBS who are also lactose intolerant, because it is digested differently than other FODMAPs. If you are lactose intolerant, stick to the lactose-free servings on the FODMAPs list and stacking will be no problem.

The low FODMAP diet is not just about eliminating certain foods; it's about balance, personalization and enjoyment. By understanding and controlling portion sizes, you can enjoy a more varied, nutritious and satisfying diet, promoting overall well-being.

3. Foods to Avoid

The low FODMAP diet's success rests not only on understanding what to include but also on what to avoid. Certain foods contain higher levels of FODMAPs and can act as triggers for those sensitive to these compounds. This chapter elucidates the high FODMAP foods and common triggers, along with suggestions for substitutes and alternatives.

A. List of high FODMAP foods and common triggers

Understanding what foods to avoid on the low FODMAP diet is essential to successfully managing digestive symptoms. Here's a detailed breakdown of high FODMAP foods and common triggers:

Fruits

- **Apples, Pears and Dates**: high in fructose.
- **Mangoes and Watermelon**: contain multiple types of FODMAPs.
- **Cherries and Blackberries**: known to trigger symptoms.
- **Peaches, Apricots, Grapefruits and Plums**: contain sorbitol, a sugar alcohol.

Vegetables

- **Onions and Garlic**: found in many dishes, high in fructans.
- **Brussels Sprouts, Asparagus and Artichokes**: also rich in fructans.
- **Savoy Cabbage and Cauliflower**: can cause issues in larger servings.
- **Mushrooms**: contain polyols, known as sugar alcohols.

Dairy Products

- **Milk**: especially cow's milk, high in lactose.
- **Soft Cheese**: includes ricotta and cottage cheese.
- **Yogurt with Lactose**: check labels carefully.
- **Ice Cream**: high in lactose and sometimes added sweeteners.

Grains

- **Wheat and Rye**: bread, pasta and pastries are typical culprits.
- **Couscous and Barley**: can lead to discomfort.
- **Certain Breakfast Cereals**: containing wheat or high-fructose corn syrup.

Legumes

- **Beans**: baked beans, kidney beans and others.
- **Lentils**: particularly in large portions.
- **Soy Products**: such as soy milk made from whole soybeans.

Sweeteners

- **Honey**: rich in fructose.
- **Agave Syrup**: even higher in fructose than honey.
- **High Fructose Corn Syrup**: common in sodas and processed foods.
- **Xylitol and Sorbitol**: often found in sugar-free gum and mints.

Beverages

- **Sodas with High Fructose**: such as those sweetened with apple juice.
- **Milk-Based Drinks**: like lattes or cappuccinos.
- **Some Alcoholic Beverages**: beer, rum and sweet wines.

Processed Foods

- **Ready-made Meals**: often contain hidden FODMAPs.
- **Sauces and Gravies**: many contain onion, garlic or wheat.
- **Certain Snacks**: such as granola bars with honey or chicory root.

Nuts and Seeds

- **Cashews**: high in FODMAPs.
- **Pistachios**: known to cause problems for some.

– IN THE BONUSES YOU WILL FIND A COMPLETE LIST OF FOODS TO AVOID, TO MAKE HEALTHIER CHOICES AND PREVENT DISCOMFORT –

B. Substitutes and alternatives

The low FODMAP diet's success doesn't mean a lifetime of bland and restrictive eating. With a bit of knowledge and creativity, one can easily replace high FODMAP foods with delicious alternatives. Here's a more detailed look at substitutes and alternatives:

Fruits

- **Instead of Apples and Pears**: use unripe bananas, strawberries, oranges or kiwi.
- **Sorbitol-rich Fruits**: replace with grapes, pineapples or cantaloupe.

Vegetables

- **For Onions and Garlic**: use garlic-infused oil or chives.
- **Instead of High-Fructan Veggies**: use carrots, green beans, potatoes or spinach.

Dairy Products

- **Instead of Milk**: lactose-free milk, almond milk or coconut milk.
- **For Soft Cheese**: hard cheeses like cheddar or lactose-free varieties.
- **Yogurt Alternatives**: lactose-free yogurt or coconut-based yogurt.

Grains

- **For Wheat and Rye**: try quinoa, rice, oats or gluten-free bread.
- **Instead of Couscous and Barley**: polenta, rice noodles or buckwheat.

Legumes

- **For Beans and Lentils**: canned and well-rinsed chickpeas or lentils in small portions.
- **Instead of Soy Products**: almond or coconut milk or tofu (firm and drained).

Sweeteners

- **Instead of Honey or High Fructose Corn Syrup**: maple syrup, pure cane sugar or stevia.
- **For Xylitol and Sorbitol**: erythritol or sugar alcohols that are tolerated better.

Beverages

- **Sodas**: opt for sodas without high fructose corn syrup.
- **Instead of Milk-Based Drinks**: black coffee, tea or using lactose-free milk.
- **Alcoholic Beverages**: stick to wine, vodka, gin or whiskey in moderation.

Processed Foods

- **Ready-made Meals**: cook using fresh, low FODMAP ingredients.
- **Sauces and Gravies**: homemade versions using safe spices and herbs.
- **Snacks**: nut butter without additives, rice cakes or suitable nuts like almonds.

Nuts and Seeds

- **Instead of Cashews and Pistachios**: walnuts, macadamia or pumpkin seeds.

Whether one is new to the diet or looking to broaden their culinary horizons, these alternatives offer a path to enjoying food fully while maintaining adherence to the dietary guidelines. By embracing these substitutes, individuals can create satisfying meals that nourish the body, please the palate and contribute to overall digestive health and well-being.

SCAN THE QR CODE

SCAN ME

OR COPY AND PASTE THE URL:

http://bit.ly/3KIK5mL

Part II: Quick & Easy Recipes

These recipes are carefully crafted to exclude high FODMAP foods and triggers while making the most of the safe ingredients and alternatives recommended for the low FODMAP diet.

Note: Nutritional values are approximate and may vary based on the specific ingredients used.

1. Quick & Easy Breakfast

French Toast with Strawberries and Lactose-Free Cream Cheese

Prep Time: 15 minutes; Cook Time: 10 minutes; Serving Size: 2 slices; Servings: 2

Ingredients:

- 4 slices gluten-free and low FODMAP bread
- 1/2 cup lactose-free cream cheese, softened (make sure it's low FODMAP)
- 2 tbsp maple syrup
- 1 tsp vanilla extract
- 2 large eggs
- 1/2 cup lactose-free milk or other low FODMAP dairy alternative
- 1/2 tsp cinnamon
- Pinch of salt
- 1 cup fresh strawberries, sliced
- Maple syrup, for serving
- Fresh mint leaves, to decorate

Instructions:

1. In a bowl, mix the soft cheese, syrup and vanilla extract until everything is well combined. This will be used as the filling for the French toast.
2. Spread the cheese mixture on two slices of bread and then put the other two slices on top to make sandwiches.
3. In a small bowl, mix the eggs, milk, cinnamon, and a bit of salt together using a whisk.
4. Dip all the sandwiches into the egg mixture and make sure to coat both sides well.
5. In a nonstick skillet or on a griddle, melt a small quantity of butter over medium heat.. Put the dipped sandwiches on the skillet and cook each side for 2-3 minutes, until they turn golden brown.
6. Serve the cooked French toast on plates. Add sliced strawberries on top and drizzle with maple syrup. Decorate the dish with fresh mint leaves.

Nutritional Facts (per serving): Calories: 360 | Total Fat: 13g | Saturated Fat: 5g | Trans Fat: 0g | Cholesterol: 160mg | Sodium: 460mg | Total Carbohydrates: 50g | Dietary Fiber: 5g | Sugars: 18g | Protein: 13g | Vitamin A: 15% | Vitamin C: 40% | Calcium: 20% | Iron: 15%

Quinoa Breakfast Bowl with Nuts and Citrus (Vegan)

Prep Time: 15 minutes; Cook Time: 15 minutes; Serving Size: 1 bowl; Servings: 2

Ingredients:
- 1 cup quinoa, rinsed
- 2 cups water
- Zest and juice of 1 orange
- 1/4 cup mixed nuts (e.g., almonds, peanuts), chopped
- 2 tbsp unsweetened shredded coconut
- 2 tbsp chia seeds
- 1 tbsp maple syrup (optional)
- Fresh berries for topping

Instructions:
1. Mix the quinoa and water in a medium-sized saucepan. Bring to a boil, then reduce the heat to low. Cover and let it simmer for approximately 15 minutes, or until the quinoa is tender and the water is fully absorbed.
2. When cooked, fluff the quinoa with a fork and stir in the orange zest and juice.
3. In a dry skillet over medium heat, toast the mixed nuts and shredded coconut until lightly golden and fragrant. Set aside.
4. In a small bowl, combine the chia seeds with 4 tablespoons water. Let sit for a few minutes until they form a gel-like consistency.
5. To assemble, divide the cooked quinoa into two serving bowls.
6. Drizzle with maple syrup if desired.
7. In each bowl, spoon the chia seed mixture over the quinoa.
8. Top with toasted nuts, shredded coconut and fresh berries.

Nutritional Facts (per bowl): Calories: 380 | Total Fat: 15g | Saturated Fat: 4g | Trans Fat: 0g | Cholesterol: 0mg | Sodium: 10mg | Total Carbohydrates: 53g | Dietary Fiber: 11g | Sugars: 11g | Protein: 12g | Vitamin D: 0% | Calcium: 10% | Iron: 20% | Potassium: 550mg

Low FODMAP Granola

Prep Time: 10 minutes; Cook Time: 20-25 minutes; Serving Size: about 1/2 cup; Servings: 8

Ingredients:
- 2 gluten-free and low FODMAP rolled oats
- 1/2 cup shredded coconut (unsweetened)
- 1/2 cup mixed nuts and seeds (e.g., almonds, walnuts, pumpkin seeds, sunflower seeds)
- 1/4 cup pure maple syrup
- 2 tbsp melted coconut oil
- 1 tsp vanilla extract
- 1/2 tsp ground cinnamon
- A pinch of salt
- 1/2 cup dried cranberries (optional, make sure it's low FODMAP)

Instructions:
1. Heat your oven to 325°F (165°C). Cover a baking sheet with parchment paper.
2. In a big bowl, put rolled oats, shredded coconut, mixed nuts, and seeds together. Stir until the ingredients are well combined.

3. Take another bowl and mix pure maple syrup, melted coconut oil, vanilla extract, ground cinnamon, and a pinch of salt.
4. Mix the wet mixture with the dry ingredients until everything is coated evenly.
5. Put the mixture on the baking sheet making sure it's spread evenly. Press the mixture lightly to create a smooth surface.
6. Put the baking sheet in the preheated oven and bake for 20 to 25 minutes until it becomes golden brown and fragrant. Stir the granola during halfway through baking to evenly brown.
7. After baking, remove the granola from the oven and allow it to cool completely on the baking sheet. The granola will become crispier as it cools.
8. Add dried cranberries to the cooled granola and mix well.

Keep the low FODMAP granola in a sealed container at room temperature for best results. Eat with lactose-free yogurt, in parfaits, or as a crunchy topping on your breakfast!

Nutritional Facts (per serving - about 1/2 cup): Calories: 220 | Total Fat: 12g | Saturated Fat: 5g | Trans Fat: 0g | Cholesterol: 0mg | Sodium: 10mg | Total Carbohydrates: 27g | Dietary Fiber: 4g | Sugars: 10g | Protein: 4g | Vitamin D: 0% | Calcium: 2% | Iron: 8% | Potassium: 120mg

Strawberry and Chia Overnight Oatmeal (Vegan)

Prep Time: 10 minutes; Serving Size: 1 jar; Servings: 2

Ingredients:
- 1 cup gluten-free and low FODMAP rolled oats
- 2 tbsp chia seeds
- 1 ½ cups unsweetened almond milk or other low FODMAP dairy alternative
- 1 cup fresh strawberries, sliced
- 1 tbsp maple syrup (optional, for sweetness)
- 1/2 tsp vanilla extract
- A pinch of salt

Instructions:
1. Combine the rolled oats, chia seeds, almond milk, vanilla extract, and a pinch of salt in a mixing bowl. Stir the mixture thoroughly.
2. Add maple syrup to the mixture, if desired, and stir to combine. Adjust the sweetness to your liking.
3. Separate the mixture into two jars or containers with airtight lids.
4. Close the containers tightly and put them in the refrigerator for at least four hours, or overnight, so that the oats and chia seeds can soak up the liquid.

Before serving:
1. Remove the containers from the fridge.
2. Mix the oats thoroughly to ensure they are even and creamy.
3. Add sliced strawberries to each serving.

Nutritional Facts (per serving): Calories: 250 | Total Fat: 8g | Saturated Fat: 1g | Trans Fat: 0g | Cholesterol: 0mg | Sodium: 80mg | Total Carbohydrates: 40g | Dietary Fiber: 10g | Sugars: 6g | Protein: 8g | Vitamin D: 0% | Calcium: 35% | Iron: 15% | Potassium: 10%

Buckwheat Porridge with Kiwi and Cinnamon (Vegan)

Prep Time: 5 minutes; Cook Time: 15 minutes; Serving Size: 1 bowl; Servings: 2

Ingredients:
- 1 cup raw buckwheat groats
- 2 cups water
- 1 cup almond milk or other low FODMAP dairy alternative
- 2 tbsp maple syrup
- 1/2 tsp ground cinnamon
- 1/4 tsp ground nutmeg (optional)
- 1/4 tsp salt
- 2 kiwis, peeled and diced
- 1/4 cup chopped nuts (e.g., walnuts, pecans), toasted
- 2 tbsp unsweetened shredded coconut (optional)

Instructions:
1. Rinse the buckwheat groats under cold water and drain.
2. Bring 2 cups of water to a boil in a saucepan. Add the rinsed buckwheat groats and reduce heat to low. Cover and simmer for about 15 minutes, or until the buckwheat is tender and the water is absorbed.
3. Stir in the almond milk, maple syrup, ground cinnamon, ground nutmeg (if using), and salt. Simmer for another 5 minutes, stirring occasionally. Remove from heat and allow to thicken for a few minutes.
4. Divide the mixture into bowls. Top each bowl with diced kiwi, a sprinkling of chopped nuts or seeds, and fresh mint leaves for a burst of freshness.

Nutritional Facts (per serving - 1 bowl): Calories: 320 | Total Fat: 7g | Saturated Fat: 0.5g | Trans Fat: 0g | Cholesterol: 0mg | Sodium: 150mg | Total Carbohydrates: 61g | Dietary Fiber: 9g | Sugars: 18g | Protein: 8g | Vitamin D: 25% | alcium: 20% | Iron: 15% | Potassium: 700mg

Mixed Berry Smoothie Bowl with Lactose-Free Yogurt

Prep Time: 10 minutes; Cook Time: 0 minutes; Servings: 2

Ingredients:
- 2 cups mixed berries (e.g., strawberries, blueberries, raspberries)
- 1 cup lactose-free yogurt (make sure it's low FODMAP)
- 2 small unripe bananas, frozen
- 1/2 cup low FODMAP granola
- 2 tbsp chia seeds
- 2 tbsp shredded coconut
- Fresh mint leaves for garnish (optional)

Instructions:
1. Place the mixed berries, yogurt and frozen banana
2. Blend carefully until the mixture is smooth and creamy. Add a small amount of water or milk if necessary to achieve the desired consistency.
3. Pour the smoothie into a bowl and serve.
4. Top with low FODMAP granola, chia seeds, shredded coconut and fresh mint leaves, if desired.

Nutritional Facts (per serving): Calories: 300 | Total Fat: 10g | Saturated Fat: 3g | Trans Fat: 0g | Cholesterol: 5mg | Sodium: 50mg | Total Carbohydrates: 47g | Dietary Fiber: 10g | Sugars: 22g | Protein: 10g | Vitamin D: 10% | Calcium: 20% | Iron: 10% | Potassium: 540mg

Muffin Tin Egg Cups with Red Bell Peppers and Zucchini (Vegetarian)

Prep Time: 15 minutes; Cook Time: 20 minutes; Serving Size: 3 egg cups; Servings: 2

Ingredients:
- 6 large eggs
- 1/4 cup lactose-free milk or other low FODMAP dairy alternative
- 1/2 cup diced red bell peppers
- 1/2 cup diced zucchini
- 1/4 cup chopped fresh chives
- Salt and pepper to taste
- 1/4 cup shredded lactose-free cheddar cheese (optional, make sure it's low FODMAP)

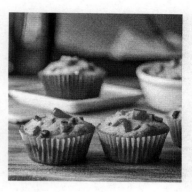

Instructions:
1. Heat the oven to 375°F (190°C). Put parchment paper cups in a muffin pan, or grease the pan.
2. Mix the eggs, milk, salt and pepper together in a bowl, using a whisk.
3. Put equal amounts of diced bell peppers and diced zucchini in each muffin cup.
4. Pour the egg mixture over the vegetables, filling each cup about 2/3 full.
5. Add some finely chopped fresh chives to the top of each egg cup.
6. If desired, add some shredded cheddar cheese to the top.
7. Bake in a preheated oven for 15-20 minutes or until the egg cups are set and slightly golden on the top.
8. Let the egg cups cool down for a few minutes before gently taking them out of the muffin tin. Serve while warm.

Nutritional Facts (per serving - 3 egg cups): Calories: 220 | Total Fat: 14g | Saturated Fat: 5g | Trans Fat: 0g | Cholesterol: 395mg | Sodium: 290mg | Total Carbohydrates: 8g | Dietary Fiber: 2g | Sugars: 4g | Protein: 15g | Vitamin D: 15% | Calcium: 20% | Iron: 10% | Potassium: 340mg

Granola Parfait with Lactose-Free Yogurt and Fresh Berries

Prep Time: 10 minutes; Serving Size: 1 glass or bowl; Servings: 2

Ingredients:
- 1 cup lactose-free yogurt (make sure it's low FODMAP)
- 1/2 cup low FODMAP granola
- 1/2 cup mixed fresh berries (e.g., strawberries, blueberries, raspberries)
- 2 tbsp maple syrup (optional)

Instructions:
1. In two glasses or bowls, begin by adding 1/4 cup of yogurt to the bottom of each.
2. Top the yogurt in each glass with 2 tablespoons of low-FODMAP granola.
3. Layer another 1/4 cup of yogurt on top of the granola in each glass.
4. Sprinkle another 2 tablespoons of granola over the yogurt in each glass.
5. Finish by topping each parfait with 1/4 cup of mixed fresh berries.
6. Drizzle with maple syrup if desired and serve.

Nutritional Facts (per parfait): Calories: 260 | Total Fat: 7g | Saturated Fat: 1g | Trans Fat: 0g | Cholesterol: 10mg | Sodium: 100mg | Total Carbohydrates: 42g | Dietary Fiber: 5g | Sugars: 19g | Protein: 9g | Vitamin D: 15% | Calcium: 30% | Iron: 10% | Potassium: 300mg

Gluten-Free Banana Pancakes with Maple Syrup

Prep Time: 15 minutes; Cook Time: 15 minutes; Servings: 2

Ingredients:
- 2 unripe bananas
- 2 large eggs
- 1/2 cup gluten-free oat flour
- 1/2 tsp baking powder
- 1/4 tsp ground cinnamon
- 1/4 tsp vanilla extract
- A pinch of salt
- Coconut oil or cooking spray, for the pan
- Pure maple syrup, for serving

Instructions:
1. Mash the unripe bananas in a bowl until they are smooth. Combine the eggs and vanilla extract with the mashed bananas. Whisk until everything is well mixed.
2. In another bowl, mix oat flour, baking powder, cinnamon, and a bit of salt.
3. Add the dry mixture to the wet mixture a little at a time, stirring until just mixed. Be careful not to mix too much, a few lumps are fine.
4. Warm a non-stick skillet or griddle over medium heat. Spread a thin layer of coconut oil or cooking spray on the surface.
5. Put about 1/4 cup of the pancake batter onto the skillet for each pancake. Cook until bubbles appear on top, then turn over and cook the other side till it becomes golden brown.
6. Repeat with the rest of the mixture.
7. Serve warm with a drizzle of pure maple syrup.

Nutritional Facts (per serving): Calories: 290 | Total Fat: 9g | Saturated Fat: 3g | Trans Fat: 0g | Cholesterol: 190mg | Sodium: 220mg | Total Carbohydrates: 45g | Dietary Fiber: 5g | Sugars: 17g | Protein: 10g | Vitamin D: 6% | Calcium: 10% | Iron: 15% | Potassium: 470mg

Chia Seed Pudding with Kiwi and Pineapple (Vegan)

Prep Time: 10 minutes; Chilling Time: 4 hours or overnight; Serving Size: 1 bowl; Servings: 2

Ingredients:
- 1/4 cup chia seeds
- 1 cup coconut milk or other low FODMAP dairy alternative
- 1 tbsp maple syrup (adjust to taste)
- 1/2 tsp vanilla extract
- 1 kiwi, peeled and diced
- 1/2 cup fresh pineapple, diced
- 1 tbsp unsweetened shredded coconut
- Fresh mint leaves to garnish (optional)

Instructions:

1. In a bowl, combine the chia seeds, coconut milk, maple syrup, and vanilla extract. Stir well until mixture is blended.
2. Cover the bowl and refrigerate for at least 4 hours or overnight to allow the chia seeds to absorb the liquid and form a pudding-like consistency.
3. Before serving, stir the chia seed pudding well to make sure even distribution.
4. Divide the chia seed pudding between two serving bowls.
5. Top with diced kiwi, pineapple and unsweetened shredded coconut.
6. Garnish with fresh mint leaves, if desired.

Nutritional Facts (per bowl): Calories: 230 | Total Fat: 10g | Saturated Fat: 4g | Trans Fat: 0g | Cholesterol: 0mg | Sodium: 15mg | Total Carbohydrates: 31g | Dietary Fiber: 12g | Sugars: 13g | Protein: 5g | Vitamin D: 0% | Calcium: 20% | Iron: 15% | Potassium: 320mg

Ham and Cheese Omelet with Fresh Herbs

Prep Time: 10 minutes; Cook Time: 10 minutes; Serving Size: 1 omelet; Servings: 2

Ingredients:

- 4 large eggs
- 1/4 cup lactose-free milk
- Salt and pepper to taste
- 1/2 cup cooked ham, diced (make sure it's low FODMAP)
- 1/2 cup shredded Cheddar cheese
- 2 tbsp fresh herbs (e.g., chives, parsley, thyme), chopped
- 1 tbsp butter or lactose-free margarine (make sure it's low FODMAP)

Instructions:

1. In a bowl, whisk together the eggs, milk, salt, and pepper until well blended.
2. Heat a nonstick skillet over medium heat. Add butter or margarine and melt.
3. Add half of the egg mixture to the skillet. Swirl to coat the bottom evenly.
4. Cook the eggs for one minute or until the edges start to firm up.
5. Sprinkle half of the diced ham, shredded cheddar and fresh herbs over one half of the omelet.
6. Fold the remaining half of the omelet over the filling gently to create a half-moon shape. Gently press down with a spatula.
7. Continue to cook until cheese is melted and omelet is cooked through, 1-2 minutes. Gently transfer the omelet to a plate.
8. Repeat to make a second omelet.

Nutritional Facts (per omelet): Calories: 250 | Total Fat: 18g | Saturated Fat: 9g | Trans Fat: 0g | Cholesterol: 370mg | Sodium: 600mg | Total Carbohydrates: 2g | Dietary Fiber: 0g | Sugars: 1g | Protein: 18g | Vitamin D: 15% | Calcium: 25% | Iron: 10% | Potassium: 210mg

Rice Cakes with Almond Butter and Banana Slides (Vegan)

Prep Time: 5 minutes; Serving Size: 2 rice cakes; Servings: 1

Ingredients:
- 2 rice cakes (make sure it's low FODMAP)
- 4 tbsp almond butter (make sure it's low FODMAP)
- 1 medium unripe banana, sliced

Instructions:
1. Place the rice cakes on a plate. Spread 2 tablespoons almond butter on top of each rice cake.
2. Place slices of unripe banana on top of each almond butter coated rice cake and serve.

Nutritional Facts (per serving - 2 rice cakes): Calories: 320 | Total Fat: 16g | Saturated Fat: 1.5g | Trans Fat: 0g | Cholesterol: 0mg | Sodium: 40mg | Total Carbohydrates: 40g | Dietary Fiber: 7g | Sugars: 15g | Protein: 9g | Vitamin D: 0% | Calcium: 10% | Iron: 8% | Potassium: 460mg

Scrambled Eggs with Spinach and Feta Cheese (Vegetarian)

Prep Time: 10 minutes; Cook Time: 15 minutes; Servings: 2

Ingredients:
- 4 large eggs
- 1 cup fresh spinach, chopped
- 1/2 cup crumbled feta cheese (make sure it's low FODMAP)
- 2 tbsp extra-virgin olive oil
- Salt and pepper, to taste
- Chopped fresh parsley for garnish (optional)

Instructions:
1. Break open the eggs and put them in a bowl. Mix them together well. Put it to the side.
2. Put a non-stick skillet on medium heat. Put olive oil in the skillet and heat it up.
3. Put the chopped spinach in the skillet and stir it for 2-3 minutes until it becomes wilted.
4. Add the beaten eggs to the skillet containing the spinach. Scramble the eggs gently and cook them for about 3-4 minutes or until slightly set.
5. Top the scrambled eggs with crumbled feta cheese. Stir the eggs and cheese gently until well combined, and let the cheese melt slightly.
6. Add salt and pepper according to your taste.
7. Take the skillet off the heat when the eggs are cooked to your liking.
8. Serve the scrambled eggs warm and add chopped fresh parsley on top, if you wish.

Nutritional Facts (per serving): Calories: 220 | Total Fat: 17g | Saturated Fat: 6g | Trans Fat: 0g | Cholesterol: 370mg | Sodium: 460mg | Total Carbohydrates: 3g | Dietary Fiber: 1g | Sugars: 1g | Protein: 14g | Vitamin D: 15% | Calcium: 15% | Iron: 10% | Potassium: 8%

2. Meat-Based Recipes

Grilled Lamb Chops with Mint Pesto and Mashed Potatoes

Prep Time: 20 minutes; Cook Time: 25 minutes; Serving Size: 2 lamb chops + mashed potatoes; Servings: 2

Ingredients:

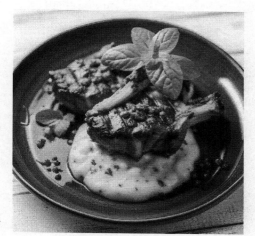

- 4 lamb chops
- 2 tbsp garlic-infused olive oil
- Salt and pepper to taste
- For Mint Pesto
    - 1 cup fresh mint leaves
    - 1/4 cup pine nuts
    - 2 tbsp grated Parmesan cheese (make sure it's low FODMAP)
    - 1 tbsp lemon juice
    - 3 tbsp garlic-infused olive oil
    - Salt and pepper, to taste
- For Mashed Potatoes
    - 2 large potatoes, peeled and diced
    - 1/4 cup lactose-free milk or other low FODMAP dairy alternative
    - 2 tbsp butter (make sure it's low FODMAP)
    - Salt and pepper, to taste

Instructions:

1. Preheat the grill to a medium-high temperature.
2. Coatthe lamb chops with garlic-infused olive oil and season to taste with salt and pepper.
3. Grill the lamb chops for 3-4 minutes on each side or longer, depending on your desired level of doneness. Take the lamb chops off the grill and set them aside to rest.
4. For Mint Pesto: in a food processor, combine the fresh mint leaves, pine nuts, grated Parmesan cheese, lemon juice, garlic-infused olive oil, salt and pepper. Blend until smooth and well combined.
5. For Mashed Potatoes: Boil the diced potatoes until they are tender. Drain them and put them back in the pot.
6. Mash the potatoes together with the milk and the butter until the mixture is smooth and creamy. Season with salt and pepper according to your taste.
7. Serve the grilled lamb chops drizzled with mint pesto and alongside the mashed potatoes. Serve warm.

Nutritional Facts (per serving - 2 lamb chops + mashed potatoes): Calories: 580 | Total Fat: 37g | Saturated Fat: 10g | Trans Fat: 0g | Cholesterol: 110mg | Sodium: 320mg | Total Carbohydrates: 30g | Dietary Fiber: 4g | Sugars: 2g | Protein: 33g | Vitamin D: 4% | Calcium: 20% | Iron: 25% | Potassium: 1180mg

Slow-Cooked Beef Stew with Root Vegetables

Prep Time: 20 minutes; Cook Time: 4 hours; Serving Size: 1 cup; Servings: 6

Ingredients:
- 1.5 lb (about 680g) beef stew meat, cubed
- 2 cups low-sodium beef broth (make sure it's low FODMAP)
- 1 cup carrots, peeled and diced
- 1 cup parsnips, peeled and diced
- 1 cup potatoes, peeled and diced
- 1 cup turnips, peeled and diced
- 1 cup green beans, trimmed and cut into 1-inch pieces
- 1 cup diced tomatoes (canned or fresh)
- 2 tbsp tomato paste
- 2 tbsp garlic-infused olive oil
- 1 tsp dried thyme
- 1 tsp dried rosemary
- Salt and pepper to taste

Instructions:
1. Heat the garlic-infused olive oil in a large skillet on medium-high heat. Add the beef stew meat and cook until browned on all sides. Move the meat to a slow cooker.
2. Put in the chopped tomatoes, tomato paste, dry thyme, dried rosemary, salt, and pepper into the slow cooker.
3. Add the beef broth to the slow cooker, making sure the meat is covered.
4. Place the slow cooker on low heat level and cook the ingredients for 3 hours.
5. After 3 hours, add the diced carrots, parsnips, potatoes, turnips, and green beans to the slow cooker.
6. Keep cooking for 1 more hour or until the meat is soft and the vegetables are cooked.
7. Taste and adjust seasonings if needed before serving. Serve warm.

Nutritional Facts (per serving - 1 cup): Calories: 280 | Total Fat: 9g | Saturated Fat: 2.5g | Trans Fat: 0g | Cholesterol: 70mg | Sodium: 220mg | Total Carbohydrates: 27g | Dietary Fiber: 6g | Sugars: 7g | Protein: 25g | Vitamin D: 10% | Calcium: 8% | Iron: 20% | Potassium: 970mg

Pork Tenderloin with Rosemary and Roasted Red Bell Peppers

Prep Time: 15 minutes; Cook Time: 25 minutes; Serving Size: 1 pork tenderloin slice; Servings: 4

Ingredients:
- 1 lb (about 450g) pork tenderloin, trimmed and sliced into 1-inch thick pieces
- 2 tbsp extra-virgin olive oil
- 1 tbsp fresh rosemary, minced
- Salt and pepper to taste
- 2 large red bell peppers, sliced
- 2 tbsp garlic-infused olive oil
- 1 tbsp balsamic vinegar
- 1 tbsp fresh parsley, chopped (for garnish)

Instructions:

1. Heat the oven to 400°F (200°C).
2. In a bowl, mix the pork tenderloin slices with olive oil, chopped rosemary, salt, and pepper. Ensure that the pork is well covered with the seasonings.
3. Heat a skillet over medium-high heat. Add a small amount of olive oil. When it's hot, cook the pork pieces for about 2-3 minutes on each side until they're golden brown. Take it out of the pan and keep it on a separate plate.
4. Mix together the cut bell peppers with olive oil and vinegar flavored with garlic. Put them evenly on a flat baking tray. Put the tray in the oven which has been already heated, and roast for 15 to 20 minutes or until they become soft and slightly burnt.
5. Put the cooked pork tenderloin slices on a plate with the bell peppers roasted before. Decorate with parsley that has been finely chopped.

Nutritional Facts (per serving - 1 pork tenderloin slice): Calories: 230 | Total Fat: 13g | Saturated Fat: 2g | Trans Fat: 0g | Cholesterol: 75mg | Sodium: 80mg | Total Carbohydrates: 6g | Dietary Fiber: 2g | Sugars: 4g | Protein: 21g | Vitamin A: 140% | Vitamin C: 280% | Calcium: 4% | Iron: 8%

Maple-Glazed Turkey Breast with Steamed Carrots

Prep Time: 10 minutes; Cook Time: 1 hour 15 minutes; Serving Size: 4 ounces turkey + steamed carrots; Servings: 4

Ingredients:

- 1.5 lb (about 680g) boneless turkey breast.
- 1/4 cup pure maple syrup
- 2 tbsp garlic-infused olive oil
- 1 tsp dried thyme
- Salt and pepper to taste
- 1 lb (about 450g) carrots, peeled and sliced
- Fresh parsley for garnish

Instructions:

1. Heat the oven to 350°F (175°C).
2. In a bowl, whisk together the maple syrup, garlic-infused olive oil, dried thyme, salt and, pepper.
3. Place the turkey breast in a roasting pan and brush it generously with the maple syrup mixture.
4. Roast the turkey breast in the preheated oven for about 1 hour, basting it with the remaining maple syrup mixture every 20 minutes, or until the internal temperature reaches 165°F (74°C) and the turkey is golden and glazed.
5. While the turkey is roasting, steam the sliced carrots until tender, about 5-7 minutes.
6. When the turkey is done, remove from the oven and let rest for a few minutes before slicing.
7. Serve the sliced maple-glazed turkey breast with the steamed carrots. Garnish with fresh parsley. Serve warm.

Nutritional Facts (per serving - 4 ounces turkey + steamed carrots): Calories: 280 | Total Fat: 7g | Saturated Fat: 1.5g | Trans Fat: 0g | Cholesterol: 80mg | Sodium: 160mg | Total Carbohydrates: 25g | Dietary Fiber: 4g | Sugars: 16g | Protein: 28g | Vitamin D: 6% | Calcium: 8% | Iron: 15% | Potassium: 810mg

Savory Roast Beef with Dijon Mustard and Parsnips

Prep Time: 15 minutes; Cook Time: 1 hour 15 minutes; Serving Size: 4 ounces beef + parsnips; Servings: 4

Ingredients:
- 1.5 pounds (about 680g) boneless beef roast (such as sirloin or tenderloin)
- 2 tbsp low FODMAP Dijon mustard
- 2 tbsp garlic-infused olive oil
- 1 tsp dried thyme
- Salt and pepper to taste
- 1 pound (about 450g) parsnips, peeled and sliced
- Fresh parsley for garnish

Instructions:
1. Preheat the oven to 375°F (190°C).
2. In a small bowl, mix together the Dijon mustard, garlic-infused olive oil, dried thyme, salt and pepper.
3. Apply the mustard mixture to the beef roast, covering the entire surface..
4. Place the beef roast on a roasting rack in an ovenproof dish.
5. Arrange the sliced parsnips around the beef roast in the baking dish.
6. Roast in the oven preheated to the desired temperature for nearly an hour, or until the internal temperature of the beef reaches your desired degree of doneness.
7. Once the beef is fully cooked, remove it from the oven, and then allow it to rest for a couple of minutes before cutting it into slices.
8. Serve the sliced roast beef alongside the roasted parsnips. Garnish with fresh parsley. Serve warm.

Nutritional Facts (per serving - 4 ounces beef + parsnips): Calories: 350 | Total Fat: 15g | Saturated Fat: 4.5g | Trans Fat: 0g | Cholesterol: 100mg | Sodium: 220mg | Total Carbohydrates: 20g | Dietary Fiber: 5g | Sugars: 5g | Protein: 35g | Vitamin D: 10% | Calcium: 8% | Iron: 20% | Potassium: 940mg

Pulled Pork Sandwiches on Gluten-Free Bread with Coleslaw

Prep Time: 15 minutes; Cook Time: 6 hours (slow cooker); Serving Size: 1 sandwich + coleslaw; Servings: 6

Ingredients:
- 3 pounds (about 1360g) boneless pork shoulder
- 1 cup low FODMAP BBQ sauce
- 1 tsp garlic-infused olive oil
- Salt and pepper to taste
- 6 gluten-free and low FODMAP hamburger buns
- For Coleslaw
  - 3 cups shredded green cabbage
  - 1 cup shredded carrots
  - 1/4 cup low FODMAP Mayonnaise
  - 2 tbsp red wine vinegar
  - 1 tsp low FODMAP Dijon mustard
  - Salt and pepper, to taste

Instructions:
1. Rub the pork shoulder with garlic-infused olive oil, salt and pepper.
2. Place the seasoned pork shoulder in a slow cooker.
3. Pour the BBQ sauce over the pork.
4. Cover and cook for about 6 hours, or until the pork is tender and easily shredded with a fork.
5. For Coleslaw: while the pork is cooking, in a bowl toss the shredded green cabbage and shredded carrots.
6. In a separate bowl, whisk together the mayonnaise, vinegar, Dijon mustard, salt and pepper. Pour the dressing over the cabbage and carrots. Toss to combine.
7. Once the pork is ready, shred it using two forks.
8. To make the sandwiches, place a generous portion of pulled pork onto each hamburger bun. Top with a scoop of coleslaw.
9. Serve the Pulled Pork Sandwiches with Coleslaw on the side.

Nutritional Facts (per serving - 1 sandwich + coleslaw): Calories: 500 | Total Fat: 20g | Saturated Fat: 5g | Trans Fat: 0g | Cholesterol: 100mg | Sodium: 550mg | Total Carbohydrates: 55g | Dietary Fiber: 6g | Sugars: 12g | Protein: 25g | Vitamin D: 4% | Calcium: 10% | Iron: 20% | Potassium: 480mg

Pan-Seared Veal Chops with Garlic Spinach

Prep Time: 10 minutes; Cook Time: 15 minutes; Serving Size: 1 veal chop + spinach; Servings: 2

Ingredients:
- 2 veal chops
- Salt and pepper, to taste
- 1 tbsp garlic-infused olive oil
- 1 tbsp fresh lemon juice
- 2 cups baby spinach leaves
- Lemon zest for garnish
- Fresh parsley for garnish

Instructions:
1. Season both sides of the veal chops with salt and pepper.
2. Heat the garlic-infused olive oil in a skillet over medium-high heat.
3. Add the veal chops to the skillet and cook each side for approximately 4-5 minutes, or until cooked to your liking.
4. While the veal chops are cooking, add a small amount of garlic-infused olive oil in a separate skillet over medium heat.
5. Add the baby spinach leaves and sauté until the spinach leaves are just beginning to wilt.
6. Drizzle fresh lemon juice over the sauteed spinach and toss to coat.
7. After cooking the veal chops, remove them from the skillet and allow them to rest for a few minutes.
8. Serve the Pan-Seared Veal Chops alongside the garlic spinach and garnish with lemon zest and fresh parsley. Serve warm.

Nutritional Facts (per serving - 1 veal chop + spinach): Calories: 280 | Total Fat: 15g | Saturated Fat: 5g | Trans Fat: 0g | Cholesterol: 150mg | Sodium: 220mg | Total Carbohydrates: 3g | Dietary Fiber: 1g | Sugars: 1g | Protein: 30g | Vitamin D: 10% | Calcium: 10% | Iron: 20% | Potassium: 480mg

Braised Chicken with Tomatoes and Oregano over Polenta

Prep Time: 15 minutes; Cook Time: 45 minutes; Serving Size: 1 chicken thigh + polenta; Servings: 4

Ingredients:

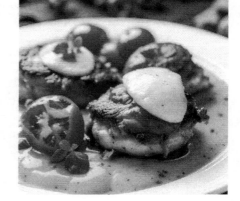

- 4 boned, skinless chicken thighs
- Salt and pepper to taste
- 1 tbsp garlic-infused olive oil
- 1 cup canned diced tomatoes (make sure they're low FODMAP)
- 1 tsp dried oregano
- 1 cup low FODMAP chicken broth
- 1 cup cornmeal
- 4 cups water
- Fresh oregano leaves for garnish

Instructions:

1. Season both sides of the chicken thighs with salt and pepper.
2. Heat garlic-infused olive oil in a large skillet over medium-high heat.
3. Add the chicken thighs and sear for approximately 3-4 minutes on each side until they turn golden brown. Remove from the skillet and keep aside.
4. Add diced tomatoes and dried oregano to the same skillet. Cook for 2-3 minutes to blend the flavors.
5. Put the seared chicken thighs back in the skillet. Pour the chicken broth over the chicken.
6. Reduce the heat to low, cover the skillet, and let the chicken simmer for approximately 30 minutes or until it is tender and fully cooked.
7. While the chicken is braising, prepare the polenta. Bring 4 cups of water to a boil in a separate pot.
8. Whisk in the cornmeal gradually and continue until the mixture thickens.
9. Lower heat to low and cook polenta, stirring occasionally, until smooth and creamy, 15 to 20 minutes.
10. Serve the Braised Chicken with Tomatoes and Oregano over a bed of creamy polenta and garnish with fresh oregano leaves. Serve warm.

Nutritional Facts (per serving - 1 chicken thigh + polenta): Calories: 400 | Total Fat: 15g | Saturated Fat: 3.5g | Trans Fat: 0g | Cholesterol: 100mg | Sodium: 500mg | Total Carbohydrates: 40g | Dietary Fiber: 3g | Sugars: 2g | Protein: 25g | Vitamin D: 4% | Calcium: 4% | Iron: 20% | Potassium: 300mg

Stir-Fried Pork with Ginger and Bok Choy

Prep Time: 15 minutes; Cook Time: 15 minutes; Serving Size: 1 cup; Servings: 4

Ingredients:
- 1 pound pork tenderloin, thinly sliced
- 2 tbsp garlic-infused olive oil
- 2 tbsp low-sodium soy sauce (make sure it's low FODMAP)
- 1 tbsp fresh ginger, minced
- 1 tsp sesame oil
- 1 bunch bok choy, washed and chopped
- 1 medium carrot, peeled and julienned
- Salt and pepper to taste
- Sesame seeds for garnish

Instructions:

1. In a bowl, combine the sliced pork, soy sauce, minced ginger and a pinch of salt and pepper. Let it marinate for about 10 minutes.
2. Warm the garlic-infused olive oil in a sizable skillet or wok over medium-high heat.
3. Incorporate the marinated pork slices and stir-fry for roughly 3-4 minutes, or until they are fully cooked and lightly browned. Extract the pork from the skillet and reserve it to the side.
4. Incorporate the sesame oil into the same skillet and add the chopped bok choy and the julienned carrot, stirring them. Stir-fry for roughly 2-3 minutes, or until the vegetables turn soft.
5. Add the cooked pork back to the skillet with the vegetables, and toss them to combine.
6. Sprinkle with sesame seeds for added flavor and serve over rice.

Nutritional Facts (per serving - 1 cup): Calories: 220 | Total Fat: 10g | Saturated Fat: 2g | Trans Fat: 0g | Cholesterol: 55mg | Sodium: 350mg | Total Carbohydrates: 8g | Dietary Fiber: 3g | Sugars: 3g | Protein: 25g | Vitamin D: 0% | Calcium: 15% | Iron: 15% | Potassium: 570mg

BBQ Ribs with Homemade low FODMAP BBQ Sauce and Grilled Corn

Prep Time: 15 minutes; Cook Time: 2.5 hours; Serving Size: 2 ribs + 1 corn; Servings: 4

Ingredients:

- For BBQ Ribs
  - 2 racks baby back pork ribs (about 4 pounds total)
  - Salt and pepper to taste
  - 1 tbsp garlic-infused olive oil
  - 1 cup low FODMAP BBQ Sauce
- For Grilled Corn
  - 4 ears of corn, husks removed
  - 1 tbsp garlic-infused olive oil
  - Salt and pepper to taste

Instructions:

- For BBQ Ribs
  1. Preheat the oven to 275°F (135°C).
  2. Season the racks of baby back ribs with salt and pepper on both sides.
  3. Wrap each rack in aluminum foil and place them on a baking sheet.
  4. Bake the ribs in the preheated oven for about 2-2.5 hours, or until they are tender.
  5. While the ribs are baking, prepare the Grilled Corn.
- For Grilled Corn
  1. Preheat the grill to medium-high heat.
  2. Brush each ear of corn with garlic-infused olive oil and season with salt and pepper.
  3. Grill the corn for about 10-12 minutes, turning occasionally, until it is slightly charred and cooked through.
- To assemble
  1. Preheat the grill to medium-high heat.
  2. Remove the ribs from the oven and carefully unwrap them.
  3. Brush the ribs generously with the BBQ Sauce.
  4. Place the sauced ribs on the grill and cook for about 3-4 minutes on each side, or until they are nicely caramelized.
  5. Serve the BBQ Ribs with Grilled Corn, brushing the corn with additional garlic-infused olive oil if desired.

Nutritional Facts (per serving - 2 ribs + 1 corn): Calories: 600 | Total Fat: 29g | Saturated Fat: 9g | Trans Fat: 0g | Cholesterol: 110mg | Sodium: 600mg | Total Carbohydrates: 60g | Dietary Fiber: 4g | Sugars: 24g | Protein: 32g | Vitamin D: 10% | Calcium: 4% | Iron: 20% | Potassium: 960mg

Lemon-Herb Grilled Chicken with Garlic-infused Olive Oil

Prep Time: 15 minutes; Cook Time: 15 minutes; Serving Size: 1 chicken breast; Servings: 4

Ingredients:
- 4 boneless, skinless chicken breasts
- 1/4 cup garlic-infused olive oil
- Juice of 1 lemon
- 2 tbsp fresh parsley, chopped
- 1 tbsp fresh rosemary, chopped
- Salt and pepper to taste

Instructions:
1. Heat the grill to moderate heat.
2. In a bowl, mix the garlic-infused olive oil, lemon juice, chopped parsley, chopped rosemary, salt and pepper.
3. Put the chicken breasts in a shallow dish and pour the marinade over them. Make sure to coat each breast evenly. Marinate them for 10-15 minutes at room temperature.
4. Take the chicken breasts out of the marinade and get rid of any extra liquid on them. Throw away the liquid in which the chicken breasts were soaking.
5. Put the chicken breasts on the heated grill and cook for around 6-8 minutes on each side until they are completely cooked and get good grill marks. Ensure that the chicken breasts have a temperature of 165°F (74°C) inside.
6. After cooking, take the chicken breasts off the grill and give them some time to cool down for some minutes before serving.

Nutritional Facts (per serving - 1 chicken breast): Calories: 250 | Total Fat: 15g | Saturated Fat: 2.5g | Trans Fat: 0g | Cholesterol: 80mg | Sodium: 350mg | Total Carbohydrates: 1g | Dietary Fiber: 0g | Sugars: 0g | Protein: 26g | Vitamin D: 4% | Calcium: 2% | Iron: 6% | Potassium: 290mg

Grilled Sausages with Sauteed Green Beans and Almonds

Prep Time: 10 minutes; Cook Time: 20 minutes; Serving Size: 2 sausages + green beans; Servings: 4

Ingredients:
- 8 low FODMAP sausages
- 1 pound (about 450g) green beans, ends trimmed
- 1/4 cup sliced almonds
- 2 tbsp garlic-infused olive oil
- Salt and pepper to taste
- Fresh parsley for garnish

Instructions:
1. Heat the grill to medium-high.
2. Cook the sausage over medium-high heat on the grill, turning them occasionally, for 12-15 minutes or until the sausage is fully cooked and has grill marks. Remove the sausage from the grill and set it aside.
3. Heat the garlic-infused olive oil in a large frying pan over medium heat.
4. Add green beans to the frying pan and sauté for 5-7 minutes, or until they are tender and crispy.
5. Add sliced almonds to the frying pan and cook for 2-3 minutes until both the beans and almonds are cooked to desired doneness. Season the green beans and almonds with salt and pepper.
6. Serve the grilled sausages alongside the toasted green beans and almonds. Garnish with fresh parsley. Serve warm.

Nutritional Facts (per serving - 2 sausages + green beans): Calories: 450 | Total Fat: 35g | Saturated Fat: 9g | Trans Fat: 0g | Cholesterol: 60mg | Sodium: 600mg | Total Carbohydrates: 14g | Dietary Fiber: 6g | Sugars: 4g | Protein: 20g | Vitamin D: 0% | Calcium: 10% | Iron: 20% | Potassium: 760mg

Low FODMAP BBQ Sauce

Prep Time: 5 minutes; Cook Time: 10 minutes; Serving Size: 2 tbsp; Servings: 4

Ingredients:
- 1 cup tomato sauce (make sure it's low FODMAP)
- 2 tbsp brown sugar
- 2 tbsp red wine vinegar
- 1 tbsp low-sodium soy sauce or tamari (make sure it's low FODMAP)
- 1 tsp smoked paprika
- 1/2 tsp ground cumin
- 1/2 tsp ground black pepper
- 1/4 tsp cayenne pepper (adjust to taste)
- Salt to taste

Instructions:
1. In a small saucepan, combine the tomato sauce, brown sugar, red wine vinegar, soy sauce, smoked paprika, ground cumin, ground black pepper and cayenne pepper.
2. Put the saucepan on a medium heat and let the mixture come to a boil.
3. Let the sauce simmer for about 5-7 minutes, stirring occasionally, until it thickens slightly and the flavors meld.
4. Taste and season with salt to your preference. Adjust cayenne pepper to the desired heat.
5. Remove the saucepan from the heat and let the BBQ sauce cool.

Nutritional Facts (per serving - 2 tbsp): Calories: 35 | Total Fat: 0g | Saturated Fat: 0g | Trans Fat: 0g | Cholesterol: 0mg | Sodium: 280mg | Total Carbohydrates: 8g | Dietary Fiber: 1g | Sugars: 6g | Protein: 1g | Vitamin D: 0% | Calcium: 2% | Iron: 2% | Potassium: 160mg

Low FODMAP Dijon Mustard

Prep Time: 5 minutes; Cook Time: 0 minutes; Serving Size: 2 tbsp; Servings: 4

Ingredients:
- 1/4 cup ground yellow mustard seeds
- 2 tbsp white wine vinegar
- 1 tbsp water
- 1 tsp maple syrup
- 1/4 tsp salt

Instructions:
1. Combine ingredients: In a small bowl, whisk together the mustard seeds, white wine vinegar, water, maple syrup and salt.
2. If the mustard is too thick for your liking, you can add a little more water to achieve the desired consistency.
3. Taste the mustard and adjust the salt and sweetness as needed, keeping in mind your personal preference.
4. Storage: pour the Dijon Mustard into a clean, airtight container. Store it in the refrigerator for up to 2 weeks.

Nutritional Facts (per serving - 1 tsp): Calories: 5 | Total Fat: 0g | Saturated Fat: 0g | Trans Fat: 0g | Cholesterol: 0mg | Sodium: 25mg | Total Carbohydrates: 1g | Dietary Fiber: 0g | Sugars: 0.5g | Protein: 0.2g | Vitamin A: 0% | Vitamin C: 0% | Calcium: 1% | Iron: 2%

Low FODMAP Chicken Broth

Prep Time: 10 minutes; Cook Time: 2 hours; Serving Size: 1 cup; Servings: 8

Ingredients:
- 1 whole chicken (about 3-4 pounds), skin removed
- 2 carrots, peeled and chopped
- 1 rosemary stem
- 1 bay leaf
- 1 tsp whole peppercorns
- 1 tsp dried thyme
- 8 cups water

Instructions:
1. Place the whole chicken in a large pot and cover it with water. Add the chopped carrots, rosemary, bay leaf, whole peppercorns and dried thyme to the pot.
2. Bring the mixture to a boil over high heat, then reduce the heat to low and let it simmer for about 2 hours, skimming off any foam that rises to the surface.
3. After simmering, strain the broth through a fine mesh strainer into another pot or container to remove the solids.
4. Let the broth cool, then refrigerate it. Once chilled, you can remove any solidified fat that rises to the top.
5. The chicken broth is now ready to use in your recipes.

Store the low FODMAP Chicken Broth in an airtight container in the refrigerator for up to 4 days or freeze it for longer storage.

Nutritional Facts (per serving - 1 cup): Calories: 10 | Total Fat: 0g | Saturated Fat: 0g | Trans Fat: 0g | Cholesterol: 0mg | Sodium: 25mg | Total Carbohydrates: 1g | Dietary Fiber: 0g | Sugars: 1g | Protein: 1g | Vitamin D: 0% | Calcium: 0% | Iron: 0% | Potassium: 25mg

3. Fish-Based Recipes

Shrimps and Scallops Skewers with Zesty Lime Marinade

Prep Time: 20 minutes; Cook Time: 10 minutes; Serving Size: 3 skewers; Servings: 4

Ingredients:

- For Marinade
  - 1/4 cup extra-virgin olive oil
  - Zest and juice of 2 limes
  - 2 tbsp fresh parsley, chopped
  - 1 tbsp maple syrup
  - 1 tsp ground cumin
  - Salt and pepper to taste
- For Finger Food Skewers
  - 12 large shrimps, peeled and deveined
  - 12 large sea scallops, tough muscle removed
  - 1/2 cup low FODMAP Fresh Basil Pesto
  - 3 slices gluten-free and low FODMAP bread
  - Bamboo skewers, soaked in water for 30 minutes

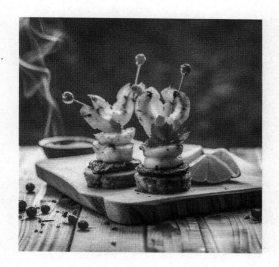

Instructions:

1. In a mixing bowl make the marinade: whisk together the olive oil, lime zest, lime juice, chopped parsley, maple syrup, ground cumin, salt, and pepper. Season to taste.
2. In a large bowl, place the shrimps and scallops. Pour the marinade over them, making sure each piece is well coated. Refrigerate for at least 30 minutes to 1 hour, covered with plastic wrap.
3. While seafood is marinating, preheat the oven to 375°F (190°C). Quarter gluten-free bread slices to make small squares. Place on a baking sheet and toast in the oven until lightly golden and crisp, about 5-7 minutes. Remove and set aside.
4. Preheat a grill or skillet over medium-high heat. Remove the shrimp and scallops from the marinade and grill them for about 2-3 minutes per side, or until they are opaque and have grill marks.
5. Place a square of toasted bread on a plate. Place a dollop (about a teaspoon) of the Fresh Basil Pesto on top of the bread. Skewer a grilled scallop, then a shrimp, and finally push the skewer through the center of the bread square so that seafood sits atop the pesto-covered bread. The bread should be at the bottom, acting as a base.
6. Arrange the finger food skewers on a serving plate. Serve warm or at room temperature.

Nutritional Facts (per serving - 3 skewers): Calories: 250 | Total Fat: 12g | Saturated Fat: 2g | Trans Fat: 0g | Cholesterol: 100mg | Sodium: 300mg | Total Carbohydrates: 12g | Dietary Fiber: 2g | Sugars: 6g | Protein: 24g | Vitamin D: 10% | Calcium: 6% | Iron: 15% | Potassium: 600mg

Baked Cod with Lemon-Dill Sauce and Sauteed Zucchini

Prep Time: 15 minutes; Cook Time: 20 minutes; Serving Size: 1 serving; Servings: 2

Ingredients:
- For Baked Cod
  - 2 cod fillets, about 6 oz (170 g) each
  - 1 tbsp extra-virgin olive oil
  - 1 tbsp lemon juice
  - 1/2 tsp dried dill
  - Salt and pepper to taste
- For Lemon-Dill Sauce
  - 1/4 cup lactose-free yogurt (make sure it's low FODMAP)
  - 1 tbsp lemon juice
  - 1 tbsp fresh dill, chopped
  - Salt and pepper to taste
- For Sautéed Zucchini
  - 2 small zucchinis, sliced
  - 1 tbsp extra-virgin olive oil
  - Salt and pepper to taste

Instructions:
1. For Baked Cod: preheat the oven to 375°F (190°C). Place the cod fillets on a baking dish. Drizzle with oil and lemon juice. Sprinkle with dried dill, salt and pepper. Bake the cod in the preheated oven for about 15-20 minutes, or until the fish flakes easily with a fork.
2. For Lemon-Dill Sauce: while the cod is baking, in a small bowl mix together yogurt, lemon juice, chopped dill, salt and pepper. Set aside.
3. For Sautéed Zucchini: in a skillet, heat oil over medium heat. Add the sliced zucchinis and cook for about 5-7 minutes, or until they are tender and slightly golden. Season to taste with salt and pepper.
4. Once the cod is cooked, remove from the oven and place on serving plates. Drizzle with the Lemon-Dill Sauce.
5. Serve the Baked Cod with Lemon-Dill Sauce alongside the sautéed zucchinis.

Nutritional Facts (per serving): Calories: 280 | Total Fat: 14g | Saturated Fat: 2g | Trans Fat: 0g | Cholesterol: 60mg | Sodium: 220mg | Total Carbohydrates: 9g | Dietary Fiber: 2g | Sugars: 4g | Protein: 28g | Vitamin D: 15% | Calcium: 15% | Iron: 10% | Potassium: 700mg

Grilled Tuna Steaks with Olive Tapenade and Steamed Green Beans

Prep Time: 15 minutes; Cook Time: 10 minutes; Serving Size: 1 tuna steak with green beans; Servings: 2

Ingredients:
- For Grilled Tuna
  - 2 tuna steaks, about 6 oz (170 g) each
  - 1 tbsp extra-virgin olive oil
  - 1 tsp lemon zest
  - Salt and pepper to taste
- For Olive Tapenade
  - 1/2 cup Kalamata olives, pitted and chopped
  - 2 tbsp fresh parsley, chopped
  - 1 tbsp capers, drained and chopped
  - 1 tbsp extra-virgin olive oil
  - 1 tsp lemon juice
  - Salt and pepper to taste

- For Steamed Green Beans
    - 2 cups green beans, trimmed
    - 1 tbsp extra-virgin olive oil
    - Salt and pepper to taste

Instructions:

1. <u>For Grilled Tuna</u>: preheat the grill to medium-high heat. Brush the tuna steaks with olive oil and sprinkle with lemon zest, salt and pepper. Grill the tuna steaks for about 4-5 minutes on each side, or until they are cooked to your desired doneness. Set aside.
2. <u>For Olive Tapenade</u>: in a bowl, mix together the chopped Kalamata olives, parsley, capers, lemon juice, olive oil, salt and pepper to make the Olive Tapenade.
3. <u>For Steamed Green Beans</u>: in a steamer, steam the green beans for about 3-4 minutes, or until tender but still crisp. Remove from the steamer and toss with olive oil, salt and pepper.
4. To serve, place a grilled tuna steak on each plate. Top with a generous spoon of Olive Tapenade. Serve with steamed green beans on the side.

Nutritional Facts (per serving - 1 tuna steak with green beans): Calories: 300 | Total Fat: 18g | Saturated Fat: 2.5g | Trans Fat: 0g | Cholesterol: 45mg | Sodium: 450mg | Total Carbohydrates: 15g | Dietary Fiber: 7g | Sugars: 4g | Protein: 26g | Vitamin D: 10% | Calcium: 10% | Iron: 15% | Potassium: 800mg

Pan-Seared Halibut with Pineapple Salsa and Wild Rice

Prep Time: 15 minutes; Cook Time: 15 minutes; Serving Size: 1 halibut fillet with rice and salsa; Servings: 4

Ingredients:

- For Pan-Seared Halibut
    - 4 halibut fillets, about 6 oz (170 g) each
    - 2 tbsp extra-virgin olive oil
    - Salt and pepper to taste
- For Pineapple Salsa
    - 1 cup fresh pineapple, diced
    - 1/4 cup red bell pepper, finely chopped
    - 2 tbsp fresh cilantro, chopped
    - 1 tbsp lime juice
    - Salt and pepper to taste
- For Wild Rice
    - 1 cup wild rice
    - 2 cups water
    - Salt to taste

Instructions:

1. <u>For Halibut</u>: pat the halibut fillets dry with paper towels. Season both sides with salt and pepper. Heat olive oil over medium heat in a large skillet. Place halibut fillets in the skillet with the skin side facing down. Cook on each side for 4-5 minutes or until the fish is fully cooked. Internal temperature should be 145°F (63°C).
2. <u>For Pineapple Salsa</u>: in a bowl, combine the diced pineapple, chopped red bell pepper, chopped cilantro, lime juice, salt and pepper. Mix well to make the salsa.
3. <u>For Wild Rice</u>: rinse wild rice in cold water. In a pot, combine the rinsed rice, water and a pinch of salt. Bring the mixture to a boil and then low down the heat. Cover the pot and let it simmer for about 45-50 minutes or until the rice is soft and the water is absorbed.
4. Serve the pan-seared halibut fillets over a portion of cooked wild rice and top with pineapple salsa.

Nutritional Facts (per serving - halibut fillet with rice and salsa): Calories: 380 | Total Fat: 12g | Saturated Fat: 2g | Trans Fat: 0g | Cholesterol: 50mg | Sodium: 300mg | Total Carbohydrates: 42g | Dietary Fiber: 4g | Sugars: 7g | Protein: 30g | Vitamin D: 10% | Calcium: 4% | Iron: 15% | Potassium: 800mg

Roasted Haddock with Spinach and Lemon Risotto

Prep Time: 15 minutes; Cook Time: 35 minutes; Serving Size: 1 fillet and 1 cup of risotto; Servings: 4

Ingredients:
- For Roasted Haddock
    - 4 haddock fillets (about 6 ounces each)
    - 2 tbsp extra-virgin olive oil
    - 1 tsp dried thyme
    - Salt and pepper to taste
- For Risotto
    - 1 cup Arborio rice
    - 2 cups low FODMAP vegetable broth
    - 1 cup fresh spinach, chopped
    - 1 lemon, zest and juice
    - 2 tbsp extra-virgin olive oil
    - 2 tbsp fresh chives, chopped
    - Salt and pepper to taste

Instructions:

- For Roasted Haddock
    1. Preheat the oven to 400°F (200°C).
    2. Place the haddock fillets on a baking sheet. Add a bit of olive oil, dried thyme, salt, and pepper on top.
    3. Roast in the preheated oven for about 15-20 minutes, or until the fish flakes easily with a fork.

- For Risotto
    1. In a medium saucepan, heat the olive oil over medium heat. Add the Arborio rice and sauté for 1-2 minutes until the rice is slightly translucent.
    2. Gradually add the vegetable broth, 1/2 cup at a time, stirring frequently. Allow the liquid to absorb before adding more. Continue until the rice is creamy and cooked to your desired texture (about 20-25 minutes).
    3. Stir in the chopped spinach, lemon zest and lemon juice into the risotto. Cook for an additional 2-3 minutes until the spinach is wilted and the flavors are well combined. Add salt and pepper according to your taste.
    4. For Serving: serve the roasted haddock fillets on top of a generous portion of spinach and lemon risotto. Garnish with fresh chives.

Nutritional Facts (per serving - 1 fillet and 1 cup of risotto): Calories: 380 | Total Fat: 14g | Saturated Fat: 2g | Trans Fat: 0g | Cholesterol: 60mg | Sodium: 520mg | Total Carbohydrates: 40g | Dietary Fiber: 2g | Sugars: 1g | Protein: 24g | Vitamin D: 15% | Calcium: 10% | Iron: 15% | Potassium: 450mg

Stuffed Squid with Rice, Olives and Tomato Sauce

Prep Time: 25 minutes; Cook Time: 40 minutes; Serving Size: 2 stuffed squid tubes; Servings: 2

Ingredients:

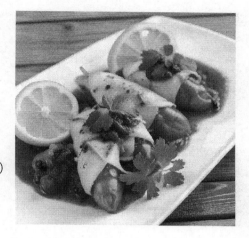

- 4 medium squid tubes, cleaned and tentacles reserved
- 1/2 cup cooked rice
- 10 Kalamata olives, pitted and chopped
- 2 tbsp fresh parsley, chopped
- 1 tbsp extra-virgin olive oil
- Salt and pepper to taste
- For Tomato Sauce
  - 1 cup canned crushed tomatoes (make sure it's low FODMAP)
  - 1 tbsp extra-virgin olive oil
  - 1/2 tsp dried oregano
  - Salt and pepper to taste

Instructions:

1. For Tomato Sauce: in a saucepan, heat 1 tbsp of olive oil over medium heat. Add the canned crushed tomatoes and dried oregano. Season with salt and pepper. Cook for about 10-15 minutes, stirring occasionally, until the sauce is heated through and slightly thickened.
2. In a bowl, combine the cooked rice, chopped Kalamata olives, chopped parsley, olive oil, salt and pepper. Mix well to create the stuffing mixture.
3. Carefully stuff each squid tube with the rice and olive mixture, leaving a little space at the top. Seal the top of each squid with a toothpick to secure the stuffing.
4. In a separate pan, heat a bit of olive oil over medium-high heat. Add the reserved squid tentacles and cook for a few minutes until they start to curl. Push the tentacles to the sides of the pan and add the stuffed squid tubes. Cook for about 3-4 minutes on each side until the squid is cooked and opaque.
5. To serve, spoon some of the tomato sauce onto a plate and place the cooked stuffed squid tubes on top. Garnish with the cooked squid tentacles.

Nutritional Facts (per serving - 2 stuffed squid tubes): Calories: 280 | Total Fat: 11g | Saturated Fat: 1.5g | Trans Fat: 0g | Cholesterol: 225mg | Sodium: 400mg | Total Carbohydrates: 24g | Dietary Fiber: 2g | Sugars: 5g | Protein: 21g | Vitamin A: 20% | Vitamin C: 40% | Calcium: 10% | Iron: 15%

Tilapia in a White Wine and Saffron Sauce with Baby Carrots

Prep Time: 10 minutes; Cook Time: 20 minutes; Serving Size: 1 fillet with sauce and carrots; Servings: 2

Ingredients:
- 2 tilapia fillets, about 6 oz (170 g) each
- Salt and pepper to taste
- 1 tbsp extra-virgin olive oil
- 1/2 cup dry white wine
- 1/4 tsp saffron threads
- 1/2 cup low FODMAP vegetable broth
- 1 tbsp lactose-free butter (make sure it's low FODMAP)
- 1 cup baby carrots, peeled and trimmed
- 1 tbsp chopped fresh parsley

Instructions:
1. <u>For Tilapia</u>: Season both sides of the tilapia fillets with salt and pepper. Heat olive oil in a large skillet over medium-high heat. Cook the tilapia fillets in the skillet for 3-4 minutes on each side or until they easily flake with a fork. Remove the fillets from the skillet and set them aside.
2. <u>For Sauce</u>: in the same skillet, pour in the dry white wine and add saffron threads. Simmer for a minute. Add the vegetable broth and let it simmer for another 2-3 minutes.
3. Add the baby carrots to the skillet and cook for about 8-10 minutes, or until the carrots are tender and the liquid has reduced by half.
4. Reduce the heat to low. Stir in the butter until melted and the sauce slightly thickens.
5. Place a tilapia fillet on each plate, spoon the saffron sauce over the fillets and arrange the baby carrots on the side. Sprinkle chopped fresh parsley over the top.

Nutritional Facts (per serving - 1 fillet with sauce and carrots): Calories: 280 | Total Fat: 12g | Saturated Fat: 3.5g | Trans Fat: 0g | Cholesterol: 50mg | Sodium: 280mg | Total Carbohydrates: 13g | Dietary Fiber: 3g | Sugars: 5g | Protein: 22g | Vitamin A: 270% | Vitamin C: 8% | Calcium: 6% | Iron: 10%

Orange and Herb Marinated Swordfish with Steamed Broccoli

Prep Time: 15 minutes; Cook Time: 10 minutes; Serving Size: 1 fillet with broccoli; Servings: 2

Ingredients:
- <u>For Marinated Swordfish</u>
  - 2 swordfish fillets
  - Zest and juice of 1 orange
  - 2 tbsp extra-virgin olive oil
  - 2 tbsp fresh parsley, chopped
  - 1 tbsp fresh thyme leaves
  - Salt and pepper to taste
- <u>For Steamed Broccoli</u>
  - 2 cups broccoli florets
  - Salt to taste

Instructions:
1. In a shallow bowl, combine the orange zest, orange juice, olive oil, chopped parsley, fresh thyme, salt and pepper. Place the swordfish fillets in the marinade, turning to coat both sides. Cover and let marinate in the refrigerator for about 15-20 minutes.
2. While the swordfish is marinating, steam the broccoli florets until tender, about 5-7 minutes. Season with a pinch of salt.
3. Heat a skillet over medium-high heat. Remove the swordfish fillets from the marinade and place them in the skillet. Cook for about 3-4 minutes on each side, or until the fish is opaque and cooked through.
4. Divide the cooked swordfish fillets and steamed broccoli between two plates.

Nutritional Facts (per serving - 1 fillet with broccoli): Calories: 300 | Total Fat: 18g | Saturated Fat: 2.5g | Trans Fat: 0g | Cholesterol: 60mg | Sodium: 300mg | Total Carbohydrates: 10g | Dietary Fiber: 4g | Sugars: 4g | Protein: 25g | Vitamin A: 40% | Vitamin C: 150% | Calcium: 15% | Iron: 20%

Oven-Poached Sole with Spinach and low FODMAP Fresh Basil Pesto

Prep Time: 15 minutes; Cook Time: 20 minutes; Serving Size: 1 fillet with spinach; Servings: 2

Ingredients:
- 2 sole fillets
- 4 cups fresh spinach leaves
- 2 tbsp low FODMAP Fresh Basil Pesto
- 2 tbsp extra-virgin olive oil
- Salt and pepper to taste
- Lime wedges, for serving

Instructions:
1. <u>For Pesto Spinach</u>: in a skillet, heat olive oil over medium heat. Add the spinach and sauté until wilted, about 2-3 minutes. Remove from heat and stir in the Fresh Basil Pesto.
2. <u>For Sole</u>: preheat the oven to 375°F (190°C). Season the sole fillets with a pinch of salt and pepper.
3. Place the seasoned sole fillets in an oven-safe dish. Top each fillet with the pesto spinach mixture.
4. Cover the dish with aluminum foil and bake in the preheated oven for about 12-15 minutes, or until the fish is opaque and flakes easily with a fork.
5. Carefully transfer the poached sole fillets with spinach to serving plates. Serve with lime wedges on the side.

Nutritional Facts (per serving - 1 fillet with spinach): Calories: 250 | Total Fat: 15g | Saturated Fat: 2g | Trans Fat: 0g | Cholesterol: 50mg | Sodium: 350mg | Total Carbohydrates: 6g | Dietary Fiber: 3g | Sugars: 1g | Protein: 24g | Vitamin A: 120% | Vitamin C: 30% | Calcium: 15% | Iron: 20%

Baked Sea Bass with Rosemary Potatoes and Glazed Parsnips

Prep Time: 20 minutes; Cook Time: 40 minutes; Serving Size: 1 sea bass fillet, potatoes and parsnips; Servings: 2

Ingredients:
- 2 sea bass fillets, about 6 oz (170 g) each
- 4 small parsnips, peeled and sliced into thin strips
- 1 cup baby potatoes, halved
- 2 tbsp extra-virgin olive oil
- 1 tbsp fresh rosemary, chopped
- Salt and pepper to taste
- <u>For Glaze</u>
  - 2 tbsp maple syrup
  - 1 tbsp low FODMAP Dijon mustard
  - 1 tbsp extra-virgin olive oil

Instructions:

<u>For Glaze</u>: Whisk the maple syrup, low FODMAP Dijon mustard, and olive oil together in a small bowl. Set the mixture aside.

<u>For Potatoes and Parsnips</u>
1. Preheat the oven to 400°F (200°C).
2. In a bowl, toss the baby potatoes with 1 tbsp of olive oil, chopped rosemary, salt and pepper. Spread the potatoes on one half of a baking sheet. On the other half, place the sliced parsnips. Pour the remaining olive oil over the parsnips, then add salt and pepper for seasoning.
3. Place the baking sheet in the preheated oven and bake for about 20-25 minutes, or until the potatoes are tender and the parsnips are glazed and slightly caramelized.

For Sea Bass

1. While the vegetables are baking, place the sea bass fillets on a separate baking sheet lined with parchment paper. Brush the fillets with the prepared glaze on both sides.
2. Bake in the oven for 12-15 minutes until the fish is thoroughly cooked and flakes effortlessly with a fork.

For Serving: divide the baked sea bass fillets, rosemary potatoes and glazed parsnips between two plates. Drizzle any remaining glaze over the fish. Serve immediately.

Nutritional Facts (per serving): Calories: 390 | Total Fat: 18g | Saturated Fat: 2.5g | Trans Fat: 0g | Cholesterol: 50mg | Sodium: 160mg | Total Carbohydrates: 41g | Dietary Fiber: 5g | Sugars: 15g | Protein: 18g | Vitamin A: 10% | Vitamin C: 40% | Calcium: 8% | Iron: 10%

Fish Tacos with Fresh Vegetables and Tangy Yogurt Sauce

Prep Time: 20 minutes; Cook Time: 15 minutes; Serving Size: 2 tacos; Servings: 2

Ingredients:
- For Fish Tacos
    - 2 white fish fillets (such as cod or haddock), about 6 oz (170 g) each
    - 1 tbsp extra-virgin olive oil
    - 1 tsp paprika
    - Salt and pepper to taste
    - 4 small gluten-free and low FODMAP tortillas
- For Taco Fillings
    - 1 cup finely shredded lettuce or mixed greens
    - 1/2 cup diced tomatoes
    - 1/4 cup chopped fresh cilantro
    - 1/4 cup sliced red bell peppers
    - 1/4 cup sliced cucumber
    - Lime wedges for serving
- For Tangy Yogurt Sauce
    - 1/2 cup lactose-free plain yogurt (make sure it's low FODMAP)
    - 1 tbsp fresh lime juice
    - 1 tsp ground cumin
    - Salt and pepper to taste

Instructions:
1. For Fish Tacos: pat the fish fillets dry and rub them with olive oil, paprika, salt and pepper. Heat a non-stick skillet over medium-high heat. Add the fish fillets and cook until the fish flakes easily with a fork, about 3-4 minutes on each side. Remove from heat and break the fish into chunks.
2. For Tangy Yogurt Sauce: in a small bowl, whisk together yogurt, fresh lime juice, ground cumin, salt and pepper until well combined.
3. Heat the tortillas according to the package instructions.
4. Spread a generous amount of the tangy yogurt sauce onto each tortilla. Place a portion of the shredded lettuce or mixed greens onto the sauce.
5. Top with chunks of the cooked fish, diced tomatoes, chopped cilantro, sliced red bell peppers and sliced cucumber.
6. Serve the fish tacos with lime wedges on the side for squeezing.

Nutritional Facts (per serving - 2 tacos): Calories: 300 | Total Fat: 10g | Saturated Fat: 2g | Trans Fat: 0g | Cholesterol: 60mg | Sodium: 350mg | Total Carbohydrates: 30g | Dietary Fiber: 7g | Sugars: 5g | Protein: 25g | Vitamin A: 40% | Vitamin C: 45% | Calcium: 15% | Iron: 15%

Grilled Mackerel with Cabbage Salad and Lemon Vinaigrette

Prep Time: 15 minutes; Cook Time: 10 minutes; Serving Size: 1 fillet with salad; Servings: 2

Ingredients:
- For Grilled Mackerel
  - 2 mackerel fillets, about 6 oz (170 g) each
  - 1 tbsp extra-virgin olive oil
  - 1 tsp dried thyme
  - Salt and pepper to taste
- For Cabbage Salad
  - 2 cups finely shredded green cabbage
  - 1/2 cup grated carrots
  - 2 tbsp chopped fresh parsley
- For Lemon Vinaigrette
  - 3 tbsp extra-virgin olive oil
  - 2 tbsp fresh lemon juice
  - 1 tsp low FODMAP Dijon mustard
  - 1 tsp maple syrup
  - Salt and pepper to taste

Instructions:
1. In a large bowl, combine the finely shredded green cabbage, grated carrots and chopped fresh parsley.
2. Combine the olive oil, fresh lemon juice, Dijon mustard, maple syrup, salt and pepper in a small bowl by whisking them together until they are well blended.
3. Drizzle the lemon vinaigrette over the cabbage salad and toss to coat.

For Grilled Mackerel
1. Preheat the grill to medium-high heat. Pat the mackerel fillets dry with paper towels.
2. Brush both sides of the fillets with olive oil and sprinkle with dried thyme, salt and pepper.
3. Place the fillets on the grill and cook each side for approximately 4 to 5 minutes, or until the fish becomes tender enough to break easily with a fork.. Remove from heat and set aside.

For Serving: divide the cabbage salad between two plates. Place a grilled mackerel fillet on each plate alongside the salad.

Nutritional Facts (per serving - 1 fillet with salad): Calories: 350 | Total Fat: 24g | Saturated Fat: 4g | Trans Fat: 0g | Cholesterol: 60mg | Sodium: 300mg | Total Carbohydrates: 10g | Dietary Fiber: 3g | Sugars: 5g | Protein: 25g | Vitamin A: 130% | Vitamin C: 60% | Calcium: 10% | Iron: 10%

Low FODMAP Vegetable Broth

Prep Time: 10 minutes; Cook Time: 1 hour 30 minutes; Serving Size: 1 cup; Servings: about 8 cups

Ingredients:
- 2 medium carrots, chopped
- 1 small zucchini, chopped
- 1 stem of rosemary
- 1 small bunch of fresh parsley
- 2 bay leaves
- 1 tsp dried thyme
- 1 tsp whole peppercorns
- 8 cups water

Instructions:
1. Rinse and clean the vegetables thoroughly. In a large pot, combine the chopped carrots, zucchini, parsley, bay leaves, rosemary, dried thyme and peppercorns. Pour in the water.
2. Bring the mixture to a boil over high heat, then reduce the heat to low and let it simmer uncovered for about 1 hour 30 minutes. This will allow the flavors to infuse into the broth.
3. Once the broth has simmered and the vegetables have released their flavors, remove the pot from the heat. Strain the broth through a fine mesh strainer or cheesecloth into a clean bowl or container. Discard the solids.
4. Let the broth cool completely before storing. You can refrigerate the broth in airtight containers for up to 4-5 days or freeze it for longer storage.

Nutritional Facts (per 1 cup serving): Calories: 10 | Total Fat: 0g | Saturated Fat: 0g | Trans Fat: 0g | Cholesterol: 0mg | Sodium: 10mg | Total Carbohydrates: 2g | Dietary Fiber: 1g | Sugars: 1g | Protein: 0g | Vitamin A: 100% | Vitamin C: 8% | Calcium: 2% | Iron: 2%

Low FODMAP Fresh Basil Pesto

Prep Time: 10 minutes; Cook Time: 0 minutes; Serving Size: 2 tbsp; Servings: about 4

Ingredients:
- 2 cups fresh basil leaves, packed
- 1/2 cup pine nuts
- 1/2 cup grated Parmesan cheese (make sure it's aged and low FODMAP)
- 1/4 cup garlic-infused olive oil
- Salt to taste

Instructions:
1. In a food processor, combine the fresh basil leaves, grated Parmesan cheese, pine nuts and olive oil.
2. Process the ingredients in quick intervals until they're thoroughly mixed to form a grainy paste.
3. You can adjust the texture by pulsing more for a smoother consistency or less for a chunkier texture.
4. Season the pesto with a pinch of salt. Remember that Parmesan cheese adds saltiness, so adjust the salt to your taste.
5. Taste the pesto and adjust the olive oil as needed to achieve the desired flavor and consistency.
6. Storage: Pour the pesto into a clean, airtight container. Cover the whole surface of the pesto with a layer of olive oil, this way it will keep better. You can store it in the refrigerator for up to 1 week or freeze it in ice cube trays for longer storage.

Nutritional Facts (per serving - 2 tbsp): Calories: 160 | Total Fat: 15g | Saturated Fat: 2.5g | Trans Fat: 0g | Cholesterol: 5mg | Sodium: 70mg | Total Carbohydrates: 3g | Dietary Fiber: 1g | Sugars: 0.5g | Protein: 4g | Vitamin A: 15% | Vitamin C: 10% | Calcium: 10% | Iron: 8%

4. Vegetable & Pasta Dishes

Spaghetti Squash Primavera with Fresh Basil Pesto

Prep Time: 15 minutes; Cook Time: 45 minutes; Serving Size: 1 plate; Servings: 4

Ingredients:

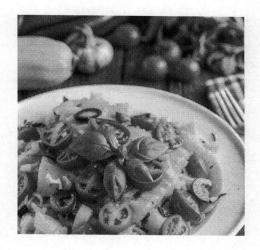

- For Spaghetti Squash
  - 1 medium spaghetti squash
  - 2 tbsp garlic-infused olive oil
  - Salt and pepper to taste
- For low FODMAP Fresh Basil Pesto: prepare for 4 servings
- For Primavera Sauce
  - 1 cup cherry tomatoes, halved
  - 1 cup zucchini, sliced
  - 1 cup red bell peppers, sliced
  - 1 cup low FODMAP vegetable broth
  - 1 tbsp extra-virgin olive oil
  - Salt and pepper, to taste

Instructions:

1. Preheat the oven to 400°F (200°C).
2. Cut the spaghetti squash in half lengthwise and scoop out the seeds. Brush the cut sides with garlic-infused olive oil and then sprinkle salt and pepper over the top.
3. Place the halves cut-side down on a baking sheet. Roast in the preheated oven for about 35-40 minutes, or until the flesh is tender and can be easily scraped into strands using a fork.
4. For Primavera Sauce: in a large skillet, heat 1 tbsp of olive oil over medium heat. Add the sliced zucchini, red bell pepper and halved cherry tomatoes. Sauté for about 5-7 minutes, until the vegetables are slightly softened.
5. Add the vegetable broth to the skillet and bring to a simmer. Stir in about 1/4 cup of the prepared fresh basil pesto and mix well.
6. Using a fork, scrape the roasted spaghetti squash into strands and add them to the skillet. Toss the squash with the primavera sauce and vegetables until well combined.
7. Divide the spaghetti squash into individual plates. Drizzle with extra fresh basil pesto if desired.

Nutritional Facts (per serving): Calories: 320 | Total Fat: 28g | Saturated Fat: 4g | Trans Fat: 0g | Cholesterol: 5mg | Sodium: 220mg | Total Carbohydrates: 15g | Dietary Fiber: 4g | Sugars: 5g | Protein: 6g | Vitamin A: 40% | Vitamin C: 80% | Calcium: 15% | Iron: 10%

Low FODMAP Fettuccine Alfredo with Roasted Chicken and Broccoli

Prep Time: 15 minutes; Cook Time: 25 minutes; Serving Size: 1 plate; Servings: 4

Ingredients:

- 12 oz (340 g) gluten-free and low FODMAP fettuccine
- 2 boneless, skinless chicken breasts
- 2 tbsp garlic-infused olive oil
- 2 cups broccoli florets
- 1 cup lactose-free heavy cream (make sure it's low FODMAP)
- 1 cup grated Parmesan cheese
- 1/2 tsp dried oregano
- Salt and pepper to taste
- Fresh parsley, chopped (for garnish)

Instructions:

For Roast Chicken and Broccoli

1. Preheat Oven: Preheat the oven to 400°F (200°C).
2. Place the chicken breasts and broccoli florets on a baking sheet.
3. Drizzle with 1 tbsp of garlic-infused olive oil and season with salt and pepper. Cook the chicken and broccoli in a preheated oven for approximately 20-25 minutes, or until the chicken is fully cooked, and the broccoli is soft.
4. After taking the chicken out of the oven, allow it to rest for a few minutes before slicing it.

For Fettuccine: Cook the fettuccine according to the package instructions in a large pot of boiling salted water. Drain the fettuccine and set it aside.

For Alfredo Sauce

1. In a separate pan, heat the remaining 1 tbsp of garlic-infused olive oil over medium heat. Add the heavy cream and bring to a gentle simmer.
2. Add the grated Parmesan cheese and dried oregano to the mixture while stirring. Continue cooking until the cheese melts and the sauce thickens to the desired consistency which takes about 3 to 4 minutes.

To assemble

1. Add the cooked fettuccine to the Alfredo sauce and toss to coat the pasta evenly. Gently fold in the sliced roasted chicken and broccoli.
2. Season with salt and pepper to taste. Arrange the fettuccine on individual plates and garnish with chopped fresh parsley.

Nutritional Facts (per serving): Calories: 520 | Total Fat: 27g | Saturated Fat: 15g | Trans Fat: 0g | Cholesterol: 135mg | Sodium: 540mg | Total Carbohydrates: 41g | Dietary Fiber: 3g | Sugars: 2g | Protein: 29g | Vitamin A: 35% | Vitamin C: 70% | Calcium: 35% | Iron: 15%

Gluten-Free Penne with Shrimps, Tomatoes and Arugula

Prep Time: 15 minutes; Cook Time: 20 minutes; Serving Size: 1 cup; Servings: 4

Ingredients:

- 8 oz (225 g) gluten-free and low FODMAP penne pasta
- 1 lb shrimps, peeled and deveined
- 1 cup cherry tomatoes, halved
- 2 cups arugula
- 2 tbsp extra-virgin olive oil
- 2 tbsp garlic-infused olive oil
- 1 tbsp lemon juice
- 1 tsp dried oregano
- Salt and pepper, to taste
- Fresh basil leaves, to garnish

Instructions:

1. Prepare penne pasta according to package instructions until it is al dente. Drain pasta and set it aside.
2. Heat olive oil over medium heat in a large skillet. Add shrimps to the skillet and cook for 2-3 minutes on each side, or until they turn pink and opaque. Remove shrimps from the skillet and set them aside.
3. Next, add halved cherry tomatoes to the same skillet and cook for 2-3 minutes, or until they begin to soften.
4. Add the cooked penne pasta, arugula, cooked shrimps and dried oregano to the skillet. Toss everything together gently.
5. In a small bowl, whisk together the garlic-infused olive oil, lemon juice, salt and pepper. Drizzle the dressing over the pasta and toss to combine.
6. Transfer the pasta to serving plates. Garnish with fresh basil leaves.

Nutritional Facts (per serving): Calories: 380 | Total Fat: 12g | Saturated Fat: 2g | Trans Fat: 0g | Cholesterol: 135mg | Sodium: 350mg | Total Carbohydrates: 43g | Dietary Fiber: 3g | Sugars: 3g | Protein: 25g

Stir-Fried Bok Choy and Tofu with Ginger-Sesame Sauce

Prep Time: 15 minutes; Cook Time: 15 minutes; Serving Size: 1 cup; Servings: 4

Ingredients:

- 1 lb firm tofu, pressed and cubed
- 2 bunches bok choy, washed and chopped
- 2 tbsp garlic-infused olive oil
- 2 tbsp low-sodium tamari or soy sauce (make sure it's low FODMAP)
- 1 tbsp sesame oil
- 1 tbsp freshly grated ginger
- 1 tbsp maple syrup
- 1 tbsp rice vinegar
- 1 tsp toasted sesame seeds
- Salt and pepper, to taste

Instructions:

1. In a large skillet or wok, heat the garlic-infused olive oil over medium-high heat.
2. Add the cubed tofu to the skillet and stir-fry until golden and crispy on all sides. Remove the tofu from the skillet and set aside.
3. In the same skillet, add the chopped bok choy and stir-fry for 2-3 minutes until wilted but still slightly crunchy.
4. In a small bowl, whisk together tamari or soy sauce, sesame oil, grated ginger, maple syrup, rice vinegar and toasted sesame seeds.
5. Return the cooked tofu to the skillet with the bok choy. Pour the ginger-sesame sauce over the tofu and bok choy. Toss to combine and heat through.
6. Season with salt and pepper to taste. Divide the stir-fried mixture among serving plates.

Nutritional Facts (per serving): Calories: 260 | Total Fat: 18g | Saturated Fat: 2.5g | Trans Fat: 0g | Cholesterol: 0mg | Sodium: 350mg | Total Carbohydrates: 14g | Dietary Fiber: 3g | Sugars: 2g | Protein: 14g

Butternut Squash Risotto with Sage and Parmesan

Prep Time: 15 minutes; Cook Time: 30 minutes; Serving Size: 1 cup; Servings: 4

Ingredients:

- 2 cups low FODMAP butternut squash, peeled, seeded and diced
- 2 tbsp garlic-infused olive oil
- 1 cup Arborio rice
- 4 cups low FODMAP vegetable broth
- 1/2 cup dry white wine
- 1 tbsp fresh sage, chopped
- 1/4 cup lactose-free Parmesan cheese, grated
- Salt and pepper, to taste

Instructions:

1. Heat garlic-infused olive oil over medium heat in a large skillet. Cook the diced butternut squash for 5-7 minutes or until it is tender and slightly golden. Remove the squash from the skillet and set it aside.
2. In the same skillet, add the Arborio rice and sauté for 2-3 minutes, stirring frequently, until the rice is lightly toasted.
3. Pour in the dry white wine and cook, stirring constantly, until it's mostly absorbed by the rice.
4. Add the vegetable broth one ladleful at a time, while stirring the rice continuously, allow the rice to absorb the broth before adding more. Repeat the process until the rice becomes creamy and has an al dente texture, which may take approximately 20 to 25 minutes.
5. Stir in the sautéed butternut squash and chopped sage during the last 5 minutes of cooking.
6. Remove the skillet from heat and stir in the Parmesan cheese until melted and incorporated. Add salt and pepper to season.
7. Divide the risotto in individual plates and serve warm.

Nutritional Facts (per serving): Calories: 320 | Total Fat: 10g | Saturated Fat: 3g | Trans Fat: 0g | Cholesterol: 10mg | Sodium: 450mg | Total Carbohydrates: 48g | Dietary Fiber: 3g | Sugars: 4g | Protein: 7g

Buckwheat Noodles with Grilled Zucchini and Sesame Seeds

Prep Time: 15 minutes; Cook Time: 10 minutes; Serving Size: 1 cup; Servings: 4

Ingredients:

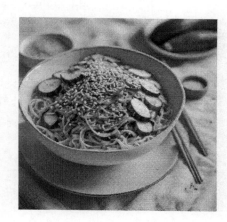

- 8 oz (225 g) buckwheat noodles
- 2 medium zucchinis, sliced lengthwise
- 2 tbsp garlic-infused olive oil
- 1 tbsp toasted sesame oil
- 1 tbsp low-sodium tamari or soy sauce (make sure it's low FODMAP)
- 1 tbsp rice vinegar
- 1 tbsp toasted sesame seeds
- 1 tsp freshly grated ginger
- Salt and pepper, to taste

Instructions:

1. Cook the buckwheat noodles according to the package instructions. Drain and set aside.
2. Preheat a grill or grill pan over medium-high heat. Brush the zucchini slices with garlic-infused olive oil and grill them until tender and slightly charred. Remove from the grill and set aside.
3. In a small bowl, whisk together the toasted sesame oil, tamari or soy sauce, rice vinegar, grated ginger and a pinch of black pepper.
4. In a large mixing bowl, combine the cooked buckwheat noodles, grilled zucchinis and toasted sesame seeds.
5. Pour the dressing over the noodles and zucchinis. Toss lightly to make sure everything is coated with the dressing.
6. Season with salt if needed and serve warm or at room temperature.

Nutritional Facts (per serving): Calories: 320 | Total Fat: 15g | Saturated Fat: 2g | Trans Fat: 0g | Cholesterol: 0mg | Sodium: 300mg | Total Carbohydrates: 42g | Dietary Fiber: 5g | Sugars: 4g | Protein: 7g

Garlic-Infused Olive Oil Spaghetti with Grilled Shrimp and Zucchini

Prep Time: 20 minutes; Cook Time: 15 minutes; Serving Size: 1 plate; Servings: 4

Ingredients:

- 8 oz (225 g) gluten-free and low FODMAP spaghetti
- 1 lb medium-sized shrimps, peeled and deveined
- 2 medium zucchinis, sliced lengthwise
- 3 tbsp garlic-infused olive oil
- 2 tbsp fresh parsley, chopped
- Salt and pepper, to taste
- Lemon wedges, for serving

Instructions:
1. Preheat the grill to medium-high heat.
2. Cook the spaghetti in a pot of salted boiling water according to the package instructions. Drain the spaghetti and set it aside.
3. Brush the sliced zucchinis with a tbsp of garlic-infused olive oil, then grill them for 2-3 minutes on each side, or until they have grill marks and are tender. Remove from the grill and set aside.
4. In a bowl, toss the peeled and deveined shrimps with a tbsp of garlic-infused olive oil, chopped parsley, salt and pepper.
5. Grill the shrimps for about 2-3 minutes on each side, or until they are opaque and cooked through. Remove from the grill.
6. In a large bowl, combine the cooked spaghetti, grilled zucchini and grilled shrimps. Drizzle the remaining garlic-infused olive oil over the mixture and toss to combine.
7. Transfer the pasta mixture to individual plates and garnish with extra chopped parsley and lemon wedges. Serve warm.

Nutritional Facts (per serving): Calories: 330 | Total Fat: 12g | Saturated Fat: 1.5g | Trans Fat: 0g | Cholesterol: 180mg | Sodium: 250mg | Total Carbohydrates: 32g | Dietary Fiber: 4g | Sugars: 4g | Protein: 25g

Grilled Salmon over Arugula Risotto

Prep Time: 15 minutes; Cook Time: 35 minutes; Serving size: 1 salmon fillet; Servings: 2

Ingredients:
- 2 salmon fillets
- 1 cup Arborio rice
- 4 cups low FODMAP vegetable broth
- 2 cups arugula leaves
- 2 tbsp garlic-infused olive oil
- 1/4 cup dry white wine
- 1 tbsp grated Parmesan cheese
- Salt and pepper to taste
- Lemon wedges, for serving

Instructions:
1. Preheat the grill to medium-high heat.
2. Season the salmon fillets with salt and pepper. Grill the salmon for about 4-5 minutes on each side, or until the fish flakes easily. Remove from the grill and set aside.
3. In a saucepan, heat the vegetable broth over medium heat. Keep it warm but not boiling.
4. In a separate large saucepan, heat 1 tbsp of garlic-infused olive oil over medium heat.
5. Add the Arborio rice to the saucepan and sauté for about 2 minutes, or until the rice is lightly toasted.
6. Pour in the dry white wine and cook for a couple of minutes until it's mostly absorbed by the rice.
7. Add the warm vegetable broth one ladleful at a time while stirring constantly. Wait for each addition to be mostly absorbed before adding more. Repeat this process. Continue the process until the rice is creamy and cooked al dente, which takes about 20-25 minutes.
8. Mix in the grated Parmesan cheese and remaining tbsp of garlic-infused olive oil.
9. Just before serving, stir in the arugula leaves. They will wilt slightly from the heat of the risotto.
10. Divide the Arugula Risotto among serving plates. Place a grilled salmon fillet on top of each plate of risotto. Serve with lemon wedges for an extra burst of flavor.

Nutritional Facts (per serving): Calories: 450 | Total Fat: 20g | Saturated Fat: 3.5g | Trans Fat: 0g | Cholesterol: 70mg | Sodium: 550mg | Total Carbohydrates: 38g | Dietary Fiber: 2g | Sugars: 1g | Protein: 28g

Slow-Cooked Beef Ragu with Gluten-Free Pappardelle and Steamed Broccoli

Prep Time: 20 minutes; Cook Time: 6 hours; Serving Size: 1 plate; Servings: 4

Ingredients:

- 8 oz (225 g) gluten-free and low FODMAP pappardelle pasta
- 2 cups steamed broccoli florets
- For Beef Ragu
  - 1.5 lbs (680g) beef chuck roast, trimmed and cut into chunks
  - 1 cup diced carrots
  - 1 cup diced red bell peppers
  - 1 cup diced canned tomatoes (make sure it's low FODMAP)
  - 1 cup low-sodium beef broth (make sure it's low FODMAP)
  - 1 tbsp garlic-infused olive oil
  - 1 tsp dried oregano
  - 1 tsp dried thyme
  - Salt and pepper, to taste

Instructions:

For Beef Ragu
1. In a slow cooker, combine the beef chunks, diced carrots, diced red bell pepper, canned tomatoes, beef broth, garlic-infused olive oil, dried oregano, dried thyme, salt and pepper.
2. Cover the slow cooker and cook on low heat for 6 hours, till the beef is soft and easily shredded with a fork.
3. Before serving, use two forks to shred the beef chunks in the slow cooker and mix well to combine all the flavors.

To assemble
1. Cook the pappardelle pasta according to the package instructions. Drain and set aside.
2. Steam the broccoli florets until tender, about 5 minutes.
3. Divide the pappardelle pasta among serving plates. Ladle the slow-cooked beef ragu over the pasta. Serve with steamed broccoli on the side.

Nutritional Facts (per serving): Calories: 550 | Total Fat: 15g | Saturated Fat: 5g | Trans Fat: 0g | Cholesterol: 85mg | Sodium: 480mg | Total Carbohydrates: 60g | Dietary Fiber: 7g | Sugars: 8g | Protein: 40g

Creamy Polenta with Sautéed Spinach and Garlic-Infused Oil

Prep Time: 10 minutes; Cook Time: 30 minutes; Serving Size: 1 plate; Servings: 2

Ingredients:
- For Creamy Polenta
  - 1 cup instant polenta (make sure it's low FODMAP)
  - 4 cups low FODMAP vegetable broth
  - 1 tbsp lactose-free butter (make sure it's low FODMAP)
  - Salt and pepper, to taste
- For Sautéed Spinach
  - 4 cups fresh spinach leaves
  - 2 tbsp garlic-infused olive oil
  - Salt and pepper, to taste

Instructions:
1. Heat the vegetable broth in a medium saucepan until it reaches the boiling point. Whisk in instant polenta slowly and continue whisking for 5-7 minutes until the mixture becomes thickened and smooth.
2. Reduce the heat to low and stir in the butter. Season with salt and pepper to taste. Continue to cook for another 5-7 minutes, stirring occasionally, until the polenta is creamy and thickened. If needed, add a little more broth or water to achieve your desired consistency.
3. While the polenta is cooking, heat the garlic-infused olive oil in a separate skillet over medium heat. Add the fresh spinach leaves and sauté for 2-3 minutes, or until wilted. Season with salt and pepper.
4. To serve, divide the creamy polenta between two plates. Top with the sautéed spinach and drizzle with a little extra garlic-infused olive oil if desired. Serve warm.

Nutritional Facts (per serving): Calories: 220 | Total Fat: 7g | Saturated Fat: 1g | Trans Fat: 0g | Cholesterol: 0mg | Sodium: 240mg | Total Carbohydrates: 34g | Dietary Fiber: 3g | Sugars: 1g | Protein: 5g

Seared Tuna Steaks with Tomato and Basil Quinoa Pasta Salad

Prep Time: 20 minutes; Cook Time: 15 minutes; Serving Size: 1 plate; Servings: 2

Ingredients:
- For Tuna Steaks
    - 2 tuna steaks
    - 2 tbsp garlic-infused olive oil
    - Salt and pepper, to taste
- For Quinoa Pasta Salad
    - 6 oz (170 g) quinoa pasta (gluten-free and low FODMAP)
    - 1 cup cherry tomatoes, halved
    - 1/4 cup fresh basil, chopped
    - 2 tbsp extra-virgin olive oil
    - 1 tbsp balsamic vinegar
    - Salt and pepper, to taste

Instructions:

For Tuna Steaks
1. Season the tuna steaks with salt and pepper.
2. In a skillet or grill pan, heat the garlic-infused olive oil over high heat.
3. Add the tuna steaks and sear for about 1-2 minutes on each side, or until they are cooked to your desired level of doneness. The center should be pink for medium-rare.

For Quinoa Pasta Salad
1. Cook the quinoa pasta according to the package instructions. Drain and set aside.
2. In a bowl, combine the cooked quinoa pasta, cherry tomatoes and chopped fresh basil.
3. In a separate bowl, whisk together the olive oil and balsamic vinegar. Season with salt and pepper to taste.
4. Drizzle the olive oil and balsamic mixture over the quinoa pasta salad. Toss gently to combine and ensure even distribution.

To assemble
1. Divide the Tomato and Basil Quinoa Pasta Salad among serving plates.
2. Place a seared tuna steak on top of each plate of salad.

Nutritional Facts (per serving): Calories: 420 | Total Fat: 18g | Saturated Fat: 2.5g | Trans Fat: 0g | Cholesterol: 35mg | Sodium: 300mg | Total Carbohydrates: 42g | Dietary Fiber: 5g | Sugars: 3g | Protein: 24g

Baked Lemon-Herb Chicken with Gluten-Free Penne and Spinach

Prep Time: 15minutes; Cook Time: 40 minutes; Serving Size: 1 plate; Servings: 4

Ingredients:

- 4 boneless, skinless chicken breasts
- Zest of 1 lemon
- Juice of 2 lemons
- 2 tbsp garlic-infused olive oil
- 1 tsp dried oregano
- 1 tsp dried thyme
- Salt and pepper to taste
- 8 oz (225 g) gluten-free and low FODMAP penne pasta
- 2 cups fresh spinach leaves

Instructions:

1. Preheat the oven to 375°F (190°C).
2. In a bowl, combine the lemon zest, lemon juice, garlic-infused olive oil, dried oregano, dried thyme, salt and pepper. Mix well.
3. Put the chicken breasts in the baking dish and pour the lemon-herb marinade over them, making sure that the marinade coats them evenly. Cover the dish and let the chicken marinate in the refrigerator for approximately 30 minutes.
4. While the chicken is marinating, prepare the penne pasta by following the instructions provided on the package. Drain the pasta and put it to the side
5. Heat a skillet over medium heat. Once hot, add the fresh spinach leaves and sauté until wilted. Remove from heat and set aside.
6. Take the chicken out of the marinade and put it in the oven, which you've already heated up. Bake the chicken for approximately 25 to 30 minutes or until it's thoroughly cooked and no longer pink in the center. To finish, slice the chicken into thin strips once it's done cooking.
7. In a large mixing bowl, combine the cooked penne pasta, sautéed spinach and sliced chicken. Toss gently to combine and ensure even distribution.
8. Serve the baked lemon-herb chicken mixture on plates or in bowls and garnish with additional lemon zest if desired.

Nutritional Facts (per serving): Calories: 320 | Total Fat: 8g | Saturated Fat: 1.5g | Trans Fat: 0g | Cholesterol: 75mg | Sodium: 160mg | Total Carbohydrates: 32g | Dietary Fiber: 3g | Sugars: 2g | Protein: 30g

5. Vegan and Vegetarian Options

Stir-Fried Tofu with Ginger and low FODMAP Vegetables (Vegan)

Prep Time: 15 minutes; Cook Time: 10 minutes; Servings: about 2

Ingredients:

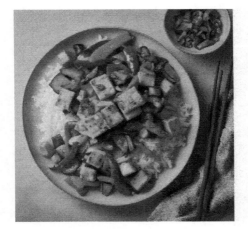

- 8 oz (225 g) firm tofu, pressed and cubed
- 1 tbsp garlic-infused olive oil
- 1 tbsp grated fresh ginger
- 1 small zucchini, sliced
- 1 cup red bell peppers, sliced
- 1 cup carrot, julienned
- 2 tbsp low-sodium soy sauce (make sure it's low FODMAP)
- 1 tbsp rice vinegar
- 1 tbsp maple syrup
- 1 tbsp sesame oil
- Sesame seeds, to garnish
- 1 cup cooked rice (optional)
- Salt and pepper, to taste

Instructions:

1. In a large skillet or wok, heat olive oil with garlic over medium-high heat. Add the diced tofu. Cook until lightly browned on all sides. Take out the tofu from the skillet and keep it aside.
2. In the same skillet, add the grated ginger and sauté for about 1 minute until fragrant.
3. Add the sliced zucchini, red bell peppers and julienned carrots to the skillet. Stir-fry for 3-4 minutes, or until the vegetables are slightly tender but still crisp.
4. Combine soy sauce, maple syrup, rice vinegar, and sesame oil in a small bowl, and whisk thoroughly. Place the vegetables along the skillet's sides, and pour the sauce in the center. Let it heat for several seconds.
5. Return the cooked tofu to the skillet, tossing gently to coat it with the sauce. Season with salt and pepper, to your liking.
6. Once everything has been heated thoroughly, remove from heat.
7. Serve the stir-fried tofu and vegetables over cooked rice or quinoa, garnished with sesame seeds, if desired.

Nutritional Facts (per serving): Calories: 280 | Total Fat: 14g | Saturated Fat: 2g | Trans Fat: 0g | Cholesterol: 0mg | Sodium: 500mg | Total Carbohydrates: 28g | Dietary Fiber: 5g | Sugars: 13g | Protein: 15g | Vitamin D: 0% | Calcium: 20% | Iron: 15% | Potassium: 25%

Grilled Eggplant and Zucchini Salad with Lemon-Herb Dressing

Prep Time: 15 minutes; Cook Time: 10 minutes; Serving Size: 1 cup; Servings: 4

Ingredients:

- 1 medium eggplant, sliced into rounds
- 2 medium zucchinis, sliced lengthwise
- 2 tbsp extra-virgin olive oil
- Salt and pepper to taste
- 2 tbsp fresh parsley, chopped
- 1 tbsp fresh chives, chopped
- For Lemon-Herb Dressing
  - 3 tbsp extra-virgin olive oil
  - 2 tbsp fresh lemon juice
  - 1 tsp fresh thyme leaves
  - Salt and pepper to taste

Instructions:

1. Preheat a grill or grill pan over medium-high heat.
2. Coat the eggplant and zucchini slices with olive oil and add salt and pepper for seasoning.
3. Grill the eggplant and zucchini slices on the grill for 3 to 4 minutes on each side, or until they are tender and you can see grill marks. Take them off the grill and let them cool down a bit.
4. Dice the grilled eggplant and zucchini into small pieces. In a bowl, combine the grilled vegetables with chopped parsley and chives.
5. For Lemon-Herb Dressing: in a separate bowl, whisk together the olive oil, fresh lemon juice, fresh thyme leaves, salt and pepper to make the lemon-herb dressing.
6. Pour the Lemon-Herb dressing over the grilled vegetables and toss gently to combine. Adjust salt and pepper to taste.
7. Serve the grilled eggplant and zucchini salad as a side dish or light meal.

Nutritional Facts (per serving - 1 cup): Calories: 120 | Total Fat: 10g | Saturated Fat: 1.5g | Trans Fat: 0g | Cholesterol: 0mg | Sodium: 10mg | Total Carbohydrates: 8g | Dietary Fiber: 4g | Sugars: 4g | Protein: 2g | Vitamin A: 20% | Vitamin C: 30% | Calcium: 4% | Iron: 4%

Baked Stuffed Red Bell Peppers with Rice and Spinach

Prep Time: 20 minutes; Cook Time: 40 minutes; Serving Size: 1 stuffed pepper; Servings: 4

Ingredients:

- 4 large red bell peppers, halved and seeds removed
- 1 cup cooked rice (such as jasmine or basmati)
- 2 cups fresh spinach, chopped
- 1 tbsp extra-virgin olive oil
- 1/2 cup lactose-free feta cheese, crumbled
- 1 tsp dried oregano
- Salt and pepper, to taste

Instructions:

1. Preheat the oven to 375°F (190°C).
2. Place the bell pepper halves in a baking dish, cut side up.
3. In a pan, heat the olive oil over medium heat. Add the chopped spinach and sauté until wilted, about 2-3 minutes. Remove from heat.
4. In a bowl, combine the cooked rice, sautéed spinach, crumbled feta cheese, dried oregano, salt and pepper. Mix well.
5. Stuff each half of the bell pepper with the rice and spinach mixture, gently pressing down on it.
6. Cover the baking dish with aluminum foil and bake it in the preheated oven for 25-30 minutes, or until the peppers become tender.
7. Remove it from the oven and allow it to cool down a bit before serving.

Nutritional Facts (per stuffed pepper): Calories: 180 | Total Fat: 6g | Saturated Fat: 2g | Trans Fat: 0g | Cholesterol: 10mg | Sodium: 350mg | Total Carbohydrates: 25g | Dietary Fiber: 4g | Sugars: 6g | Protein: 8g | Vitamin A: 140% | Vitamin C: 210% | Calcium: 15% | Iron: 10%

Roasted Root Vegetable Medley with Garlic-Infused Olive Oil

Prep Time: 15 minutes; Cook Time: 40 minutes; Serving Size: 1 cup; Servings: 6

Ingredients:

- 2 cups carrots, peeled and cut into sticks
- 2 cups parsnips, peeled and cut into sticks
- 2 cups turnips, peeled and cut into chunks
- 2 cups rutabaga, peeled and cut into chunks
- 2 tbsp garlic-infused olive oil
- Salt and pepper to taste
- Fresh thyme leaves for garnish

Instructions:

1. Preheat the oven to 400°F (200°C).
2. In a large mixing bowl, combine the carrots, parsnips, turnips and rutabaga. Drizzle the garlic-infused olive oil over the vegetables and toss to coat them evenly.
3. Sprinkle the vegetables with salt and pepper according to taste.
4. Place the vegetables in a solitary layer on a baking sheet. Roast in the preheated oven for approximately 35-40 minutes, or until the vegetables become tender and acquire a golden-brown texture. Stir the vegetables halfway through the roasting time for even cooking.
5. Transfer the roasted root vegetable medley to a serving dish. Garnish with fresh thyme leaves.

Nutritional Facts (per serving): Calories: 120 | Total Fat: 4g | Saturated Fat: 0.5g | Trans Fat: 0g | Cholesterol: 0mg | Sodium: 70mg | Total Carbohydrates: 22g | Dietary Fiber: 7g | Sugars: 6g | Protein: 2g | Vitamin A: 240% | Vitamin C: 30% | Calcium: 8% | Iron: 6%

Vegetable Sushi Rolls with Wasabi and low FODMAP Soy Sauce Substitute (Vegan)

Prep Time: 40 minutes; Cook Time: 20 minutes; Serving Size: 2 rolls; Servings: 2 rolls

Ingredients:

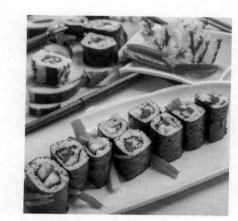

- For Sushi Rice
    - 1 cup sushi rice
    - 2 cups water
    - 2 tbsp rice vinegar
    - 1 tbsp maple syrup
    - 1/2 tsp salt
- For Sushi Rolls
    - 2 sheets nori (seaweed) wraps
    - 1 small cucumber, julienned
    - 1 small carrot, julienned
    - 1/4 cup thinly sliced red bell pepper
    - 1/4 cup pineapple, cutted into very little sticks
    - low-sodium soy sauce substitute made from tamari (make sure it's low FODMAP)
    - Wasabi paste (make sure it's low FODMAP)
    - Pickled ginger (make sure it's low FODMAP)

Instructions:

For the Sushi Rice

1. Flush the sushi rice under cold water and continue rinsing it until the water runs clear. Drain thoroughly.
2. In a saucepan, combine the rinsed sushi rice and water. Bring to a boil, then reduce the heat to low, cover and simmer for about 15-18 minutes, or until the rice is cooked and the water is absorbed.
3. In a small bowl, mix together the rice vinegar, maple syrup and salt.
4. Once the rice is cooked, transfer it to a large bowl. Gradually add the vinegar mixture while gently folding the rice with a wooden spatula. Allow the rice to cool to room temperature.

For the Sushi Rolls

1. Place a bamboo sushi rolling mat on a clean surface and put a sheet of plastic wrap on top of the mat.
2. Place a sheet of nori, shiny side down, on top of the plastic wrap.
3. Wet your fingers with water to prevent the rice from sticking. Spread a thin, even layer of sushi rice over the nori, allowing about 1 inch from the nori surface to remain uncovered..
4. Arrange the julienned cucumber, carrot, red bell pepper and pineapple sticks in a row across the center of the rice.
5. Carefully lift the bamboo mat's edge and start rolling the nori and rice over the filling. Roll tightly but gently, using the mat to shape the roll.
6. Moisten the top edge of the nori with a bit of water to seal the roll.
7. Continue rolling the mat until the roll is complete. Press gently to secure.
8. Repeat the process to make the second roll.
9. Using a sharp knife dipped in water, slice each roll into bite-sized pieces.

For Serving: serve the vegetable sushi rolls with soy sauce substitute, a small portion of wasabi paste and pickled ginger.

Nutritional Facts (per serving, includes 2 rolls): Calories: 280 | Total Fat: 4g | Saturated Fat: 0.5g | Trans Fat: 0g | Cholesterol: 0mg | Sodium: 600mg | Total Carbohydrates: 60g | Dietary Fiber: 5g | Sugars: 7g | Protein: 4g | Vitamin D: 0% | Calcium: 2% | Iron: 6% | Potassium: 8%

Potato and Kale Hash with Poached Eggs and Chives

Prep Time: 15 minutes; Cook Time: 30 minutes; Serving Size: 1 plate; Servings: 2

Ingredients:

- 2 medium potatoes, peeled and diced
- 2 cups chopped kale (stems removed)
- 2 tbsp garlic-infused olive oil
- 1 tsp paprika
- Salt and pepper, to taste
- 4 large eggs
- Fresh chives, chopped, for garnish

Instructions:

1. Preheat the oven to 400°F (200°C).
2. Coat the diced potatoes in a mixing bowl with 1 tbsp of garlic-infused olive oil, paprika, salt, and pepper.
3. Spread the potatoes evenly on a parchment paper-lined baking sheet. Roast in the preheated oven for 20 to 25 minutes, or until it becomes tender and slightly crispy.
4. Heat the remaining 1 tbsp of garlic-infused olive oil over medium heat in a large skillet. Sauté the chopped kale for 3-4 minutes or until it wilts. Season with salt and pepper to taste.
5. To poach the eggs, fill a medium-sized saucepan with water and bring it to a gentle simmer. Add a splash of vinegar to the water. Crack each egg into a small bowl, then gently slide it into the simmering water. Poach the eggs for about 3-4 minutes for a runny yolk.
6. Using a slotted spoon, carefully remove the poached eggs from the water and place them on a plate lined with a paper towel to drain off excess water.
7. To assemble, divide the roasted sweet potato and sautéed kale between two plates. Top with the poached eggs and garnish with chopped fresh chives and serve.

Nutritional Facts (per serving): Calories: 320 | Total Fat: 14g | Saturated Fat: 2.5g | Trans Fat: 0g | Cholesterol: 185mg | Sodium: 230mg | Total Carbohydrates: 38g | Dietary Fiber: 6g | Sugars: 7g | Protein: 14g

Roasted Butternut Squash Soup with Fresh Herbs (Vegan)

Prep Time: 15 minutes; Cook Time: 40 minutes; Serving Size: 1 bowl; Servings: 4

Ingredients:

- 1 medium low FODMAP butternut squash, peeled, seeded and cubed
- 2 carrots, peeled and chopped
- 1 potato, peeled and chopped
- 1 tbsp garlic-infused olive oil
- 4 cups low FODMAP vegetable broth
- 1 tsp dried thyme
- 1 tsp dried rosemary
- Salt and pepper to taste
- Fresh parsley, chopped, for garnish

Instructions:
1. Preheat the oven to 400°F (200°C).
2. Arrange cubed butternut squash, chopped carrots, and chopped potatoes on a baking sheet. Drizzle the vegetables with garlic-infused olive oil and toss to ensure they are evenly coated.
3. Roast the vegetables in the preheated oven for 25 to 30 minutes or until they become tender and slightly browned.
4. In a large pot, combine the roasted vegetables, vegetable broth, dried thyme and dried rosemary.
5. Bring the mixture to a simmer over medium heat. Let it simmer for about 10 minutes to allow the flavors to meld.
6. Use an immersion blender to puree the soup until smooth and creamy. Alternatively, carefully transfer the soup in batches to a regular blender and blend until smooth. ensure to blend in batches and allow the steam to escape to avoid splattering. Season the soup with salt and pepper to taste.
7. Ladle the Soup into serving bowls and garnish with chopped fresh parsley. Serve warm.

Nutritional Facts (per serving): Calories: 180 | Total Fat: 3.5g | Saturated Fat: 0.5g | Trans Fat: 0g | Cholesterol: 0mg | Sodium: 300mg | Total Carbohydrates: 36g | Dietary Fiber: 6g | Sugars: 6g | Protein: 3g

Gluten-Free Pasta Salad with Roasted Tomatoes and Olives (Vegan)

Prep Time: 15 minutes; Cook Time: 25 minutes; Serving Size:1 plate; Servings: 4

Ingredients:
- 8 oz (225 g) gluten-free and low FODMAP pasta
- 2 cups cherry tomatoes, halved
- 1/2 cup black olives, sliced
- 2 tbsp extra-virgin olive oil
- 1 tsp dried oregano
- Salt and pepper, to taste
- 1 cup baby spinach leaves
- 1/4 cup fresh basil leaves, chopped
- For Dressing
  - 3 tbsp extra-virgin olive oil
  - 2 tbsp balsamic vinegar
  - 1 tsp low FODMAP Dijon mustard
  - 1 tsp maple syrup
  - Salt and pepper, to taste

Instructions:
1. Preheat the oven to 400°F (200°C).
2. In a bowl, toss the halved cherry tomatoes with 2 tbsp of olive oil, dried oregano, salt and pepper. Spread them on a baking sheet and roast in the preheated oven for about 20-25 minutes, or until the tomatoes are slightly caramelized.
3. While the tomatoes are roasting, cook the pasta according to the package instructions. Drain and rinse the pasta with cold water to stop the cooking process. Set aside.
4. In a large mixing bowl, combine the cooked pasta, roasted tomatoes, sliced black olives, baby spinach and chopped basil.
5. For Dressing: Make the dressing in a separate bowl by whisking together extra-virgin olive oil, Dijon mustard, maple syrup, balsamic vinegar, salt, and pepper.
6. Pour the dressing over the pasta mixture and gently toss to coat everything evenly.
7. Adjust the seasoning with more salt and pepper if needed.
8. Serve the pasta salad immediately, or refrigerate it for a few hours to allow the flavors to meld together before serving.

Nutritional Facts (per serving): Calories: 325 | Total Fat: 14g | Saturated Fat: 2g | Trans Fat: 0g | Cholesterol: 0mg | Sodium: 250mg | Total Carbohydrates: 46g | Dietary Fiber: 6g | Sugars: 6g | Protein: 6g | Vitamin D: 0% | Calcium: 6% | Iron: 15% | Potassium: 10%

Eggplant and Zucchini Casserole with Vegan Cheese (Vegan)

Prep Time: 20 minutes; Cook Time: 40 minutes; Servins: about 2

Ingredients:

- 1 medium eggplant, sliced into rounds
- 2 medium zucchinis, sliced into rounds
- 2 tbsp garlic-infused olive oil
- 1 tsp dried oregano
- Salt and pepper, to taste
- 1 cup low FODMAP tomato sauce
- 1 cup vegan mozzarella cheese (make sure it's low FODMAP), shredded
- 2 tbsp chopped fresh basil
- 2 tbsp chopped fresh parsley
- For Vegan Cheese Sauce
  - 1 cup cooked and peeled potatoes, diced
  - 1/4 cup nutritional yeast
  - 2 tbsp lemon juice
  - 1/2 cup unsweetened almond milk or other low FODMAP plant-based milk
  - Salt and pepper, to taste

Instructions:

1. Preheat the oven to 375°F (190°C).
2. Place the sliced eggplant and zucchini rounds on a baking sheet. Brush both sides with garlic-infused olive oil and sprinkle with dried oregano, salt and pepper.
3. Roast the eggplant and zucchini in the preheated oven for about 15-20 minutes, or until they are tender and slightly golden. Remove from the oven and set aside.
4. For Vegan Cheese Sauce: In a blender, combine the cooked potatoes, nutritional yeast, lemon juice, unsweetened almond milk, salt and pepper. Blend until smooth and creamy. Adjust the seasoning to taste.
5. Spread a thin layer of tomato sauce in a greased baking dish. Place half of the roasted eggplant and zucchini rounds on top of the tomato sauce. Spread half of the vegan cheese sauce on top. Top with half of the shredded vegan mozzarella.
6. Repeat the layering process with the remaining eggplant, zucchini, vegan cheese sauce and vegan mozzarella.
7. Bake in a preheated oven for 20 minutes, covered with aluminum foil.
8. Remove the aluminum foil and bake for another 10 minutes, or until the cheese is melted and bubbling.
9. Remove from the oven and let it cool slightly before serving and garnish with chopped fresh basil and parsley before serving.

Nutritional Facts (per serving): Calories: 220 | Total Fat: 10g | Saturated Fat: 2g | Trans Fat: 0g | Cholesterol: 0mg | Sodium: 480mg | Total Carbohydrates: 26g | Dietary Fiber: 8g | Sugars: 7g | Protein: 10g | Vitamin D: 0% | Calcium: 15% | Iron: 10% | Potassium: 25%

Quinoa and Roasted Vegetable Bowl with Lemon-Tahini Dressing (Vegan)

Prep Time: 15 minutes; Cook Time: 25 minutes; Serving Size: 1 bowl; Servings: 2

Ingredients:

- 2 cups mixed salad greens (lettuce, spinach, arugula)
- 1/4 cup chopped fresh herbs (such as parsley or cilantro)
- 1/4 cup chopped peanuts
- For Roasted Vegetables
    - 1 cup red bell peppers, sliced
    - 1 cup zucchini, sliced
    - 1 cup carrots, sliced
    - 2 tbsp garlic-infused olive oil
    - Salt and pepper, to taste
    - For the Quinoa
    - 1/2 cup quinoa, rinsed
    - 1 cup water or low FODMAP vegetable broth
- For Lemon-Tahini Dressing
    - 2 tbsp tahini
    - 2 tbsp fresh lemon juice
    - 1 tbsp water
    - 1 tsp maple syrup
    - Salt and pepper, to taste

Instructions:

1. For Roasted Vegetables: preheat the oven to 400°F (200°C). Toss the sliced bell peppers, zucchini and carrots with garlic-infused olive oil, salt and pepper. Spread them on a baking sheet in a single layer. Roast the vegetables in a preheated oven for about 20-25 minutes, or until they are tender and slightly caramelized. Remove from the oven and set aside.
2. For Quinoa: Bring the water or vegetable broth to a boil in a saucepan. Add the rinsed quinoa, reduce the heat to low, cover, and simmer for around 15 minutes or until the quinoa is fully cooked and has absorbed all the liquid. Fluff the quinoa with a fork and set aside.
3. For Lemon-Tahini Dressing: in a small bowl, whisk together the tahini, fresh lemon juice, water, maple syrup, salt and pepper until smooth and well combined.
4. In serving bowls, layer the mixed salad greens, cooked quinoa and roasted vegetables.
5. Drizzle the lemon-tahini dressing over the bowl. Sprinkle with chopped fresh herbs and chopped peanuts.

Nutritional Facts (per serving): Calories: 380 | Total Fat: 23g | Saturated Fat: 3g | Trans Fat: 0g | Cholesterol: 0mg | Sodium: 150mg | Total Carbohydrates: 35g | Dietary Fiber: 7g | Sugars: 9g | Protein: 10g | Vitamin D: 0% | Calcium: 10% | Iron: 15% | Potassium: 20%

Grilled Vegetable Skewers with low FODMAP Chimichurri Sauce (Vegan)

Prep Time: 30 minutes; Cook Time: 15 minutes; Servings: about 2

Ingredients:

- 2 zucchinis, sliced into rounds
- 2 red bell peppers, cut into chunks
- 1 eggplant, cut into chunks
- 1 firm tofu block, cut into cubes
- 2 tbsp garlic-infused olive oil
- Salt and pepper to taste
- For low FODMAP Chimichurri Sauce
    - 1 cup fresh parsley, finely chopped
    - 1/4 cup fresh chives, finely chopped
    - 1/4 cup garlic-infused olive oil
    - 2 tbsp red wine vinegar
    - 1/4 tsp red pepper flakes (adjust to taste)
    - 1 tsp dried oregano
    - Salt and pepper, to taste

Instructions:

For Grilled Vegetable Skewers

1. Preheat the grill to medium-high temperature.
2. Arrange sliced zucchinis, red bell pepper chunks, eggplant chunks, and tofu cubes onto skewers, alternating between the vegetables and tofu.
3. Coat the vegetable and tofu skewers with garlic-infused olive oil and add salt and pepper for seasoning.
4. Grill the skewers for about 10-15 minutes, turning occasionally, until the vegetables become tender and moderately charred with the tofu having a golden brown color.

For low FODMAP Chimichurri Sauce: in a bowl, combine the finely chopped fresh parsley, finely chopped fresh chives, garlic-infused olive oil, red wine vinegar, dried oregano, red pepper flakes, salt and pepper. Mix well to combine.

To assemble

1. Remove the grilled vegetable skewers from the grill and place them on a serving platter.
2. Pour the chimichurri sauce over the skewers or serve it on the side as a dipping sauce.

Nutritional Facts (per serving): Calories: 250 | Total Fat: 15g | Saturated Fat: 2g | Trans Fat: 0g | Cholesterol: 0mg | Sodium: 220mg | Total Carbohydrates: 18g | Dietary Fiber: 6g | Sugars: 8g | Protein: 12g

Stuffed Acorn Squash with Quinoa, Kale and Fresh Cranberries (Vegan)

Prep Time: 20 minutes; Cook Time: 50 minutes; Serving Size: ½ acorn squash; Servings: 2

Ingredients:

- 1 medium acorn squash, halved and seeds removed
- 1/2 cup quinoa, rinsed
- 1 cup water or low FODMAP vegetable broth
- 2 cups kale, chopped
- 1/4 cup fresh cranberries, chopped
- 2 tbsp pumpkin seeds
- 1 tbsp extra-virgin olive oil
- 1 tsp maple syrup
- 1/2 tsp ground cinnamon
- Salt and pepper, to taste

Instructions:

1. Preheat the oven to 375°F (190°C).
2. Place the acorn squash halves cut side down on a baking sheet. Roast in the preheated oven for approximately 30-35 minutes, or until the flesh is soft enough to be pierced easily with a fork. Take out of the oven and set aside.
3. Rinse the quinoa under cold water while roasting the squash. Boil the water or vegetable broth in a saucepan. Add quinoa to the saucepan, reduce the heat to low, cover, and simmer for roughly 15 minutes until the quinoa is cooked and the liquid is absorbed. Fluff the quinoa with a fork and set it aside.
4. Heat the olive oil in a skillet over medium heat. Sauté the chopped kale in the skillet for 2-3 minutes or until it wilts and becomes slightly tender. Season to taste with salt and pepper.
5. In a bowl, combine the cooked quinoa, sautéed kale, chopped fresh cranberries, pumpkin seeds, maple syrup, ground cinnamon and additional salt and pepper if needed. Mix well to combine.
6. Flip the roasted acorn squash halves over so they're cut side up. Divide the quinoa mixture evenly between the halves, pressing it down gently to pack it.
7. Place the stuffed acorn squash back in the oven and bake for an additional 15-20 minutes, or until the stuffing is heated through and slightly golden. Serve warm.

Nutritional Facts (per serving): Calories: 380 | Total Fat: 12g | Saturated Fat: 1.5g | Trans Fat: 0g | Cholesterol: 0mg | Sodium: 60mg | Total Carbohydrates: 64g | Dietary Fiber: 11g | Sugars: 10g | Protein: 10g | Vitamin D: 0% | Calcium: 15% | Iron: 20% | Potassium: 35%

6. Soups Recipes

Seafood Chowder with Scallops, Shrimps and Potatoes (Lactose-Free Cream)

Prep Time: 20 minutes; Cook Time: 40 minutes; Serving Size: 1 bowl; Servings: 4

Ingredients:

- 1 tbsp garlic-infused olive oil
- 1 cup diced potatoes
- 1 cup diced carrots
- 2 cups low FODMAP vegetable broth
- 1 tsp dried thyme
- Salt and pepper, to taste
- 1 lb (450 g) scallops, cleaned and halved
- 1/2 lb (225 g) shrimps, peeled and deveined
- 2 cups lactose-free yogurt (make sure it's low FODMAP)
- 2 tbsp fresh chives, chopped
- Fresh parsley leaves, to garnish

Instructions:

1. In a large pot, heat the garlic-infused olive oil over medium heat.
2. Add the diced potatoes and carrots to the pot. Sauté for a few minutes until the vegetables start to soften. Pour in the vegetable broth. The broth should cover the vegetables.
3. Add the dried thyme, salt and pepper to the pot. Stir to combine.
4. Heat the mixture until it boils, then lower the heat. Cover the pot and cook the vegetables on low heat for 15 to 20 minutes, or until they are soft.
5. Put the halved scallops and peeled shrimps in the pot. Allow them to cook for 3 to 4 minutes or until they are properly cooked and opaque.
6. Stir in the yogurt and let the chowder simmer for another 5 minutes to heat through. Taste the chowder and adjust the seasoning if needed.
7. Ladle the seafood chowder and garnish each bowl with chopped fresh chives and fresh parsley leaves before serving.

Nutritional Facts (per serving): Calories: 320 | Total Fat: 15g | Saturated Fat: 8g | Trans Fat: 0g | Cholesterol: 120mg | Sodium: 800mg | Total Carbohydrates: 20g | Dietary Fiber: 2g | Sugars: 4g | Protein: 25g | Vitamin D: 20% | Calcium: 15% | Iron: 10% | Potassium: 25%

Chilled Cucumber Soup with Dill and Lemon

Prep Time: 15 minutes; Cook Time: 0 minutes; Chilling Time: 2 hours;Serving Size: 1 bowl;Servings: 4

Ingredients:

- 3 large cucumbers, peeled, seeded and chopped
- 1 cup lactose-free yogurt (make sure it's low FODMAP)
- 1/4 cup fresh dill, chopped
- 1 tbsp lemon juice
- 1/2 tsp garlic-infused olive oil
- Salt and pepper to taste
- Fresh dill sprigs to garnish

Instructions:

1. Peel the cucumbers, cut them in half lengthwise and scoop out the seeds. Chop the cucumber flesh into small pieces.
2. In a blender, combine the chopped cucumbers, yogurt, fresh dill, lemon juice and garlic-infused olive oil. Blend until smooth and creamy.
3. Season the soup with salt and pepper according to taste. Blend again to incorporate the seasoning.
4. Transfer the cucumber soup to a bowl and cover it. Place the bowl in the refrigerator and chill for at least 2 hours to allow the flavors to meld and the soup to become cold.
5. When ready to serve, use a ladle to transfer the chilled cucumber soup into bowls. Garnish with fresh dill sprigs.

Nutritional Facts (per serving): Calories: 70 | Total Fat: 2.5g | Saturated Fat: 0.5g | Trans Fat: 0g | Cholesterol: 5mg | Sodium: 40mg | Total Carbohydrates: 9g | Dietary Fiber: 2g | Sugars: 5g | Protein: 3g | Vitamin A: 10% | Vitamin C: 15% | Calcium: 10% | Iron: 2%

Fragrant Thai Chicken Soup with Lemongrass and Lime Leaves

Prep Time: 20 minutes; Cook Time: 30 minutes; Serving Size: 1 bowl; Servings: 4

Ingredients:

- 1 lb (450 g) boneless, skinless chicken breasts, thinly sliced
- 1 tbsp garlic-infused olive oil
- 1 tbsp fresh ginger, minced
- 2 lemongrass stalks, bruised and cut into segments
- 4 cups low FODMAP chicken broth
- 1 cup canned coconut milk (make sure it's low FODMAP)
- 1 small zucchini, sliced
- 1 red bell pepper, thinly sliced
- 1 tbsp fish sauce or soy sauce (make sure it's low FODMAP)
- Juice of 1 lime
- Salt and pepper, to taste
- Fresh cilantro leaves, to garnish

Instructions:

1. Heat garlic-infused olive oil in a large pot over medium heat.
2. Add minced ginger and sliced chicken to the pot. Cook until the chicken is no longer pink and is completely cooked. Remove the chicken from the pot and set it aside.
3. Add the lemongrass to the pot and sauté for a minute to release its fragrance. Pour the chicken broth into the pot and bring it to a simmer.
4. Add the coconut milk from the can to the pot. Allow the soup to simmer for approximately ten minutes to let the flavors blend.
5. Take out and throw away the sections of lemongrass from the pot.
6. Return the cooked chicken to the pot. Add the sliced zucchini and red bell pepper to the pot. Let the soup simmer for another 5-7 minutes until the vegetables are tender.
7. Stir in the fish sauce (or soy sauce) and lime juice. Add salt and pepper to the soup as per your taste.
8. Ladle the fragrant Thai chicken soup into bowls. Garnish each bowl with fresh cilantro leaves. Serve warm.

Nutritional Facts (per serving): Calories: 280 | Total Fat: 12g | Saturated Fat: 6g | Trans Fat: 0g | Cholesterol: 65mg | Sodium: 750mg | Total Carbohydrates: 10g | Dietary Fiber: 2g | Sugars: 4g | Protein: 30g | Vitamin D: 6% | Calcium: 4% | Iron: 15% | Potassium: 25%

Hearty Carrot and Ginger Soup with Chives

Prep Time: 15 minutes; Cook Time: 30 minutes; Serving Size: 1 bowl; Servings: 4

Ingredients:

- 1 lb (450 g) carrots, peeled and chopped
- 1 potato, peeled and chopped
- 1 tbsp garlic-infused olive oil
- 1 tbsp fresh ginger, minced
- 4 cups low FODMAP vegetable broth
- 1 tsp ground turmeric
- 2 tbsp chopped fresh chives
- Salt and pepper, to taste

Instructions:

1. In a large pot, heat the garlic-infused olive oil over medium heat.
2. Add the chopped carrots and the potato to the pot and sauté for about 5 minutes, stirring occasionally.
3. Stir in the minced ginger and ground turmeric and cook for another 1-2 minutes until fragrant.
4. Add the vegetable broth to the pot and bring the mixture to a boil.
5. Reduce the heat to low, cover the pot and let the soup simmer for 20 to 25 minutes or until the carrots and potato are tender.
6. Puree the soup until smooth using an immersion blender. Alternatively, carefully transfer the soup in batches to a blender and blend until smooth. Take care when handling hot liquids. Add salt and pepper to the soup according to your preference.
7. Ladle the carrot and ginger soup into bowls, garnish each bowl with chopped fresh chives and serve warm.

Nutritional Facts (per serving): Calories: 140 | Total Fat: 3g | Saturated Fat: 0.5g | Trans Fat: 0g | Cholesterol: 0mg | Sodium: 600mg | Total Carbohydrates: 27g | Dietary Fiber: 5g | Sugars: 7g | Protein: 2g | Vitamin D: 0% | Calcium: 6% | Iron: 6% | Potassium: 20%

Creamy Potato and Parsley Soup with Crumbled Bacon (Lactose-Free)

Prep Time: 15 minutes; Cook Time: 30 minutes; Serving Size: 1 bowl; Servings: 4

Ingredients:

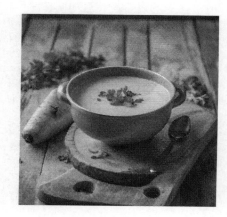

- 4 slices bacon
- 1 tbsp garlic-infused olive oil
- 4 cups diced potatoes
- 2 cups diced carrots
- 4 cups low FODMAP chicken broth
- 1 tsp dried thyme
- Salt and pepper, to taste
- 1 cup coconut milk
- 1/4 cup fresh parsley leaves, chopped
- Additional fresh parsley leaves, for garnish

Instructions:

1. Cook the bacon until crispy in a large pot. Take out the bacon from the pot, crumble it, and put it aside for garnish.
2. Heat the olive oil, infused with garlic, in the same pot over medium heat.
3. Add the diced potatoes and carrots to the pot. Sauté the vegetables until they start to soften, which should take just a few minutes. Add the chicken broth to the pot. Make sure the vegetables are covered by the broth. Put the dried thyme, salt, and pepper in the pot. Stir the mixture to combine the ingredients.
4. Boil the mixture and then reduce the heat to low. Simmer the vegetables in a covered pot for 15-20 minutes or until they become tender.
5. Make the soup smooth by blending it with an immersion blender or a regular blender.
6. Put the blended soup back in the pot. Mix in coconut milk and freshly chopped parsley leaves.
7. Bring the soup back to a simmer over medium heat. Let it simmer for another 5 minutes to heat through. Taste the soup and adjust the seasoning if needed.
8. Ladle the creamy potato and parsley soup into bowls and garnish each bowl with crumbled bacon and additional fresh parsley leaves before serving.

Nutritional Facts (per serving): Calories: 250 | Total Fat: 12g | Saturated Fat: 5g | Trans Fat: 0g | Cholesterol: 10mg | Sodium: 800mg | Total Carbohydrates: 30g | Dietary Fiber: 4g | Sugars: 6g | Protein: 5g | Vitamin D: 0% | Calcium: 4% | Iron: 15% | Potassium: 20%

Roasted Tomato and Basil Soup with Garlic-Infused Oil

Prep Time: 15 minutes; Cook Time: 40 minutes; Serving Size: 1 bowl; Servings: 4

Ingredients:
- 2 lbs (900 g) ripe tomatoes, halved
- 1 tbsp garlic-infused olive oil
- 1 tbsp fresh basil leaves, chopped
- 2 cups low FODMAP vegetable broth
- 1 tsp dried oregano
- Salt and pepper, to taste
- 1 tbsp garlic-infused olive oil (for drizzling)
- Fresh basil leaves, for garnish

Instructions:

1. Preheat the oven to 400°F (200°C).
2. Place the halved tomatoes on a baking sheet, cut side up. Drizzle with 1 tbsp of garlic-infused olive oil. Roast the tomatoes in the preheated oven for about 25-30 minutes, or until they are softened and slightly caramelized.
3. In a blender or food processor, combine the roasted tomatoes (including any juices), chopped fresh basil and vegetable broth. Blend until smooth.
4. Pour the tomato mixture into a pot. Add the dried oregano, salt and pepper.
5. Simmer the soup over medium heat. Simmer for around 10 minutes to allow the flavors to blend. Taste for seasoning and season to taste if necessary.
6. Ladle the roasted tomato and basil soup into bowls and drizzle each bowl with a little more garlic-infused olive oil. Garnish with fresh basil leaves before serving.

Nutritional Facts (per serving): Calories: 90 | Total Fat: 5g | Saturated Fat: 0.5g | Trans Fat: 0g | Cholesterol: 0mg | Sodium: 500mg | Total Carbohydrates: 12g | Dietary Fiber: 4g | Sugars: 8g | Protein: 2g | Vitamin D: 0% | Calcium: 4% | Iron: 6% | Potassium: 20%

Shrimp and Zucchini Noodle Soup in a Light Tomato Broth

Prep Time: 15 minutes; Cook Time: 20 minutes; Serving Size: 1 bowl; Servings: 2

Ingredients:

- 8 oz (225 g) shrimps, peeled and deveined
- 2 medium zucchinis, spiralized into noodles
- 2 cups low FODMAP vegetable broth
- 1 cup canned diced tomatoes (make sure they're low FODMAP)
- 1 tbsp garlic-infused olive oil
- 1 tsp dried basil
- 1/2 tsp dried oregano
- Salt and pepper, to taste
- Fresh basil leaves, for garnish

Instructions:

1. On a pot, warm up the garlic-infused olive oil on medium heat.
2. Include the dried basil and dried oregano in the pot. Sauté for about 60 seconds until it smells fragrant.
3. Empty the canned diced tomatoes and the chicken broth in the pot. Bring the mixture to a boiling point and reduce the heat to low.
4. Put the deveined and peeled shrimps into the broth that's already simmering. Cook them for 3 to 4 minutes, or until they turn pink and opaque.
5. With a slotted spoon, remove the cooked shrimps from the broth and set them aside.
6. Add zucchini noodles to the broth that's simmering. Cook the vegetables for about 2 to 3 minutes, or until they become tender but remain slightly crisp. Add salt and pepper to the broth in accordance with personal preference.
7. Divide the zucchini noodles and broth between serving bowls. Arrange the cooked shrimps on top of the zucchini noodles and garnish each bowl with fresh basil leaves before serving. Serve warm.

Nutritional Facts (per serving): Calories: 180 | Total Fat: 7g | Saturated Fat: 1g | Trans Fat: 0g | Cholesterol: 150mg | Sodium: 800mg | Total Carbohydrates: 10g | Dietary Fiber: 3g | Sugars: 5g | Protein: 20g | Vitamin D: 10% | Calcium: 8% | Iron: 15% | Potassium: 25%

Oven-Roasted Red Bell Pepper and Tomato Bisque with Fresh Basil

Prep Time: 15 minutes; Cook Time: 45 minutes; Serving Size: 1 bowl; Servings: 4

Ingredients:

- 3 red bell peppers, halved and seeds removed
- 6 medium tomatoes, halved
- 1 tbsp garlic-infused olive oil
- 1 tbsp fresh basil leaves, chopped
- 4 cups low FODMAP vegetable broth
- 1 tsp dried oregano
- Salt and pepper, to taste
- Fresh basil leaves, to garnish

Instructions:

1. Preheat the oven to 400°F (200°C).
2. Arrange the red bell pepper halves and tomato halves, sliced side up, on a baking sheet. Drizzle garlic-infused olive oil over the vegetables. Roast the red bell peppers and tomatoes in a preheated oven for 30-35 minutes or until they are tender and lightly caramelized.
3. Take the baking sheet out of the oven and let the roasted vegetables cool briefly. After cooling, peel the skin off of the roasted red bell peppers.
4. Combine the roasted red bell peppers, roasted tomatoes (including their juices), fresh basil (chopped), and vegetable broth in a blender or food processor. Blend until the mixture is smooth.
5. Pour the blended mixture into a pot. Add the dried oregano, salt, and pepper.
6. Simmer the soup over medium heat. Allow the soup to simmer for around 10 minutes to let the flavors blend. Taste the bisque and adjust the seasoning according to your preference, if necessary.
7. Ladle the oven-roasted red bell pepper and tomato bisque into bowls and garnish each bowl with fresh basil leaves before serving. Serve warm.

Nutritional Facts (per serving): Calories: 90 | Total Fat: 3.5g | Saturated Fat: 0.5g | Trans Fat: 0g | Cholesterol: 0mg | Sodium: 800mg | Total Carbohydrates: 12g | Dietary Fiber: 4g | Sugars: 8g | Protein: 2g | Vitamin D: 0% | Calcium: 6% | Iron: 10% | Potassium: 15%

Hearty Winter Vegetable Soup with Thyme and Oregano

Prep Time: 20 minutes; Cook Time: 40 minutes; Serving Size: 1 bowl; Servings: 4

Ingredients:

- 1 tbsp garlic-infused olive oil
- 2 medium carrots, peeled and diced
- 2 medium parsnips, peeled and diced
- 1 cup diced turnips
- 1 cup diced zucchini
- 1 cup diced butternut squash
- 6 cups low FODMAP vegetable broth
- 1 tsp dried thyme
- 1/2 tsp dried oregano
- Salt and pepper, to taste
- Fresh thyme leaves, for garnish

Instructions:

1. In a large pot, heat the garlic-infused olive oil over medium heat.
2. Add the diced carrots, parsnips, turnips, zucchini and butternut squash to the pot. Sauté for a few minutes until the vegetables start to soften. Pour in the vegetable broth. The broth should cover the vegetables.
3. Add the dried thyme and dried oregano to the pot. Stir to combine.
4. Bring the soup to a boil, then reduce the heat to low. Cover the pot and let the soup simmer for about 30-35 minutes, or until the vegetables are tender. Season the soup with salt and pepper to taste.
5. Ladle the soup into bowls and garnish each bowl with fresh thyme leaves before serving. Serve warm.

Nutritional Facts (per serving): Calories: 120 | Total Fat: 2.5g | Saturated Fat: 0.5g | Trans Fat: 0g | Cholesterol: 0mg | Sodium: 800mg | Total Carbohydrates: 25g | Dietary Fiber: 6g | Sugars: 6g | Protein: 2g | Vitamin D: 0% | Calcium: 6% | Iron: 10% | Potassium: 20%

Warm Sorghum and Roasted Vegetable Soup with Fresh Parsley

Prep Time: 15 minutes; Cook Time: 45 minutes; Serving Size: 1 bowl; Servings: 4

Ingredients:

- 1 cup sorghum grains, rinsed and drained
- 2 cups diced carrots
- 2 cups diced zucchini
- 1 red bell pepper, diced
- 1 tbsp garlic-infused olive oil
- 4 cups low FODMAP vegetable broth
- 1 tsp dried thyme
- Salt and pepper, to taste
- Fresh parsley leaves, chopped, for garnish

Instructions:

1. In a pot, bring 2 cups of water to a boil. Add the rinsed sorghum grains and cook according to package instructions, usually about 25-30 minutes. Drain any excess water and set the cooked sorghum aside.
2. Preheat the oven to 400°F (200°C).
3. Arrange the carrots, zucchini, and red bell pepper dices on a baking sheet. Drizzle garlic-infused olive oil over the vegetables and toss them to coat evenly.
4. Bake in the preheated oven for about 20-25 minutes, or until the vegetables are tender and caramelized.
5. In a pot, bring the vegetable broth to a simmer. Add the roasted vegetables, cooked sorghum, dried thyme, salt and pepper to the simmering broth. Let the soup simmer for about 10 minutes to allow the flavors to meld. Taste the soup and adjust the seasoning if needed.
6. Ladle the soup into bowls and garnish each bowl with chopped fresh parsley before serving.

Nutritional Facts (per serving): Calories: 280 | Total Fat: 4.5g | Saturated Fat: 0.5g | Trans Fat: 0g | Cholesterol: 0mg | Sodium: 800mg | Total Carbohydrates: 56g | Dietary Fiber: 10g | Sugars: 8g | Protein: 7g | Vitamin D: 0% | Calcium: 6% | Iron: 20% | Potassium: 15%

Lemon and Dill-infused Sea Bass Soup with Spinach

Prep Time: 15 minutes; Cook Time: 25 minutes; Serving Size: 1 bowl + 1 fillet; Servings: 2

Ingredients:

- 2 sea bass fillets
- 1 lemon, zest and juice
- 1 tbsp garlic-infused olive oil
- 4 cups low FODMAP vegetable broth
- 1 tsp dried dill
- Salt and pepper, to taste
- 2 cups fresh spinach leaves
- Fresh dill sprigs, for garnish

Instructions:

1. Pat the sea bass fillets dry with paper towels and sprinkle salt and pepper on top.
2. In a bowl, combine the lemon zest, lemon juice and garlic-infused olive oil. Brush this mixture over both sides of the sea bass fillets. Set aside to marinate for a few minutes.
3. Bring the vegetable broth to a simmer in a saucepan. Add the dried dill to the simmering broth. Stir to infuse the flavors. Carefully place the marinated sea bass fillets into the simmering broth. Let them cook for about 4-5 minutes on each side, or until the fish is opaque and flakes easily with a fork. Take out the fish fillets from the broth and place them separately.
4. Add the fresh spinach leaves to the simmering broth. Let them wilt for about 1-2 minutes.
5. Taste the broth and adjust the seasoning with salt and pepper if needed.
6. Ladle the soup with spinach into bowls and place a cooked sea bass fillet on top of each bowl. Garnish each bowl with fresh dill sprigs before serving.

Nutritional Facts (per serving): Calories: 220 | Total Fat: 9g | Saturated Fat: 1.5g | Trans Fat: 0g | Cholesterol: 60mg | Sodium: 800mg | Total Carbohydrates: 6g | Dietary Fiber: 2g | Sugars: 2g | Protein: 30g | Vitamin D: 10% | Calcium: 15% | Iron: 15% | Potassium: 30%

Savory Beef Stew with Root Vegetables (low FODMAP Selection)

Prep Time: 20 minutes; Cook Time: 2 hours; Serving Size: 1 bowl; Servings: 4

Ingredients:

- 1 lb (450 g) beef stew meat, cubed
- 2 tbsp garlic-infused olive oil
- 2 cups low-sodium beef broth (make sure it's low FODMAP)
- 2 cups diced potatoes
- 1 cup diced carrots
- 1 cup diced parsnips
- 1 cup diced turnips
- 1 tsp dried thyme
- Salt and pepper, to taste
- Chopped fresh parsley, for garnish

Instructions:

1. In a large pot, heat the garlic-infused olive oil over medium-high heat.
2. Add the cubed beef stew meat to the pot. Brown the meat on all sides, then remove it from the pot and set it aside.
3. In the same pot, add the diced potatoes, carrots, parsnips and turnips. Sauté for a few minutes until the vegetables start to soften.
4. Return the browned beef stew meat to the pot with the sautéed vegetables and pour in the beef broth. The broth should cover the meat and vegetables.
5. Add the dried thyme, salt and pepper to the pot. Stir to combine.
6. Heat the pot with the stew until it boils, and then lower the heat to a simmer. Cover the pot and allow the stew to simmer for about 1.5 to 2 hours or until the meat has become tender and the flavors have combined. Savor the stew and modify the seasoning as required.
7. Ladle the savory beef stew with root vegetables into bowls and garnish each bowl with chopped fresh parsley before serving. Serve warm.

Nutritional Facts (per serving): Calories: 350 | Total Fat: 12g | Saturated Fat: 4g | Trans Fat: 0g | Cholesterol: 80mg | Sodium: 800mg | Total Carbohydrates: 35g | Dietary Fiber: 6g | Sugars: 7g | Protein: 25g | Vitamin D: 6% | Calcium: 8% | Iron: 20% | Potassium: 30%

7. Quick Meals and Lunches for Work

Rice Paper Rolls with Tofu, Mint and low FODMAP Dipping Sauce (Vegan)

Prep Time: 20 minutes ; Cook Time: 10 minutes ; Serving Size: 2 rolls; Servings: 1

Ingredients:

- For Rice Paper Rolls
  - 4 rice paper wrappers
  - 4 oz (about 115 g) firm tofu, sliced into thin strips
  - 1 cup shredded lettuce
  - 1 cup julienned carrots
  - 1/2 cup fresh mint leaves
- For low FODMAP Dipping Sauce
  - 2 tbsp low-sodium soy sauce (make sure it's low FODMAP)
  - 1 tbsp pure maple syrup
  - 1 tbsp rice vinegar
  - 1 tsp sesame oil
  - 1/2 tsp grated fresh ginger

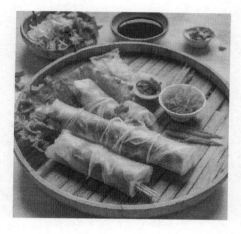

Instructions:

1. Start by preparing the tofu. Heat a non-stick skillet over medium heat. Lightly spray it with oil. Add the tofu slices and cook for about 2-3 minutes on each side, or until they are golden and slightly crispy. Remove from the heat and set aside.
2. Fill a shallow dish or a large plate with warm water. Dip one rice paper wrapper into the water for about 10-15 seconds, or until it becomes soft and pliable. Carefully place it on a clean surface, like a cutting board.
3. On the lower third of the rice paper, place a few strips of cooked tofu, followed by some shredded lettuce, julienned carrots and fresh mint leaves. Be sure not to overfill the wrapper.
4. Fold the sides of the rice paper over the filling, then gently roll up from the bottom, tucking the sides in as you go, to form a tight roll. Repeat this process with the remaining ingredients to make the remaining rolls.
5. For Dipping sauce: Combine soy sauce, pure maple syrup, rice vinegar, sesame oil, and freshly grated ginger in a small bowl, whisk together until well combined.
6. Serve the rice paper rolls with the dipping sauce.

Nutritional Facts (per serving): Calories: 230 | Total Fat: 7g | Saturated Fat: 1g | Cholesterol: 0mg | Sodium: 570mg | Total Carbohydrates: 34g | Dietary Fiber: 4g | Sugars: 10g | Protein: 10g | Calcium: 180mg | Iron: 2.5mg | Potassium: 480mg

Grilled Chicken Salad with Spinach and low FODMAP Vinaigrette

Prep Time: 15 minutes; Cook Time: 10 minutes; Serving Size: 1 plate; Servings: 2

Ingredients:

- For Grilled Chicken
    - 2 boneless, skinless chicken breasts
    - 1 tbsp garlic-infused olive oil
    - Salt and pepper, to taste
- For Salad
    - 4 cups fresh baby spinach
    - 1 cup cherry tomatoes, halved
    - 1/2 cucumber, sliced
    - 1/4 cup sliced carrots
    - 2 tbsp chopped scallion green tops
- For low FODMAP Vinaigrette
    - 3 tbsp extra-virgin olive oil
    - 2 tbsp white wine vinegar
    - 1 tsp low FODMAP Dijon mustard
    - 1 tsp maple syrup or other low FODMAP sweetener
    - Salt and pepper, to taste

Instructions:
1. For Grilled Chicken: preheat the grill or grill pan over medium-high heat. Coat the chicken breasts with garlic-infused olive oil and sprinkle them with salt and pepper. Grill the chicken breasts for about 4-5 minutes on each side, or until cooked through and no longer pink in the center. Remove from the grill and let them rest for a few minutes before slicing.
2. For Salad: in a large bowl, combine the baby spinach, cucumber, cherry tomatoes, sliced carrots and chopped scallion green tops.
3. For low FODMAP Vinaigrette: Combine olive oil, white wine vinegar, Dijon mustard, maple syrup, salt, and pepper in a small bowl. Whisk them together to make the vinaigrette.
4. Drizzle the vinaigrette dressing evenly over the ingredients of the salad, then toss them gently to combine.
5. Divide the salad mixture between two plates and top each salad with sliced grilled chicken.

Nutritional Facts (per serving): Calories: 350 | Total Fat: 20g | Saturated Fat: 3g | Trans Fat: 0g | Cholesterol: 70mg | Sodium: 400mg | Total Carbohydrates: 20g | Dietary Fiber: 4g | Sugars: 8g | Protein: 25g | Vitamin D: 8% | Calcium: 10% | Iron: 20% | Potassium: 25%

Baked Potatoes with Tuna Salad and Chives

Prep Time: 10 minutes; Cook Time: 45 minutes; Serving Size: 1 potato; Servings: 2

Ingredients:

- 2 medium potatoes
- 1 can (5 oz/140 g) canned tuna, drained (make sure it's low FODMAP)
- 2 tbsp low FODMAP Mayonnaise
- 1 tbsp low FODMAP Dijon mustard
- 1 tbsp chopped fresh chives
- Salt and pepper, to taste

Instructions:

1. Preheat the oven to 400°F (200°C). Scrub the potatoes clean and pierce them several times with a fork.
2. Put the potatoes on a baking sheet and bake them in the preheated oven for approximately 40 to 45 minutes or until you can poke them tenderly with a fork.
3. While the potatoes are baking, prepare the tuna salad. In a bowl, mix the drained canned tuna, Mayonnaise, Dijon mustard, chopped fresh chives, salt and pepper. Stir to combine.
4. Once the potatoes are cooked, remove them from the oven and let them cool slightly.
5. Cut a slit in the top of each potato and gently press the ends to open the potatoes.
6. Spoon the tuna salad mixture into the opened potatoes and garnish with additional chopped chives, if desired.

Nutritional Facts (per serving): Calories: 280 | Total Fat: 9g | Saturated Fat: 1.5g | Trans Fat: 0g | Cholesterol: 30mg | Sodium: 400mg | Total Carbohydrates: 35g | Dietary Fiber: 5g | Sugars: 10g | Protein: 15g | Vitamin D: 10% | Calcium: 6% | Iron: 15% | Potassium: 25%

Rice Noodles with Stir-Fried Shrimps and Red Bell Peppers

Prep Time: 15 minutes; Cook Time: 15 minutes; Serving Size: 2 servings

Ingredients:

- 8 oz (225 g) rice noodles (make sure they are low FODMAP)
- 8 oz (225 g) shrimps, peeled and deveined
- 1 red bell pepper, thinly sliced
- 2 tbsp garlic-infused olive oil
- 2 tbsp low-sodium soy sauce (make sure it's low FODMAP)
- 1 tbsp rice vinegar
- 1 tsp sesame oil
- 1 tsp grated fresh ginger
- 2 tbsp chopped scallion green tops
- Sesame seeds, to garnish

Instructions:

1. Cook the rice noodles according to the package instructions. Drain and set aside.
2. In a bowl, marinate the shrimps with 1 tbsp of garlic-infused olive oil, soy sauce and rice vinegar for about 10 minutes.
3. In a wok or large skillet, heat the remaining tbsp of garlic-infused olive oil over medium-high heat.
4. Add the marinated shrimps to the wok and stir-fry for about 2-3 minutes, or until they turn pink and opaque. Remove the shrimps from the wok and set them aside.
5. In the same wok, add the thinly sliced red bell pepper and grated fresh ginger. Stir-fry for about 2 minutes, or until the bell pepper starts to soften.
6. Add the cooked rice noodles and cooked shrimps back to the wok.
7. Drizzle the sesame oil over the noodles and toss everything together to combine. Stir in the chopped scallion green tops.
8. Divide the rice noodle and shrimp mixture between two plates and garnish with sesame seeds before serving.

Nutritional Facts (per serving): Calories: 400 | Total Fat: 12g | Saturated Fat: 1.5g | Trans Fat: 0g | Cholesterol: 160mg | Sodium: 800mg | Total Carbohydrates: 55g | Dietary Fiber: 3g | Sugars: 4g | Protein: 20g | Vitamin D: 8% | Calcium: 6% | Iron: 15% | Potassium: 10%

Gluten-Free Turkey Wrap with Lettuce, Carrots and low FODMAP Mayo

Prep Time: 10 minutes; Cook Time: 0 minutes; Servings: 1 wrap

Ingredients:
- 1 gluten-free and low FODMAP tortilla or wrap
- 3-4 slices of cooked turkey breast
- 1 large lettuce leaf
- 1/4 cup shredded carrots
- 2 tbsp low FODMAP Mayonnaise
- Salt and pepper, to taste

Instructions:
1. Lay the tortilla or wrap flat on a clean surface and place the lettuce leaf in the center of the tortilla.
2. Layer the cooked turkey slices on top of the lettuce and sprinkle the shredded carrots evenly over the turkey.
3. Drizzle the Mayonnaise over the carrots and season with a pinch of salt and pepper, if desired.
4. Fold the sides of the tortilla over the fillings, then roll it up tightly from the bottom to form a wrap. Slice the wrap in half diagonally if desired.

Nutritional Facts (per serving-1 wrap): Calories: 350 | Total Fat: 18g | Saturated Fat: 3.5g | Trans Fat: 0g | Cholesterol: 45mg | Sodium: 700mg | Total Carbohydrates: 30g | Dietary Fiber: 4g | Sugars: 5g | Protein: 20g | Vitamin D: 2% | Calcium: 10% | Iron: 15% | Potassium: 10%

Cold Pasta Salad with Grilled Chicken, Tomatoes and Basil

Prep Time: 15 minutes; Cook Time: 15 minutes; Serving Size: 1 plate; Servings: 4

Ingredients:
- 8 oz (225 g) gluten-free and low FODMAP pasta
- 2 boneless, skinless chicken breasts, grilled and sliced
- 1 cup cherry tomatoes, halved
- 1/4 cup fresh basil leaves, chopped
- 1/4 cup lactose-free feta cheese, crumbled
- 2 tbsp garlic-infused olive oil
- 2 tbsp balsamic vinegar
- Salt and pepper, to taste

Instructions:
1. Cook the pasta according to the package instructions. Drain and rinse under cold water to stop the cooking process. Set aside.
2. In a large bowl, combine the cooked pasta, sliced grilled chicken, cherry tomato halves and torn basil leaves.
3. In a small bowl, whisk together the garlic-infused olive oil and balsamic vinegar to make the dressing.
4. Pour the dressing over the pasta mixture and toss gently to combine, ensuring all ingredients are coated with the dressing.
5. Refrigerate the pasta salad for at least 30 minutes to allow the flavors to meld.
6. Before serving, give the salad a final toss to redistribute the dressing. Garnish with additional fresh basil leaves if desired.

Nutritional Facts (per serving): Calories: 350 | Total Fat: 12g | Saturated Fat: 2,5g | Trans Fat: 0g | Cholesterol: 70mg | Sodium: 200mg | Total Carbohydrates: 35g | Dietary Fiber: 3g | Sugars: 3g | Protein: 25g | Vitamin D: 6% | Calcium: 6% | Iron: 20% | Potassium: 15%

Mason Jar Salad with Layered Veggies and Quinoa (Vegan)

Prep Time: 15 minutes; Cook Time: 20 minutes; Serving Size: 1 mason jar salad; Servings: 1

Ingredients:

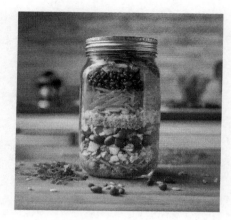

- 1/2 cup cooked quinoa
- 1/4 cup sliced cucumbers
- 1/4 cup shredded carrots
- 1/4 cup diced red bell pepper
- 1/4 cup baby spinach leaves
- 5 basil leaves, chopped
- 2 tbsp cup olives
- 2 tbsp mixed nuts (e.g., pine nuts, walnuts), chopped
- 2 tbsp sunflower seeds
- 2 tbsp low FODMAP Vinaigrette

Instructions:

1. In a mason jar, start layering the salad ingredients. Begin with the cooked quinoa as the base.
2. Layer the sliced cucumbers, shredded carrots, diced red bell pepper, olives, chopped mixed nuts, sunflower seeds, baby spinach and basil leaves on top of the quinoa in separate layers.
3. Screw the lid on the mason jar to seal the salad.
4. When ready to eat, pour the Vinaigrette dressing over the layered veggies and quinoa in the jar.
5. Shake the mason jar vigorously to distribute the dressing and mix the ingredients.
6. Remove the lid and enjoy the vegan mason jar salad straight from the jar or transfer it to a plate.

Nutritional Facts (per serving - 1 mason jar salad): Calories: 250 | Total Fat: 5g | Saturated Fat: 0.5g | Trans Fat: 0g | Cholesterol: 0mg | Sodium: 150mg | Total Carbohydrates: 45g | Dietary Fiber: 8g | Sugars: 5g | Protein: 8g | Vitamin D: 0% | Calcium: 6% | Iron: 15% | Potassium: 10%

Egg and Cheddar Breakfast Muffins with Spinach (Vegetarian)

Prep Time: 10 minutes; Cook Time: 20 minutes; Serving Size: 1 muffin; Servings: 6 muffins

Ingredients:

- 6 large eggs
- 1/4 cup lactose-free milk or other low FODMAP dairy alternative
- 1 cup fresh baby spinach, chopped
- 1/2 cup shredded cheddar cheese
- 1/4 tsp garlic-infused olive oil
- Salt and pepper, to taste
- Cooking spray, for greasing

Instructions:
1. Preheat the oven to 350°F (175°C). Grease a muffin tin with cooking spray.
2. In a bowl, whisk together the eggs and milk until well combined.
3. Stir in the chopped baby spinach and shredded cheddar cheese into the egg mixture.
4. Add the garlic-infused olive oil, salt and pepper. Mix well.
5. Divide the egg and spinach mixture evenly among the muffin tin cups.
6. Place the muffins in the oven that has been preheated and set the timer for about 15-20 minutes, or until the muffins are cooked and the tops are golden brown.
7. After baking, remove the muffins from the oven and let them cool slightly before serving. Serve the muffins while still warm.

Nutritional Facts (per serving - 1 muffin): Calories: 120 | Total Fat: 8g | Saturated Fat: 3.5g | Trans Fat: 0g | Cholesterol: 190mg | Sodium: 150mg | Total Carbohydrates: 2g | Dietary Fiber: 0g | Sugars: 0g | Protein: 9g | Vitamin D: 10% | Calcium: 10% | Iron: 4% | Potassium: 90mg

Grilled Fish Tacos with Cabbage Slaw and Eggplant Cream

Prep Time: 15 minutes; Cook Time: 15 minutes; Serving Size: 2 tacos; Servings: 1

Ingredients:
- For Tacos
    - 8 oz (225 g) white fish fillets (such as cod or haddock)
    - 1 tbsp garlic-infused olive oil
    - 1 tsp ground cumin
    - Salt and pepper, to taste
    - 4 small low FODMAP corn tortillas
- For Cabbage Slaw
    - 1 cup shredded green cabbage
    - 1 tbsp lime juice
    - Salt and pepper, to taste
- For Eggplant Cream
    - 1/2 cup cooked eggplant puree (grilled or roasted)
    - 2 tbsp lactose-free plain yogurt (make sure it's low FODMAP)
    - 1 tbsp fresh lemon juice
    - Salt and pepper, to taste

Instructions:
1. Preheat the grill or grill pan over medium-high heat.
2. In a bowl, mix the garlic-infused olive oil, ground cumin, salt and pepper. Coat the white fish fillets with this mixture.
3. Grill the fish fillets on the grill for 3 to 4 minutes on each side until they are cooked through and flaky. Take off the heat and set aside.
4. For Cabbage Slaw: in a separate bowl, combine the shredded green cabbage, chopped cilantro, lime juice, salt and pepper to make the cabbage slaw. Toss to mix well.
5. For Eggplant Cream: blend the cooked eggplant puree, plain yogurt, fresh lemon juice, salt and pepper in a blender until smooth. Adjust the seasoning to taste.
6. Heat the corn tortillas in a dry skillet or on the grill for a minute on each side.
7. To assemble the tacos, spread a layer of eggplant cream on each tortilla.
8. Top with grilled fish fillets and a generous portion of cabbage slaw.

Nutritional Facts (per serving - 2 tacos): Calories: 300 | Total Fat: 12g | Saturated Fat: 2g | Trans Fat: 0g | Cholesterol: 45mg | Sodium: 400mg | Total Carbohydrates: 25g | Dietary Fiber: 5g | Sugars: 2g | Protein: 25g | Vitamin D: 10% | Calcium: 8% | Iron: 15% | Potassium: 20%

Zucchini Noodles with Fresh Basil Pesto and Cherry Tomatoes (Vegan)

Prep Time: 15 minutes; Cook Time: 5 minutes; Serving Size: 1 plate; Servings: 2

Ingredients:
- 2 medium zucchinis, spiralized into noodles
- 1 tbsp garlic-infused olive oil
- Salt and pepper, to taste
- 4 tbsp low FODMAP Fresh Basil Pesto
- 1 cup cherry tomatoes, halved
- Vegan and low FODMAP Parmesan cheese, to garnish (optional)

Instructions:
1. In a large bowl, toss the spiralized zucchini noodles with garlic-infused olive oil, salt and pepper. Set aside.
2. Pour the fresh basil pesto over the zucchini noodles and toss the noodles to evenly coat them.
3. Heat a large skillet over medium heat. Add the cherry tomato halves. Cook for 2 to 3 minutes or until they begin to soften.
4. Divide the zucchini noodles with pesto between two plates. Top with sautéed cherry tomatoes and garnish with vegan parmesan cheese, if desired. Serve warm.

Nutritional Facts (per serving): Calories: 250 | Total Fat: 20g | Saturated Fat: 2g | Trans Fat: 0g | Cholesterol: 0mg | Sodium: 150mg | Total Carbohydrates: 15g | Dietary Fiber: 4g | Sugars: 7g | Protein: 6g | Vitamin D: 0% | Calcium: 10% | Iron: 15% | Potassium: 15%

Roast Beef Sandwich with Gluten-Free Bread and Mustard

Prep Time: 10 minutes; Cook Time: 15 minutes; Serving Size: 1 sandwich; Servings: 1

Ingredients:
- 2 slices of gluten-free and low FODMAP bread
- 3-4 oz (about 85-115 g) thinly sliced roast beef (make sure it's low FODMAP)
- 1 tbsp low FODMAP Mustard
- 1/4 cup arugula or spinach leaves
- 2-3 slices of tomato
- Salt and pepper to taste

Instructions:
1. Preheat the oven or toaster oven to 350°F (175°C). Place the roast beef slices on a baking sheet and heat them in the oven for about 5-7 minutes, just until they're slightly heated.
2. While the roast beef is warming, lightly toast the bread slices using a toaster or oven until they are crispy and golden brown.
3. Spread the mustard on one side of each toasted bread slice. On one slice of bread, layer the warmed roast beef slices evenly.
4. Top the roast beef with arugula or spinach leaves and tomato slices. Season with a pinch of salt and pepper, if desired. Place the second slice of toasted bread with mustard on top to make a sandwich.
5. Slice the sandwich in half, if desired, and serve warm.

Nutritional Facts (per serving): Calories: 280 | Total Fat: 7g | Saturated Fat: 2g | Cholesterol: 45mg | Sodium: 600mg | Total Carbohydrates: 32g | Dietary Fiber: 3g | Sugars: 5g | Protein: 23g | Calcium: 100mg | Iron: 2.5mg | Potassium: 420mg

Buckwheat Pancakes with Blueberries and Maple Syrup (Vegetarian)

Prep Time: 10 minutes ; Cook Time: 15 minutes ; Serving Size: 2 pancakes; Servings: 1

Ingredients:

- 1/2 cup buckwheat flour
- 1/2 tsp baking powder
- 1/4 tsp salt
- 1/2 cup lactose-free milk or other low FODMAP dairy alternative
- 1 tbsp vegetable oil
- 1 tbsp pure maple syrup
- 1/2 tsp vanilla extract
- 1/4 cup fresh blueberries
- Cooking spray or additional oil for cooking

Instructions:

1. In a mixing bowl, whisk together the buckwheat flour, baking powder and salt.
2. Add milk, vegetable oil, pure maple syrup and vanilla extract to the dry ingredients. Mix until just combined, taking care not to overmix. The batter will be slightly thicker than traditional pancake batter.
3. Gently fold in the fresh blueberries.
4. Heat a non-stick skillet or griddle over medium heat. Lightly grease it with cooking spray or a small amount of oil.
5. Pour 1/4 cup of the pancake batter onto the skillet for each pancake. Use the back of a spoon to spread the batter into a round shape.
6. Cook the pancakes for about 2-3 minutes on each side, or until they are golden brown and cooked through.
7. Once cooked, transfer the pancakes to a plate and keep them warm while cooking the remaining batter.
8. Serve the buckwheat pancakes with a drizzle of pure maple syrup and additional fresh blueberries, if desired.

Nutritional Facts (per serving - 2 pancakes): Calories: 290 | Total Fat: 8g | Saturated Fat: 1g | Cholesterol: 0mg | Sodium: 390mg | Total Carbohydrates: 48g | Dietary Fiber: 6g | Sugars: 11g | Protein: 6g | Calcium: 180mg | Iron: 2.5mg | Potassium: 330mg

8. Drink and Desserts

Pineapple and Coconut Mocktail (Vegan)

Prep Time: 5 minutes ; Cook Time: 0 minutes ; Serving Size: 1 mocktail; Servings: 1

Ingredients:

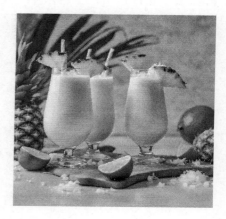

- 1/2 cup fresh pineapple chunks
- 1/2 cup coconut milk (make sure it's low FODMAP)
- 1/4 cup water
- 1 tbsp fresh lime juice
- 1 tsp pure maple syrup (optional)
- Ice cubes
- Pineapple wedge or lime slice to garnish (optional)

Instructions:

1. In a blender, combine the fresh pineapple chunks, coconut water, coconut milk, fresh lime juice and pure maple syrup (if using).
2. Add a handful of ice cubes to the blender to make the mocktail cold and refreshing.
3. Blend all the ingredients on high speed until well combined and smooth. Taste the mocktail and adjust sweetness, if desired, by adding more pure maple syrup.
4. Pour the mocktail into a glass and garnish with a pineapple wedge or lime slice, if using.

Nutritional Facts (per serving): Calories: 110 | Total Fat: 3g | Saturated Fat: 2g | Cholesterol: 0mg | Sodium: 40mg | Total Carbohydrates: 21g | Dietary Fiber: 2g | Sugars: 15g | Protein: 1g | Calcium: 20mg | Iron: 0.6mg | Potassium: 310mg

Iced Ginger-Infused Green Tea (Vegan)

Prep Time: 5 minutes ; Cook Time: 5 minutes ; Serving Size: 1 glass; Servings: 1

Ingredients:
- 1 green tea bag
- 1/2 inch fresh ginger, peeled and sliced
- 1 cup boiling water
- 1 tsp pure maple syrup (optional)
- Ice cubes
- Lemon slices or mint leaves to garnish (optional)

Instructions:

1. Place the green tea bag and sliced ginger in a heatproof glass or mug. Pour tea bag and ginger over boiling water. Steep for 3-4 minutes to allow the flavors to infuse.
2. Remove the tea bag and ginger slices, pressing the tea bag gently to release any excess liquid. Discard the tea bag and ginger.
3. If desired, stir in the pure maple syrup while the tea is still warm to sweeten it slightly. You can adjust the amount of sweetener based on your preference.
4. Let the infused tea cool down to room temperature, then refrigerate it until chilled.
5. Fill a glass with ice cubes and pour the chilled ginger-infused green tea over the ice and garnish with lemon slices or mint leaves, if desired.

Nutritional Facts (per serving): Calories: 5 | Total Fat: 0g | Saturated Fat: 0g | Cholesterol: 0mg | Sodium: 5mg | Total Carbohydrates: 1g | Dietary Fiber: 0g | Sugars: 0g | Protein: 0g | Calcium: 10mg | Iron: 0.2mg | Potassium: 20mg

Strawberry, Banana and Kiwi Smoothie with Lactose-Free Yogurt

Prep Time: 5 minutes ; Cook Time: 0 minutes ; Serving Size: 1 smoothie; Servings: 1

Ingredients:

- ½ unripe banana, peeled and sliced
- 1 kiwi, peeled and sliced
- 1/2 cup fresh strawberries, hulled and halved
- 1/2 cup lactose-free yogurt (make sure it's low FODMAP)
- 1/2 cup lactose-free milk or other low FODMAP dairy alternative
- 1 tbsp pure maple syrup (optional, for added sweetness)
- Ice cubes

Instructions:

1. Place the sliced kiwi and banana, halved strawberries, yogurt and milk in a blender. If using, add the pure maple syrup for added sweetness.
2. Add a handful of ice cubes to the blender to make the smoothie cold and refreshing.
3. Blend all the ingredients on high speed until smooth and creamy.
4. Taste the smoothie and adjust sweetness, if necessary, by adding more pure maple syrup. Pour the smoothie into a glass and serve.

Nutritional Facts (per serving): Calories: 230 | Total Fat: 4g | Saturated Fat: 0g | Cholesterol: 0mg | Sodium: 150mg | Total Carbohydrates: 45g | Dietary Fiber: 4g | Sugars: 25g | Protein: 6g | Calcium: 350mg | Iron: 0.8mg | Potassium: 600mg

Hot Chocolate with Cocoa and Almond Milk (Vegan)

Prep Time: 5 minutes ; Cook Time: 5 minutes ; Serving Size: 1 cup; Servings: 1

Ingredients:

- 1 cup unsweetened almond milk or other low FODMAP dairy alternative
- 2 tbsp unsweetened cocoa powder
- 1 tbsp pure maple syrup (adjust to taste)
- 1/4 tsp vanilla extract
- Pinch of salt

Instructions:

1. In a small saucepan, heat the unsweetened almond milk over medium heat until it's warm but not boiling.
2. In a separate bowl, whisk together the unsweetened cocoa powder and a splash of the warm almond milk to create a smooth paste.
3. Gradually whisk the cocoa paste into the saucepan with the warm almond milk. Continue whisking until the cocoa is fully incorporated and the mixture is smooth.
4. Stir in the pure maple syrup, vanilla extract and a pinch of salt. Taste and adjust sweetness, if desired.
5. Continue to heat the mixture over medium heat, stirring occasionally, until it's hot and steamy. Be careful not to bring it to a boil.
6. Once hot, remove the saucepan from the heat and pour the vegan hot chocolate into a cup.

Nutritional Facts (per serving - 1 cup): Calories: 70 | Total Fat: 3.5g | Saturated Fat: 0g | Cholesterol: 0mg | Sodium: 160mg | Total Carbohydrates: 10g | Dietary Fiber: 2g | Sugars: 6g | Protein: 1g | Calcium: 300mg | Iron: 1.5mg | Potassium: 140mg

Low FODMAP Cheesecake with Blueberry Compote

Prep Time:20 minute; Cook Time: 50minutes; Chilling Time: 4 hours; Serving Size: 1 slice; Servings: 8

Ingredients:

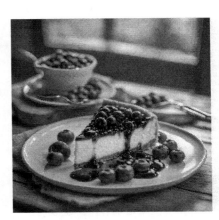

- For Cheesecake
    - 1 ½ cups gluten-free graham cracker crumbs (make sure it's low FODMAP)
    - 1/4 cup melted coconut oil
    - 16 oz (450 g) lactose-free cream cheese, softened (make sure it's low FODMAP)
    - 1/2 cup pure maple syrup
    - 2 large eggs
    - 1 tsp vanilla extract
    - Zest of 1 lemon
    - Pinch of salt
- For Blueberry Compote
    - 1 cup fresh blueberries
    - 2 tbsp pure maple syrup
    - 1 tbsp lemon juice

Instructions:

1. Preheat the oven to 325°F (160°C) and grease a 9-inch springform pan.
2. Combine the graham cracker crumbs and melted coconut oil in a mixing bowl. Create the crust by pressing the mixture firmly into the bottom of the prepared pan.
3. In a separate bowl beat cream cheese until smooth. Add the pure maple syrup, eggs, vanilla extract, lemon zest and a pinch of salt. Beat until the mixture is creamy and well combined.
4. Add the cream cheese mixture to the crust in the springform pan. Even out the top surface with a spatula.
5. Bake the cheesecake in the preheated oven for approximately 45 to 50 minutes, or until the edges are solidified and the center is slightly shaky.
6. Turn off the oven and leave the cheesecake in the oven with the door ajar for about 1 hour to cool gradually.
7. Once cooled, refrigerate the cheesecake for at least 4 hours, or until it's fully chilled and set.
8. For Blueberry Compote: in a saucepan, combine the fresh blueberries, pure maple syrup and lemon juice. Cook over low heat for about 5-7 minutes, or until the blueberries soften and release their juices. Remove from heat and let the compote cool.
9. When ready to serve, remove the cheesecake from the springform pan. Top each slice with a spoonful of blueberry compote.

Nutritional Facts (per serving - 1 slice with blueberry compote): Calories: 320 | Total Fat: 20g | Saturated Fat: 13g | Cholesterol: 75mg | Sodium: 250mg | Total Carbohydrates: 31g | Dietary Fiber: 1g | Sugars: 19g | Protein: 5g | Calcium: 70mg | Iron: 0.8mg | Potassium: 110mg

Gluten-Free Almond Cookies with Lemon Zest (Vegan)

Prep Time: 15 minutes ; Cook Time: 12 minutes ; Serving Size: 2 cookies; Servings: 12 cookies

Ingredients:

- 1 cup almond flour
- 1/4 cup maple syrup
- 1 tbsp coconut oil, melted
- Zest of 1 lemon
- 1/2 tsp vanilla extract
- 1/4 tsp baking soda
- Pinch of salt

Instructions:

1. Preheat the oven to 350°F (175°C) and line a baking sheet with parchment paper.
2. In a mixing bowl, combine the almond flour, maple syrup, melted coconut oil, lemon zest, vanilla extract, baking soda and a pinch of salt. Mix well until the ingredients form a dough-like consistency.
3. Using your hands, roll small portions of the dough into balls and place them on the prepared baking sheet. Flatten each ball slightly with your palm or the back of a fork to create a cookie shape.
4. Bake the cookies in the preheated oven for about 10-12 minutes, or until they are golden around the edges.
5. Remove the cookies from the oven and let them cool on the baking sheet for a few minutes before transferring them to a wire rack to cool completely.
6. Once the cookies are completely cooled, they are ready to be enjoyed.

Nutritional Facts (per serving - 2 cookies): Calories: 160 | Total Fat: 12g | Saturated Fat: 2.5g | Cholesterol: 0mg | Sodium: 50mg | Total Carbohydrates: 10g | Dietary Fiber: 2g | Sugars: 6g | Protein: 4g | Calcium: 50mg | Iron: 0.8mg | Potassium: 40mg

Chilled Strawberry Sorbet with Fresh Mint (Vegan)

Prep Time: 10minutes; Cook Time: 0minutes; Chilling Time: 4 hours; Serving Size: 1/2cup; Servings:4

Ingredients:

- 2 cups fresh strawberries, hulled and halved
- 1/4 cup pure maple syrup
- 1 tbsp fresh lemon juice
- 1 tbsp fresh lime juice
- 1 tbsp fresh mint leaves, chopped
- Fresh mint leaves for garnish

Instructions:

1. Place the fresh strawberries, pure maple syrup, fresh lemon juice and fresh lime juice in a blender.
2. Blend the ingredients on high speed until the mixture is smooth and well combined.
3. Add the chopped fresh mint leaves to the blender and pulse a few times to incorporate them into the mixture.
4. Taste the sorbet mixture and adjust sweetness, if needed, by adding more pure maple syrup.
5. Pour the sorbet mixture into a shallow container or ice cream maker.
6. If using an ice cream maker, follow the manufacturer's instructions to churn the sorbet until it reaches a frozen and smooth consistency. If you are not using an ice cream maker, skip to the next step.
7. Put the container, which contains the sorbet mixture, in the freezer and keep it there for no less than 4 hours until it becomes solid.
8. Before you serve, give the sorbet some time at room temperature. This will soften it slightly. Scoop out the sorbet and serve it in bowls. Add fresh mint leaves to garnish.

Nutritional Facts (per serving - 1/2 cup): Calories: 100 | Total Fat: 0g | Saturated Fat: 0g | Cholesterol: 0mg | Sodium: 5mg | Total Carbohydrates: 25g | Dietary Fiber: 2g | Sugars: 20g | Protein: 1g | Calcium: 30mg | Iron: 0.6mg | Potassium: 180mg

Chocolate-Covered Strawberries with Dark Chocolate (Vegan)

Prep Time: 15minutes; Cook Time:5 minutes; Chilling Time: 30 minutes; Servings: 5

Ingredients:
- 10 fresh strawberries, washed and dried
- 1/2 cup dark chocolate chips (make sure it's low FODMAP)
- 1 tsp coconut oil
- Crushed nuts or coconut flakes for topping (optional)

Instructions:
1. Line a tray or plate with parchment paper and set it aside.
2. Combine the dark chocolate chips and coconut oil in a bowl that is safe to use in a microwave oven. Place the bowl in the microwave and heat it for 20 seconds at a time, stirring the mixture after each interval until the chocolate is completely melted and smooth.
3. Hold each strawberry by the stem and dip it into the melted chocolate. Swirl the chocolate around to cover most of the surface of the strawberry.
4. Allow any excess chocolate to drip off, then place the chocolate-covered strawberries on the prepared parchment paper.
5. If desired, sprinkle the tops of the strawberries with crushed nuts or coconut flakes while the chocolate is still wet.
6. Repeat the dipping process with the remaining strawberries.
7. Once all the strawberries are dipped and decorated, place the tray or plate in the refrigerator for about 30 minutes to allow the chocolate to set.
8. Once the chocolate has set, the vegan chocolate-covered strawberries are ready to be enjoyed.

Nutritional Facts (per serving - 2 strawberries): Calories: 120 | Total Fat: 7g | Saturated Fat: 4g | Cholesterol: 0mg | Sodium: 0mg | Total Carbohydrates: 16g | Dietary Fiber: 3g | Sugars: 11g | Protein: 2g | Calcium: 30mg | Iron: 2mg | Potassium: 200mg

Carrot Cake with Cream Cheese Frosting (Vegetarian)

Prep Time: 20 minutes; Cook Time: 30 minutes; Serving Size: 1 slice; Servings: 12

Ingredients:

- For Carrot Cake
    - 1 ½ cups gluten-free all-purpose flour (make sure it's low FODMAP)
    - 1/2 cup almond flour
    - 1 tsp baking powder
    - 1/2 tsp baking soda
    - 1/2 tsp ground cinnamon
    - 1/4 tsp ground nutmeg
    - 1/4 tsp ground ginger
    - 1/4 tsp salt
    - 1/2 cup coconut oil, melted
    - 1/2 cup pure maple syrup
    - 2 large eggs
    - 1 tsp vanilla extract
    - 2 cups grated carrots
- For Cream Cheese Frosting
    - 8 oz (225 g) lactose-free cream cheese, softened (make sure it's low FODMAP)
    - 1/4 cup powdered sugar
    - 1/4 cup unsalted butter, softened
    - 1 tsp vanilla extract

Instructions:

1. Preheat the oven to 350°F (175°C) and grease a round 9-inch cake pan.
2. In a mixing bowl, whisk together the all-purpose flour, almond flour, baking powder, baking soda, ground cinnamon, ground nutmeg, ground ginger and salt.
3. In a separate bowl, whisk together the melted coconut oil, pure maple syrup, eggs and vanilla extract until well combined.
4. Gradually add the wet ingredients to the dry ingredients and mix until just combined.
5. Fold in the grated carrots until evenly distributed throughout the batter.
6. Transfer the batter into the cake pan that has been greased and floured, then even out the surface.
7. Place in the oven that has already been preheated to 375°F and bake for 25-30 minutes or until the toothpick inserted into the cake's center comes out clean.
8. Let the cake cool in the pan for approximately 10 minutes, then transfer it to a wire rack to cool completely.
9. For Cream Cheese Frosting: in a mixing bowl, beat the softened cream cheese and unsalted butter until smooth and creamy. Add the powdered sugar and vanilla extract and continue to beat until well combined.
10. Spread the cream cheese frosting on the top of the cake after it has cooled completely.

Nutritional Facts (per serving - 1 slice with frosting): Calories: 380 | Total Fat: 25g | Saturated Fat: 15g | Cholesterol: 80mg | Sodium: 220mg | Total Carbohydrates: 33g | Dietary Fiber: 3g | Sugars: 16g | Protein: 6g | Calcium: 80mg | Iron: 1.5mg | Potassium: 230mg

Lemon-Poppy Seed Muffins (Gluten-Free)

Prep Time: 15 minutes; Cook Time: 20 minutes; Serving Size: 1 muffin; Servings: 12 standard-sized

Ingredients:
- 1 ½ cups gluten-free all-purpose flour (make sure it's low FODMAP)
- 1/4 cup almond flour
- 1/4 cup coconut flour
- 1/2 cup granulated sugar
- 2 tsp baking powder
- 1/2 tsp baking soda
- 1/4 tsp salt
- Zest of 1 lemon
- 2 tbsp poppy seeds
- 1/2 cup lactose-free milk or other low FODMAP dairy alternative
- 1/4 cup melted coconut oil
- 2 large eggs
- 1 tsp vanilla extract
- 1/4 cup fresh lemon juice

Instructions:
1. Preheat the oven to 375°F (190°C) and line a muffin tin with paper liners.
2. In a large bowl, whisk together the all-purpose flour, almond flour, coconut flour, granulated sugar, baking powder, baking soda, salt, lemon zest and poppy seeds.
3. In a separate bowl, whisk together milk, melted coconut oil, eggs, vanilla extract and fresh lemon juice.
4. Gradually add the wet ingredients to the dry ingredients and mix until just combined. Be careful not to overmix.
5. Divide the muffin batter evenly among the prepared muffin cups, filling each cup about 3/4 full.
6. Bake in the preheated oven for about 18-20 minutes, or until a toothpick inserted into the center of a muffin comes out clean.
7. Allow the muffins to cool in the muffin tin for a few minutes before transferring them to a wire rack to cool completely.

Nutritional Facts (per serving - 1 muffin): Calories: 200 | Total Fat: 10g | Saturated Fat: 6g | Cholesterol: 35mg | Sodium: 180mg | Total Carbohydrates: 24g | Dietary Fiber: 3g | Sugars: 9g | Protein: 4g | Calcium: 70mg | Iron: 1.2mg | Potassium: 110mg

Orange and Almond Cake with Orange Glaze (Gluten-Free)

Prep Time: 20 minutes; Cook Time: 40 minute; Serving Size: 1 slice; Servings: 8

Ingredients:
- For Cake
    - 1/4 cup gluten-free all-purpose flour (make sure it's low FODMAP)
    - 1 cup almond flour
    - 1/4 cup coconut flour
    - 1/2 tsp baking soda
    - 1 tsp baking powder
    - 1/4 tsp salt
    - Zest of 1 orange
    - 1/2 cup granulated sugar
    - 1/4 cup melted coconut oil
    - 2 large eggs
    - 1/2 cup fresh orange juice
    - 1 tsp vanilla extract

- For Orange Glaze
    - 1/2 cup powdered sugar
    - 2 tbsp fresh orange juice
    - Zest of 1 orange

Instructions:

1. Preheat the oven to 350°F (175°C) and grease an 8-inch round cake pan.
2. In a bowl, mix together the almond, all-purpose, and coconut flours, baking powder, baking soda, salt, and orange zests.
3. In a separate bowl, whisk together the granulated sugar, melted coconut oil, eggs, fresh orange juice, and vanilla extract. Whisk until well combined.
4. Gradually add the wet ingredients to the dry ingredients, mixing the mixture until just combined.
5. Pour the cake batter into the greased cake pan and smooth the top.
6. Bake in a preheated oven for approximately 35-40 minutes or until a toothpick inserted in the center comes out clean.
7. For orange glaze: while the cake is baking, whisk powdered sugar, fresh orange juice, and orange zest in a bowl until the glaze is smooth.
8. Once the cake is baked, let it cool in the pan for about 10 minutes before transferring it to a wire rack.
9. Drizzle the orange glaze over the cooled cake.

Nutritional Facts (per serving - 1 slice with glaze): Calories: 220 | Total Fat: 13g | Saturated Fat: 7g | Cholesterol: 35mg | Sodium: 160mg | Total Carbohydrates: 24g | Dietary Fiber: 2g | Sugars: 18g | Protein: 3g | Calcium: 40mg | Iron: 0.7mg | Potassium: 80mg

Maple-Pecan Rice Pudding (Vegetarian)

Prep Time: 5minutes; Cook Time: 25minutes; Chilling Time: 2 hours;Serving Size: 1/2cup; Servings: 2

Ingredients:

- 1/2 cup Arborio rice (short-grain rice)
- 2 cups lactose-free milk or other low FODMAP dairy alternative
- 1/4 cup pure maple syrup
- 1/4 tsp ground cinnamon
- 1/4 tsp vanilla extract
- 1/4 cup chopped pecans
- Pinch of salt

Instructions:

1. In a medium saucepan, combine the Arborio rice and milk. Bring the mixture to a gentle simmer over medium heat.
2. Reduce the heat to low and let the rice simmer, stirring occasionally, for about 20-25 minutes, or until the rice is tender and has absorbed most of the milk. Make sure to keep an eye on it to prevent sticking or burning.
3. Stir in the pure maple syrup, ground cinnamon, vanilla extract and a pinch of salt. Continue to cook the rice pudding for an additional 2-3 minutes to allow the flavors to meld.
4. Remove the saucepan from the heat and let the rice pudding cool slightly.
5. Stir in the chopped pecans, reserving some for garnish.
6. Transfer the rice pudding to a container and cover it. Refrigerate the pudding for at least 2 hours, or until it's chilled and set.
7. Before serving, give the rice pudding a good stir. Scoop the rice pudding into serving bowls and garnish with the reserved chopped pecans.

Nutritional Facts (per serving - 1/2 cup): Calories: 240 | Total Fat: 8g | Saturated Fat: 1g | Cholesterol: 0mg | Sodium: 100mg | Total Carbohydrates: 39g | Dietary Fiber: 1g | Sugars: 19g | Protein: 4g | Calcium: 180mg | Iron: 1mg | Potassium:130mg

Part III: The 28-Day Meal Plan

1. Introduction to the Meal Plan

Embarking on the low FODMAP diet journey can seem daunting, but this 28-day meal plan has been carefully designed to make it simple and enjoyable. This plan is more than just a collection of recipes; it's a guide to help you learn how to incorporate low FODMAP foods into your daily life and see noticeable improvements in your digestive health.

A. Explanation of how to follow the 28-day plan

Following this 28-day meal plan is easy, with clear and detailed instructions. Each day, you will find new recipes that adhere to the low FODMAP guidelines. This plan provides a varied and balanced diet, incorporating different flavors and cooking techniques and catering to both vegetarian and non-vegetarian preferences.

Each week of the 28-day plan offers a variety of breakfasts, lunches, dinners and snacks or dessert that utilize the delicious and nutritious recipes provided in the previous chapters. Feel free to adjust portion sizes or switch meals around to suit your preferences and dietary requirements.

The goal is to provide you with satisfying meals that nourish your body while adhering to the principles of the low FODMAP diet. By the end of the 28 days, you should feel more in control of your digestive health and equipped with the knowledge to continue this diet on your own.

Whether you're a novice or experienced cook, this guide is here to support you in your journey to achieve better health and well-being. Enjoy!

B. Detailed daily menus, utilizing recipes from the book

Day 1:

- **Breakfast:** Quinoa Breakfast Bowl with Nuts and Citrus (Vegan)
- **Lunch:** Grilled Salmon over Arugula Risotto
- **Dinner:** Grilled Lamb Chops with Mint Pesto and Mashed Potatoes
- **Snack/Dessert:** Strawberry and Kiwi Smoothie with Lactose-Free Yogurt

Day 2:

- **Breakfast:** Gluten-Free Banana Pancakes with Maple Syrup
- **Lunch:** Baked Stuffed Red Bell Peppers with Rice and Spinach
- **Dinner:** Pan-Seared Halibut with Pineapple Salsa and Wild Rice
- **Snack/Dessert:** Lemon-Poppy Seed Muffins (Gluten-Free)

Day 3:

- **Breakfast:** Ham and Cheese Omelet with Fresh Herbs
- **Lunch:** Rice Noodles with Stir-Fried Shrimp and Red Bell Peppers
- **Dinner:** Maple-Glazed Turkey Breast with Steamed Carrots
- **Snack/Dessert:** Chocolate-Covered Strawberries with Dark Chocolate (Vegan)

Day 4:

- **Breakfast:** Chia Seed Pudding with Kiwi and Pineapple (Vegan)
- **Lunch:** Vegetable Sushi Rolls with Wasabi and Low FODMAP Soy Sauce Substitute (Vegan)
- **Dinner:** Stir-Fried Pork with Ginger and Bok Choy
- **Snack/Dessert:** Gluten-Free Almond Cookies with Lemon Zest (Vegan)

Day 5:

- **Breakfast:** Muffin Tin Egg Cups with Red Bell Peppers and Zucchini (Vegetarian)
- **Lunch:** Baked Potatoes with Tuna Salad and Chives
- **Dinner:** Roasted Haddock with Spinach and Lemon Risotto
- **Snack/Dessert:** Low-FODMAP Cheesecake with Blueberry Compote

Day 6:

- **Breakfast:** Buckwheat Porridge with Kiwi and Cinnamon (Vegan)
- **Lunch:** Grilled Eggplant and Zucchini Salad with Lemon-Herb Dressing
- **Dinner:** Savory Roast Beef with Dijon Mustard and Parsnips
- **Snack/Dessert:** Chilled Strawberry Sorbet with Fresh Mint (Vegan)

Day 7:

- **Breakfast:** French Toast with Strawberries and Lactose-Free Cream Cheese
- **Lunch:** Spaghetti Squash Primavera with Fresh Basil Pesto
- **Dinner:** Mason Jar Salad with Layered Veggies and Quinoa (Vegan)
- **Snack/Dessert:** Carrot Cake with Cream Cheese Frosting (Vegetarian)

Day 8:

- **Breakfast:** Mixed Berry Smoothie Bowl with Lactose-Free Yogurt
- **Lunch:** Zucchini Noodles with Pesto and Cherry Tomatoes (Vegan)
- **Dinner:** Baked Cod with Lemon-Dill Sauce and Sauteed Zucchini
- **Snack/Dessert:** Iced Ginger-Infused Green Tea (Vegan)

Day 9:

- **Breakfast:** Granola Parfait with Lactose-Free Yogurt and Fresh Berries
- **Lunch:** Garlic-Infused Olive Oil Spaghetti with Grilled Shrimp and Zucchini
- **Dinner:** Pulled Pork Sandwiches on Gluten-Free Bread with Coleslaw
- **Snack/Dessert:** Pineapple and Coconut Mocktail (Vegan)

Day 10:

- **Breakfast:** Strawberry and Chia Overnight Oatmeal (Vegan)
- **Lunch:** Rice Paper Rolls with Tofu, Mint, and Low-FODMAP Dipping Sauce (Vegan)
- **Dinner:** Grilled Tuna Steaks with Olive Tapenade and Steamed Green Beans
- **Snack/Dessert:** Hot Chocolate with Cocoa and Almond Milk (Vegan)

Day 11:

- **Breakfast:** Quinoa Breakfast Bowl with Nuts and Citrus (Vegan)
- **Lunch:** Grilled Fish Tacos with Cabbage Slaw and Eggplant Cream
- **Dinner:** Braised Chicken with Tomatoes and Oregano over Polenta
- **Snack/Dessert:** Low-FODMAP Cheesecake with Blueberry Compote

Day 12:

- **Breakfast:** Egg and Cheddar Breakfast Muffins with Spinach (Vegetarian)
- **Lunch:** Oven-Poached Sole with Spinach and Low FODMAP Fresh Basil Pesto
- **Dinner:** Slow-Cooked Beef Stew with Root Vegetables
- **Snack/Dessert:** Gluten-Free Almond Cookies with Lemon Zest (Vegan)

-

Day 13:

- **Breakfast:** Buckwheat Porridge with Kiwi and Cinnamon (Vegan)
- **Lunch:** Creamy Polenta with Sautéed Spinach and Garlic-Infused Oil
- **Dinner:** Oven-Roasted Red Bell Pepper and Tomato Bisque with Fresh Basil
- **Snack/Dessert:** Lemon-Poppy Seed Muffins (Gluten-Free)

Day 14:

- **Breakfast:** French Toast with Strawberries and Lactose-Free Cream Cheese
- **Lunch:** Butternut Squash Risotto with Sage and Parmesan
- **Dinner:** Grilled Sausages with Sauteed Green Beans and Almonds
- **Snack/Dessert:** Chocolate-Covered Strawberries with Dark Chocolate (Vegan)

Day 15:

- **Breakfast:** Quinoa Breakfast Bowl with Nuts and Citrus (Vegan)
- **Lunch:** Grilled Eggplant and Zucchini Salad with Lemon-Herb Dressing
- **Dinner:** Maple-Glazed Turkey Breast with Steamed Carrots
- **Snack/Dessert:** Strawberry and Kiwi Smoothie with Lactose-Free Yogurt

Day 16:

- **Breakfast:** Ham and Cheese Omelet with Fresh Herbs
- **Lunch:** Baked Stuffed Red Bell Peppers with Rice and Spinach
- **Dinner:** Garlic-Infused Olive Oil Spaghetti with Grilled Shrimp and Zucchini
- **Snack/Dessert:** Carrot Cake with Cream Cheese Frosting (Vegetarian)

Day 17:

- **Breakfast:** Gluten-Free Banana Pancakes with Maple Syrup
- **Lunch:** Baked Potatoes with Tuna Salad and Chives
- **Dinner:** Pan-Seared Halibut with Pineapple Salsa and Wild Rice
- **Snack/Dessert:** Chilled Strawberry Sorbet with Fresh Mint (Vegan)

Day 18:

- **Breakfast:** Chia Seed Pudding with Kiwi and Pineapple (Vegan)
- **Lunch:** Eggplant and Zucchini Casserole with Vegan Cheese (Vegan)
- **Dinner:** Savory Roast Beef with Dijon Mustard and Parsnips
- **Snack/Dessert:** Low-FODMAP Cheesecake with Blueberry Compote

Day 19:

- **Breakfast:** Muffin Tin Egg Cups with Red Bell Peppers and Zucchini (Vegetarian)
- **Lunch:** Roasted Root Vegetable Medley with Garlic-Infused Olive Oil
- **Dinner:** Shrimp and Scallop Skewers with Zesty Lime Marinade
- **Snack/Dessert:** Lemon-Poppy Seed Muffins (Gluten-Free)

Day 20:

- **Breakfast:** Buckwheat Porridge with Kiwi and Cinnamon (Vegan)
- **Lunch:** Potato and Kale Hash with Poached Eggs and Chives
- **Dinner:** Stuffed Squid with Rice, Olives, and Tomato Sauce
- **Snack/Dessert:** Chocolate-Covered Strawberries with Dark Chocolate (Vegan)

Day 21:

- **Breakfast:** French Toast with Strawberries and Lactose-Free Cream Cheese
- **Lunch:** Rice Noodles with Stir-Fried Shrimp and Red Bell Peppers
- **Dinner:** Pork Tenderloin with Rosemary and Roasted Bell peppers
- **Snack/Dessert:** Gluten-Free Almond Cookies with Lemon Zest (Vegan)

Day 22:

- **Breakfast:** Granola Parfait with Lactose-Free Yogurt and Fresh Berries
- **Lunch:** Mason Jar Salad with Layered Veggies and Quinoa (Vegan)
- **Dinner:** Grilled Tuna Steaks with Olive Tapenade and Steamed Green Beans
- **Snack/Dessert:** Hot Chocolate with Cocoa and Almond Milk (Vegan)

Day 23:

- **Breakfast:** Strawberry and Chia Overnight Oatmeal (Vegan)
- **Lunch:** Cold Pasta Salad with Grilled Chicken, Tomatoes, and Basil
- **Dinner:** Roasted Haddock with Spinach and Lemon Risotto
- **Snack/Dessert:** Iced Ginger-Infused Green Tea (Vegan)

Day 24:

- **Breakfast:** Mixed Berry Smoothie Bowl with Lactose-Free Yogurt
- **Lunch:** Vegetable Sushi Rolls with Wasabi and Low FODMAP Soy Sauce Substitute (Vegan)
- **Dinner:** Grilled Sausages with Sauteed Green Beans and Almonds
- **Snack/Dessert:** Pineapple and Coconut Mocktail (Vegan)

Day 25:

- **Breakfast:** French Toast with Strawberries and Lactose-Free Cream Cheese
- **Lunch:** Buckwheat Noodles with Grilled Zucchini and Sesame Seeds
- **Dinner:** Oven-Poached Sole with Spinach and Low FODMAP Fresh Basil Pesto
- **Snack/Dessert:** Low-FODMAP Cheesecake with Blueberry Compote

Day 26:

- **Breakfast:** Egg and Cheddar Breakfast Muffins with Spinach (Vegetarian)
- **Lunch:** Spaghetti Squash Primavera with Fresh Basil Pesto
- **Dinner:** Pulled Pork Sandwiches on Gluten-Free Bread with Coleslaw
- **Snack/Dessert:** Lemon-Poppy Seed Muffins (Gluten-Free)

Day 27:

- **Breakfast:** Ham and Cheese Omelet with Fresh Herbs
- **Lunch:** Zucchini Noodles with Pesto and Cherry Tomatoes (Vegan)
- **Dinner:** Grilled Lamb Chops with Mint Pesto and Mashed Potatoes
- **Snack/Dessert:** Strawberry and Kiwi Smoothie with Lactose-Free Yogurt

Day 28:

- **Breakfast:** Muffin Tin Egg Cups with Red Bell Peppers and Zucchini (Vegetarian)
- **Lunch:** Grilled Chicken Salad with Spinach and Low-FODMAP Vinaigrette
- **Dinner:** Chilled Cucumber Soup with Dill and Lemon
- **Snack/Dessert:** Carrot Cake with Cream Cheese Frosting (Vegetarian)

Part IV: Managing Your Diet

1. A Sustainable and Gradual Approach

Strategies for Easing into the Low FODMAP Diet

Starting with research is an essential aspect of the low FODMAP diet. Understanding the principles of the diet, including which foods are allowed and which ones are to be avoided, sets the foundation for a smooth transition. Familiarizing yourself with different categories of FODMAPs and knowing what to look for on food labels will empower you in making wise food choices.

Gradual elimination is the key to success. Rather than removing all high FODMAP foods at once, it's advisable to start by eliminating one group of high FODMAP foods, assess how your body reacts and then gradually remove others. This step-by-step approach minimizes shock to the system and allows for careful observation of the body's response. Seeking professional guidance from a registered dietitian with experience in the low FODMAP diet can provide personalized recommendations based on specific needs. Their insights can be invaluable in tailoring the diet to your individual requirements.

Lastly, utilizing resources such as low FODMAP apps, guides and cookbooks can make the transition more manageable. They offer a wide range of information and support to help identify suitable foods and plan enjoyable meals.

Managing Stress Related to Dietary Changes

A crucial aspect of adapting to the low FODMAP diet is managing stress related to dietary changes. Focusing on what you can eat, rather than what you can't, turns the diet into a positive experience. Embracing the vast array of delicious foods still available and celebrating new flavors and culinary experiences can make the journey enjoyable. Communication with friends and family about dietary changes is vital. Support from loved ones can ease the transition and foster a supportive environment. Practicing mindful eating, paying attention to how your body reacts to different foods and keeping a food diary can also aid in identifying specific triggers. It's essential not to be too hard on yourself. Mistakes and slip-ups may happen, but acknowledging them, learning from them and moving on is vital. Stress can exacerbate digestive symptoms, so practicing self-compassion and understanding that errors are part of the learning process is crucial.

Tips for Long-term Success and Maximizing Effectiveness

The path to long-term success in the low FODMAP diet includes several strategic approaches. The reintroduction phase, guided by a healthcare professional, helps in systematically reintroducing high FODMAP foods, identifying specific triggers and creating a more personalized, flexible diet. Considering your lifestyle is also key. The low FODMAP diet should align with aspects such as travel and dining out. Developing strategies that fit these aspects can lead to a more balanced and sustainable approach. Regular monitoring and check-ins with healthcare providers ensure that your dietary approach remains optimal for your specific symptoms and overall health.

The low FODMAP diet offers a promising solution for many people struggling with digestive disorders. Its success lies in a sustainable and gradual approach. By easing into the diet, managing stress and implementing strategies for long-term success, you set the stage for a more comfortable and effective experience with this specialized dietary approach. It's a journey of self-discovery, empowerment and wellness, guided by mindful choices and a commitment to your well-being.

2. Tips for Eating Out or at Restaurants

It's natural to feel overwhelmed when initially starting the low FODMAP diet. Navigating the world of dining out on a low FODMAP diet may seem daunting, but with the right approach and preparation, you can still enjoy food without compromising your diet.

Dining out is not just about food, but the experience. So, while it's crucial to be informed and prepared, don't forget to enjoy the company and ambiance. Whether you're an adult or helping a child, you've got this!
Let's dive into how adults can enjoy eating out and how parents can ensure their children remain symptom-free, even in social settings. Let's get started!

A. Strategies for eating out for Grown-Ups

1. Plan Ahead:

- **Restaurants**: most modern restaurants post their menus online or on rating apps. This allows you to spot potential meals that fit with low FODMAP guidelines or even restaurants that accommodate dietary requirements (indicators such as "We cater to dietary needs").
- **Friends' or Relatives' Houses**: let the host know about your dietary requirements in advance. Offer to bring a dish that you can eat and share with others.
- **Business Lunches**: suggest restaurants that you know have low FODMAP options, or have a snack before the meal so you can choose lighter, simpler dishes during the business lunch.

2. Prevent Stress:

- Anxiety can exacerbate IBS symptoms for some. By calling the restaurant ahead (during off-peak hours), you can discuss your dietary needs and see how flexible they are with menu changes. Chefs often appreciate a heads-up and are more than willing to accommodate.

3. Choosing the Right Restaurant

- A restaurant with a "scratch kitchen," where dishes are made from fresh ingredients, can be particularly accommodating. Health-focused restaurants or those catering to gluten or dairy-free needs might also be more adaptive to your requirements.

4. Choose Simple Dishes:

- **Beware of the Dips & Sauces**: These often hide ingredients like garlic and onion. Request that they're served separately.
- **Side Dishes are Your Best Friends**: When ordering, opt for dishes with fewer ingredients. This reduces the chances of hidden FODMAPs sneaking in. If the main dishes don't seem FODMAP-friendly, consider ordering sides or requesting plain protein with vegetables (or salad). Remember: grilled, steamed, or roasted dishes are usually safer bets.

5. Consider Portion Size:

- **Balance Your FODMAP Intake**: If you're planning to eat out in the evening, ensure your breakfast and lunch are strictly low in FODMAPs to avoid excessive FODMAP intake. It allows to reduce the chances of symptoms later.
- Even low FODMAP foods can become high FODMAP in large portions. **Be mindful of serving sizes** and consider sharing dishes if they are large.

6. **Communicating your dietary needs:**

- **Don't forget your Dining Out Card**: one of the precious bonus contents of this book is the DINING OUT CARD. Always keep this handy card in your wallet. It succinctly lists down your dietary requirements, ensuring there's no room for misunderstanding. Just hand it over to the staff when you're ordering.

- **Be Specific Before Ordering**: clearly mention "no onion, garlic, or other high FODMAP ingredients" you're wary of. Some cuisines, like Italian or Indian, can be especially tricky. So, be assertive, but polite.

- If you frequently dine with the same group of people, consider **educating** them about the low FODMAP diet. Share resources, articles, or even this guide to help them understand better.

7. **Offer to Help or Bring Your Own Dish:**

- When dining at a friend's or relative's house, offer to help with cooking or bring your dish. It eases the burden on the host and ensures you have something safe to eat.

8. **When You Can't Choose:**

- If attending an event at a pre-decided venue:
  1. Preview the menu if possible.
  2. Have a low FODMAP snack before heading out if options seem limited.
  3. Aim to adhere to your diet at the restaurant but don't stress. If you deviate, just resume your diet the next day.

By planning ahead, understanding common high FODMAP foods, choosing simple dishes and effectively communicating your needs, you can continue to enjoy dining out. Whether it's a formal business lunch, a casual dinner at a restaurant, or a family gathering, these strategies can support your dietary journey without isolating you from social connections and enjoyable culinary experiences.

Remember, it's a LOW, not NO FODMAP diet. So, relax and soak in the dining experience. Stay informed, ask questions confidently, and most importantly, enjoy your meal. And if you ever feel overwhelmed, our handy DINING OUT CARD has got your back!

B. Strategies for eating out tasting a Variety of Popular Cuisines

This chapter dives into popular cuisines from around the world, providing insights and tips to help you maintain your diet without compromising on flavor or missing out on cultural experiences.

Dining out on the low FODMAP diet across diverse cuisines is a journey of discovery. With these guidelines in hand, you can confidently explore and savor the world of gastronomy. Remember, it's all about balance and making informed choices without compromising the joy of dining out.

1. Italian Cuisine:

Italian food is much more than just pizza and pasta. Here's how you can indulge in Italian cuisine without straying from your low FODMAP guidelines:

- **Gluten-free alternatives**: opt for gluten-free pizza bases and pasta as they lack wheat, which can be high in FODMAPs. And, if possible, create your own pizza topping with low FODMAP ingredients!

- **Sauces**: inquire if tomato passata (used on pizzas and pasta) is made without garlic or onion. Traditional recipes might only use tomatoes and salt.

- **Bianco bases**: some pizzas use a white base of olive oil and garlic. If ordered fresh, chefs might omit garlic.

- **Cheeses**: go for harder cheeses like cheddar and parmesan, which have lower lactose content.

- **Risottos**: a potential low FODMAP choice, but ensure the stock used doesn't contain onion or garlic.

2. Chinese Cuisine:

While Chinese cuisine can be heavy on sauces and garnishes, there are ways to enjoy it while maintaining a low FODMAP diet:

- **Sauces:** clarify the ingredients of sauces, ensure don't have garlic, onion, or artificial sweeteners. Opt for those like soy or oyster that don't contain high FODMAP ingredients.
- **Garnishes:** spring onion is frequently used. Stick to the green parts or exclude them altogether.
- **Carbs:** choose rice-based dishes over wheat-based ones (such as Hokkien or Chow Mein noodles).

3. French Cuisine:

French dishes exude sophistication. Enjoying them FODMAP-friendly requires a few tweaks:

- **Steak Frites:** are your best bet! This classic dish usually comes with a sauce. Choose mustard and ensure the salad is dressed with only oil and vinegar.
- **Salads:** both Salade Lyonnaise and Nicoise salad can be modified to fit the diet. Ensure you check and omit any high FODMAP ingredients (ensure it's without garlic or onion sauces).

4. Indian Cuisine:

Indian food is rich and varied, but it often contains garlic and onion. Here's how to relish it:

- **Base Ingredients:** vegetarian and seafood dishes, which might be prepared fresh without heavy marinating (making them potentially safer).
- **Curry Bases:** they often contain shallots and other onions. Pre-calling the restaurant to discuss options can be helpful.

5. Greek Cuisine:

Choose plain meat or fish dishes served with fresh salads or veggies. Greek food offers many delicious and low FODMAP options:

- **Cheeses:** both Saganaki and Haloumi are fantastic choices.
- **Salads:** Elliniki Salata can be enjoyed with modifications (ensure it's without garlic or onion).
- **Main Courses:** chargrilled fish, scallops, and Htapodi (chargrilled octopus) are mouth-watering low FODMAP choices.

6. Vietnamese & Thai Cuisine:

Both these cuisines offer refreshing dishes that can easily be made low FODMAP:

- **Vietnamese:** rice vermicelli and rice paper rolls are often safe bets, but always inquire about the contents.
- **Thai:** opt for stir-fries without onion or garlic and served with steamed jasmine rice.

7. Japanese Cuisine:

A cuisine that's already relatively simple and fresh, making low FODMAP choices is quite easy:

- **Grilled Dishes**: grilled tofu, seafood, or meat with steamed rice are often safe choices.
- **Raw Delicacies**: plain raw tuna or salmon are low FODMAP delights.
- **Noodles**: Opt for rice noodles with your choice of meat and veggies.

When exploring other cuisines, aim for dishes that are less sauced or spiced and prioritize plain meat, fish, or rice dishes with fresh salads or steamed veggies.

C. Strategies for eating out for Little Ones (a little bit of the extra Bonus)

When it comes to kids, their world revolves around school, playdates, parties, and family gatherings. Each of these scenarios presents its own set of challenges for a parent, especially when your child is on a specific diet like FODMAP. As a guiding beacon for parents, this chapter is all about making sure your little one doesn't miss out on any fun, all the while ensuring their tummy is content and happy.

Throughout this chapter, the aim is to equip you with strategies and tools, ensuring your child enjoys all aspects of their vibrant life while maintaining their dietary needs.

And if you're craving even more insights, don't fret! This is just a taste of what's to come. As an **Additional Bonus Content**, there will be a dedicated section entirely focused on managing children's eating out scenarios. So, let's dive in and make this journey smooth and enjoyable for both you and your child.

1. School Lunches:

- Educate teachers and cafeteria staff about your child's dietary needs. **Provide** them with **a list of safe** foods and potential substitutes.
- Some schools even allow you to send special lunches for your child. If that's the case **homemade pre-packed FODMAP-friendly lunches are gold!**

2. Playdates and Parties:

- **Always inform the hosting parents** about your child's dietary needs. Most hosts will appreciate the heads-up and might even prepare something special!
- **Offering to send a packed meal or snacks** can be a practical solution. This ensures your child doesn't feel left out and their gut remains happy.

3. Holidays with Family and Friends:

- Make sure to **inform relatives in advance**. Brief them about the diet and you might also want to bring a few safe dishes to share.
- If you're staying for an extended period, maybe even **cook a meal together?** This way, you ensure there's something FODMAP-friendly on the table, and It's both bonding and enlightening!

4. Traveling & Outings:

- Whether it's the local zoo or a theme park, **packed FODMAP-friendly snacks are your best friend**. Think rice cakes, lactose-free yogurt, or FODMAP-friendly granola bars. This way, they can munch away without worries. And remember, if they have a slip-up, it's okay. They can get back on track the next meal.

5. Child's Dining Out Card:

- A child's dining out card is like a magic wand. Just like the adult version, this card simplifies dining out. It's an easy reference for others to understand their dietary needs. It's tailored for children, ensuring they get to enjoy their meal and the outing without any hiccups.

Conclusion

Recap of Key Takeaways

Understanding the low FODMAP diet is more than grasping a list of allowed and disallowed foods; it's about recognizing a scientific approach aimed at minimizing certain fermentable carbohydrates that can cause digestive discomfort. The diet requires an initial phase of elimination, followed by a careful reintroduction of foods to personalize the diet to an individual's unique needs.

Meal planning and preparation are paramount, as they aid in a smooth transition into this dietary lifestyle. Planning a 28-day meal program, shopping with organized lists and using specific low FODMAP recipes can enhance the culinary experience without compromising taste or nutrition.

The emphasis on sustainability and adaptability is significant in long-term success with the diet. It requires a gradual approach and effective stress management techniques. The tips for dining outside the home are not just about maintaining the diet but about enjoying social life and business engagements without anxiety or hassle.

Community and support also play an indispensable role. Friends, family and low FODMAP communities offer encouragement and understanding, strengthening your resolve and ensuring that you are not alone in this journey.

Enjoy the Journey Ahead

Embarking on the low FODMAP diet is not just about following a set of dietary rules but about embracing personal empowerment. It's a journey of understanding your body's unique needs and nourishing it accordingly. It's not a restriction but a path to better health and well-being.

Patience, flexibility and an open mind are your allies. Mistakes and challenges are natural parts of this journey and learning from them will foster growth and success. Seek professional guidance if needed and don't hesitate to engage with dietitians or healthcare providers specializing in the low FODMAP diet.

Celebrate your progress, no matter how small and enjoy the process of discovery, cooking and social dining within the low FODMAP framework. Acknowledge the progress, enjoy the culinary creativity and cherish the connections with those who support you.

The low FODMAP diet is not a one-size-fits-all approach, nor is it a quick fix. It's a carefully designed method to personal well-being that necessitates a deep connection to how food affects your body. This guide has aimed to equip you with the knowledge, resources and motivation to embark on this journey confidently.

May the recipes, strategies and insights shared here inspire you and ease your path as you navigate this unique dietary landscape. Your journey to better digestive health begins now and with perseverance and positivity, the rewards will be well worth the effort.

Glossary of Terms

Here's a collection of terms often encountered throughout the low FODMAP diet journey. Understanding these terms will help guide your comprehension and execution of the diet.

1. FODMAP: An acronym that stands for Fermentable Oligo-, Di-, Mono-saccharides And Polyols. These are types of carbohydrates that may be poorly absorbed in the small intestine, leading to digestive discomfort in some individuals.

2. Low FODMAP Diet: A dietary approach that emphasizes the temporary reduction and then controlled reintroduction of FODMAPs to alleviate gastrointestinal symptoms.

3. IBS (Irritable Bowel Syndrome): A common digestive disorder that can result in symptoms like bloating, gas, diarrhea, and constipation. The low FODMAP diet may be used as a management strategy.

4. Elimination Phase: The initial phase of the low FODMAP diet where high FODMAP foods are removed from the diet for a period to assess their impact on digestive health.

5. Reintroduction Phase: A controlled phase of the low FODMAP diet where individual FODMAPs are reintroduced to determine personal tolerance levels.

6. Monash University: An Australian university that has played a leading role in researching and developing the low FODMAP diet.

7. Dietitian: A healthcare professional specializing in diet and nutrition who may guide individuals in the proper implementation of the low FODMAP diet.

8. Lactose: A type of sugar found in milk and dairy products and considered a disaccharide, part of the FODMAP group.

9. Fructose: A monosaccharide sugar found in many fruits and honey that may be poorly absorbed by some individuals.

10. Gluten-Free: Refers to food products without gluten, a protein found in wheat, barley, and rye. Though not synonymous with low FODMAP, some gluten-free products may fit within the diet.

11. Polyols: A type of carbohydrate that includes sugar alcohols like sorbitol and mannitol, often found in artificial sweeteners and some fruits and vegetables.

12. Prebiotics: Compounds that feed beneficial gut bacteria. Some high FODMAP foods are prebiotic, and care is needed to ensure that a low FODMAP diet maintains a healthy gut microbiome.

13. Gastroenterologist: A doctor specializing in the digestive system who may recommend the low FODMAP diet to patients with specific digestive issues.

14. Fermentation: The process by which bacteria in the large intestine break down undigested carbohydrates, potentially producing gas and discomfort.

15. Soluble Fiber: A type of fiber that dissolves in water, forming a gel-like substance. Some forms of soluble fiber may be high in FODMAPs.

This glossary is by no means exhaustive but serves as a foundational reference point for the terms you may encounter while exploring or following the low FODMAP diet. If in doubt, always consult with a healthcare professional or dietitian specializing in the low FODMAP diet.

References

I. Morariu, L. Avasilca, M. Vieriu, et al. (2023). Effects of a Low-FODMAP Diet on Irritable Bowel Syndrome in Both Children and Adults-A Narrative Review. Nutrients, 15(10): 2295.

C. J. Black, H. M. Staudacher, A. C. Ford (2022). Efficacy of a low FODMAP diet in irritable bowel syndrome: systematic review and network meta-analysis. Gut, 71(6):1117-1126

A. Stróżyk, A. Horvath, H. Szajewska (2021). A Low-FODMAP Diet in the Management of Children With Functional Abdominal Pain Disorders: A Protocol of a Systematic Review. Journal of Pediatric Gastroenterology and Nutrition, 2(2):e065.

C. Tuck, E. Ly, A. Bogatyrev, I. Costetsou, P. R. Gibson, J. Barrett, J. Muir (2018). Fermentable short chain carbohydrate (FODMAP) content of common plant-based foods and processed foods suitable for vegetarian- and vegan-based eating patterns. Journal of Human Nutrition and Dietetics, 31(3):422-435.

J. Varney, J. Barrett, K. Scarlata, P. Catsos, P. R. Gibson, J. G. Muir (2017). FODMAPs: food composition, defining cutoff values and international application. Journal of Gastroenterology and Hepatology, 32 (1), 53-61.

Marsh, A., Eslick, E. M., & Eslick, G. D. (2016). Does a diet low in FODMAPs reduce symptoms associated with functional gastrointestinal disorders? A comprehensive systematic review and meta-analysis. European Journal of Nutrition, 55(3), 897-906.

Halmos, E. P., Power, V. A., Shepherd, S. J., Gibson, P. R., & Muir, J. G. (2014). A diet low in FODMAPs reduces symptoms of irritable bowel syndrome. Gastroenterology, 146(1), 67-75:e05.

Gibson, P. R., & Shepherd, S. J. (2010). Evidence-based dietary management of functional gastrointestinal symptoms: The FODMAP approach. Journal of Gastroenterology and Hepatology, 25(2), 252-258.

By Cabot Health, Bristol Stool Chart - http://cdn.intechopen.com/pdfs-wm/46082.pdf, CC BY-SA 3.0, https://commons.wikimedia.org/w/index.php?curid=84257571 (used for the Bonus "Daily Symptoms Tracker")

https://www.monashfodmap.com

Printed in Great Britain
by Amazon

31521383R00059

France

Paris – North
Normandy – Brittany

EXPLORAMA

A photographic travel to France

Part 1

PARIS & AROUND

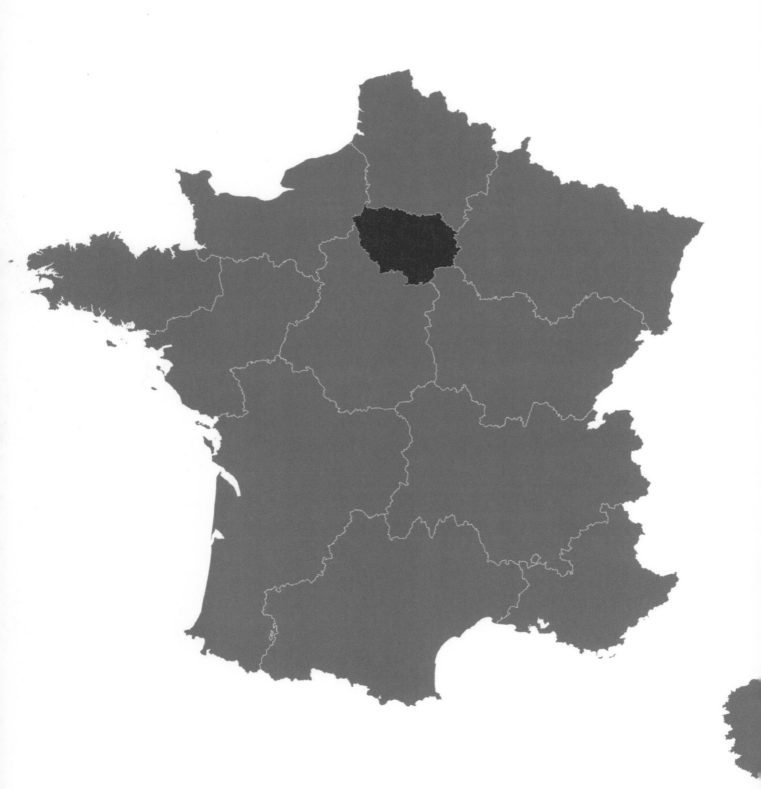

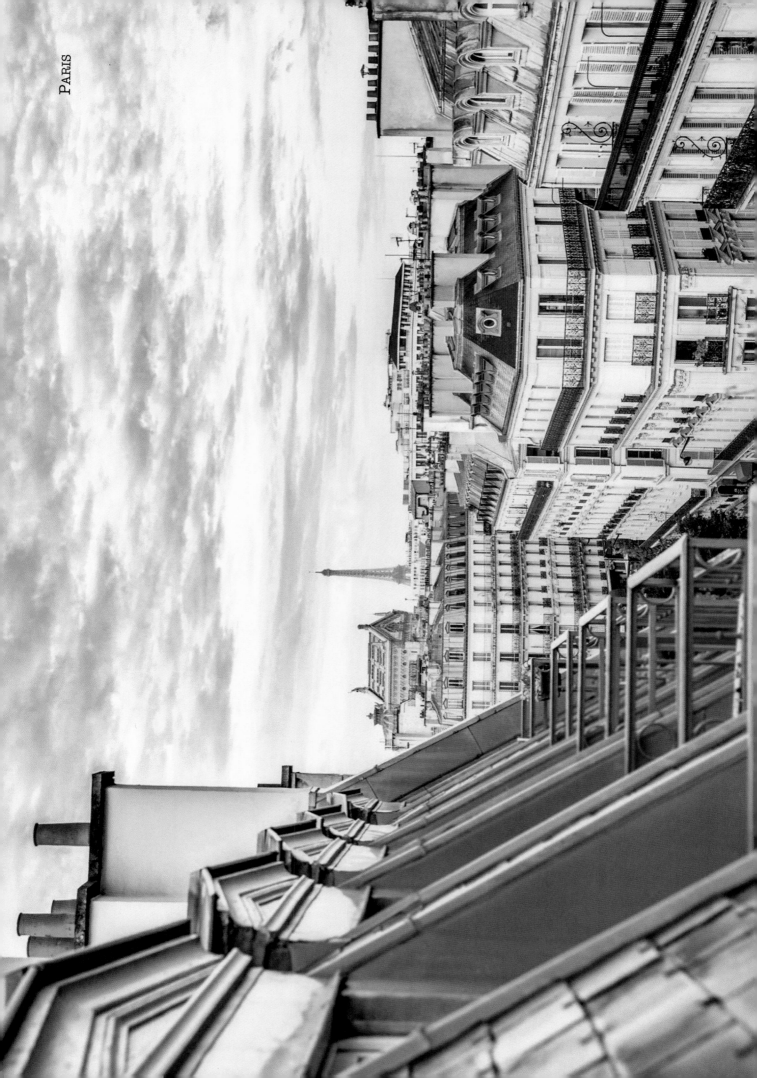

PARIS

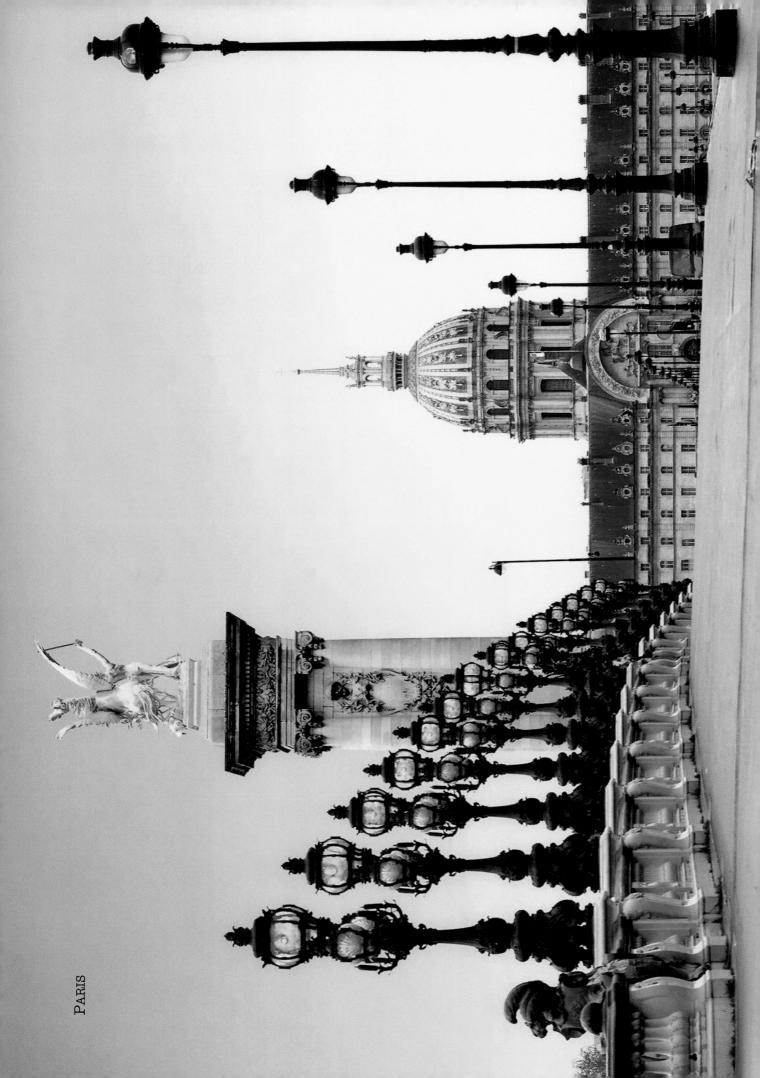

PARIS

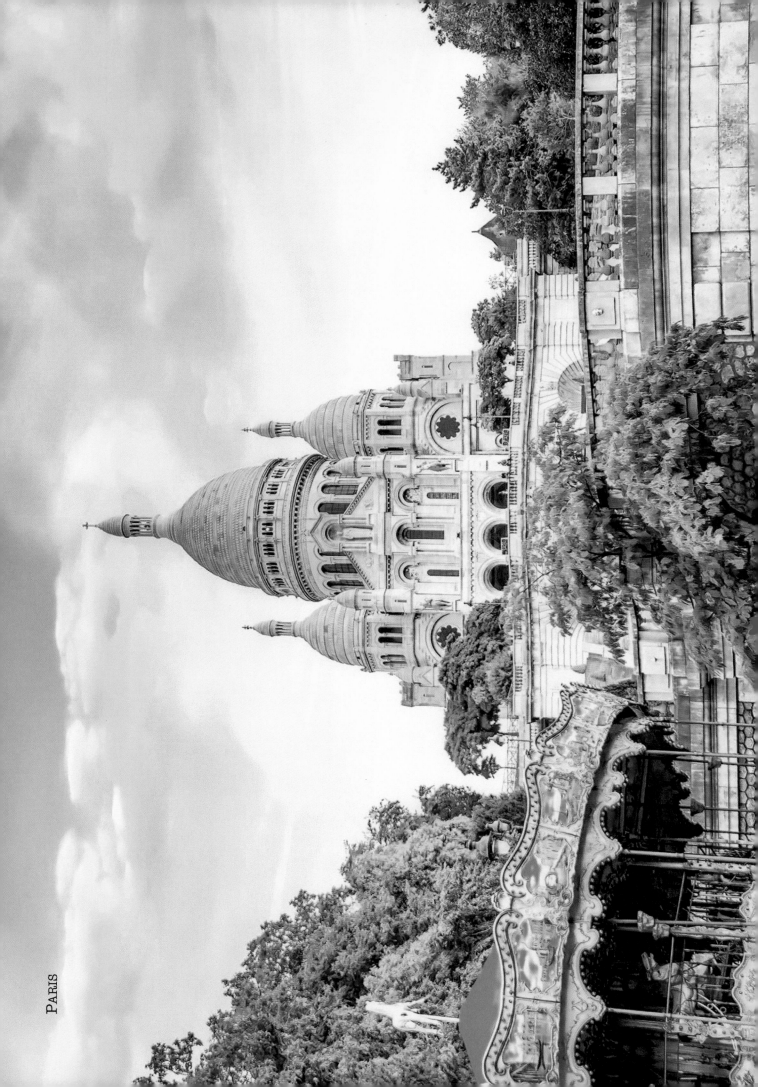

PARIS

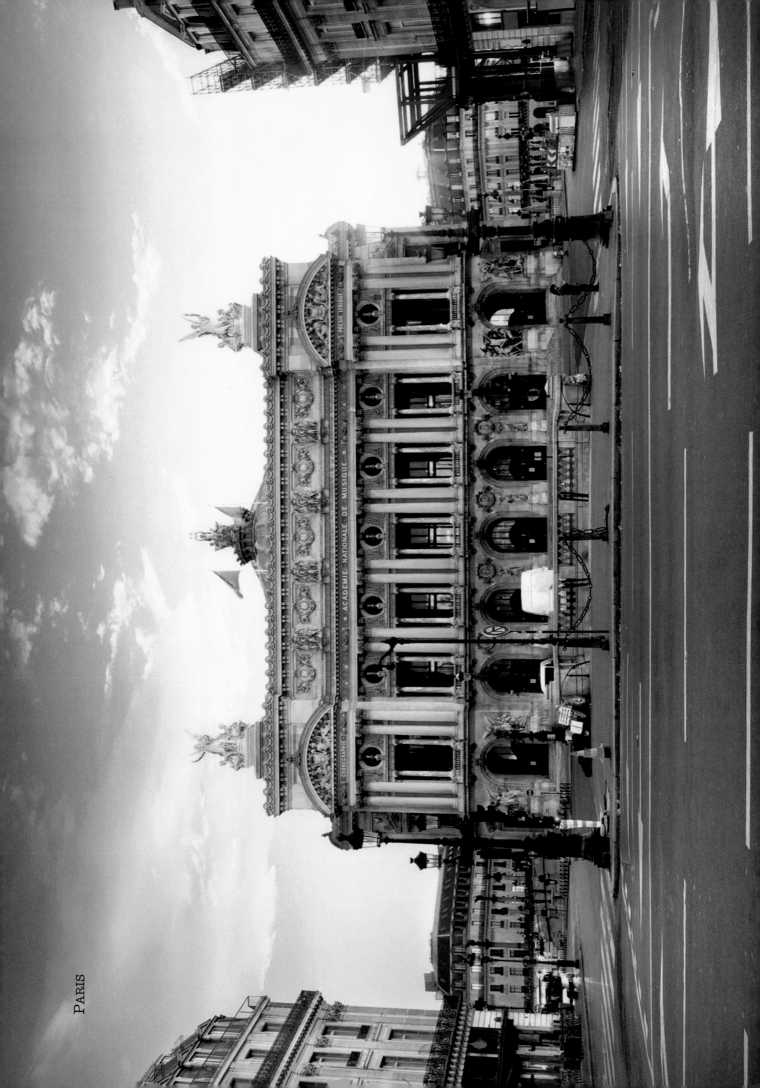

PARIS

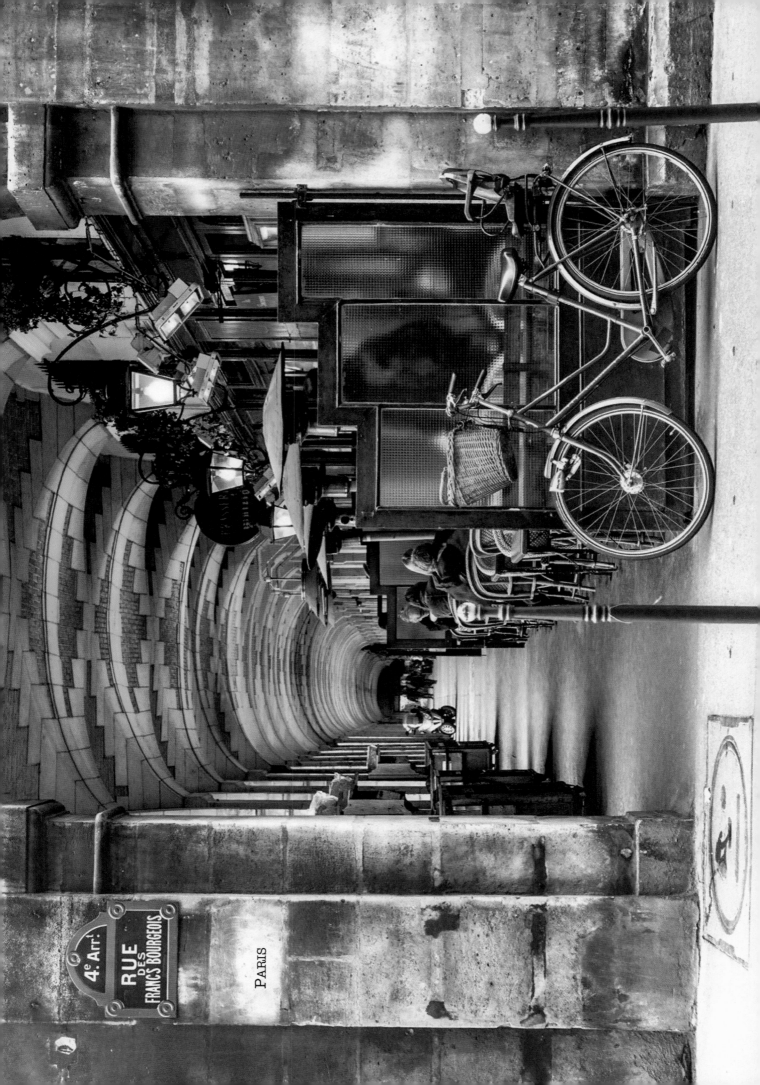

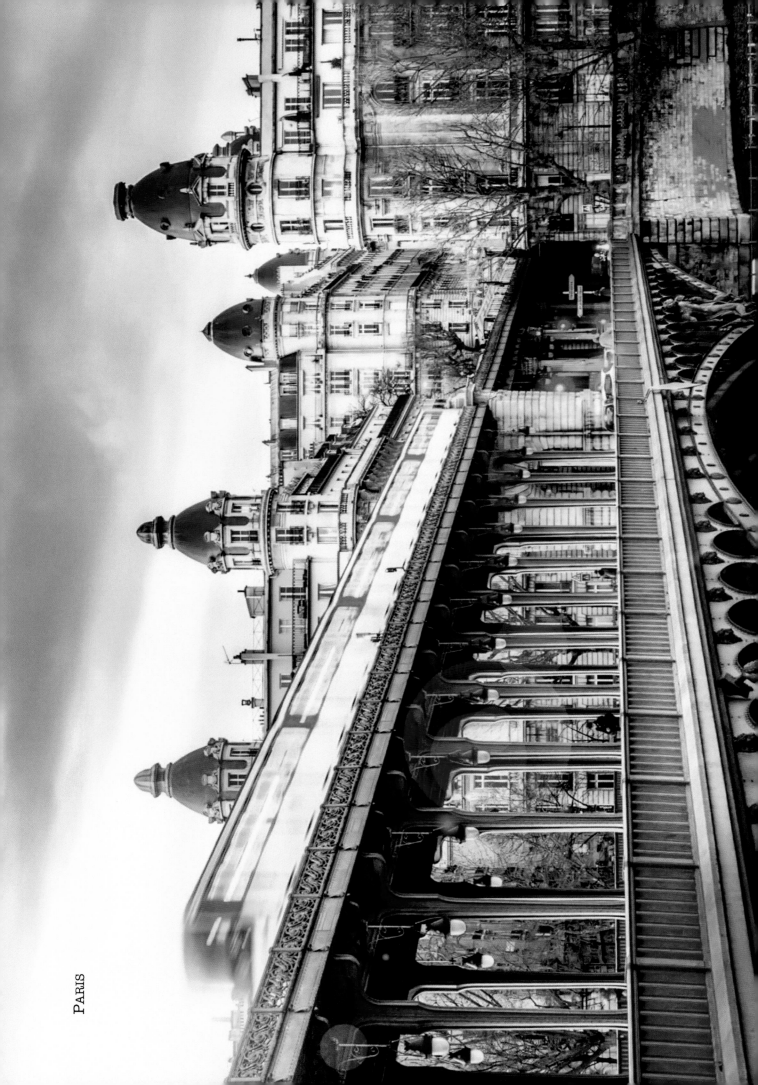

PARIS

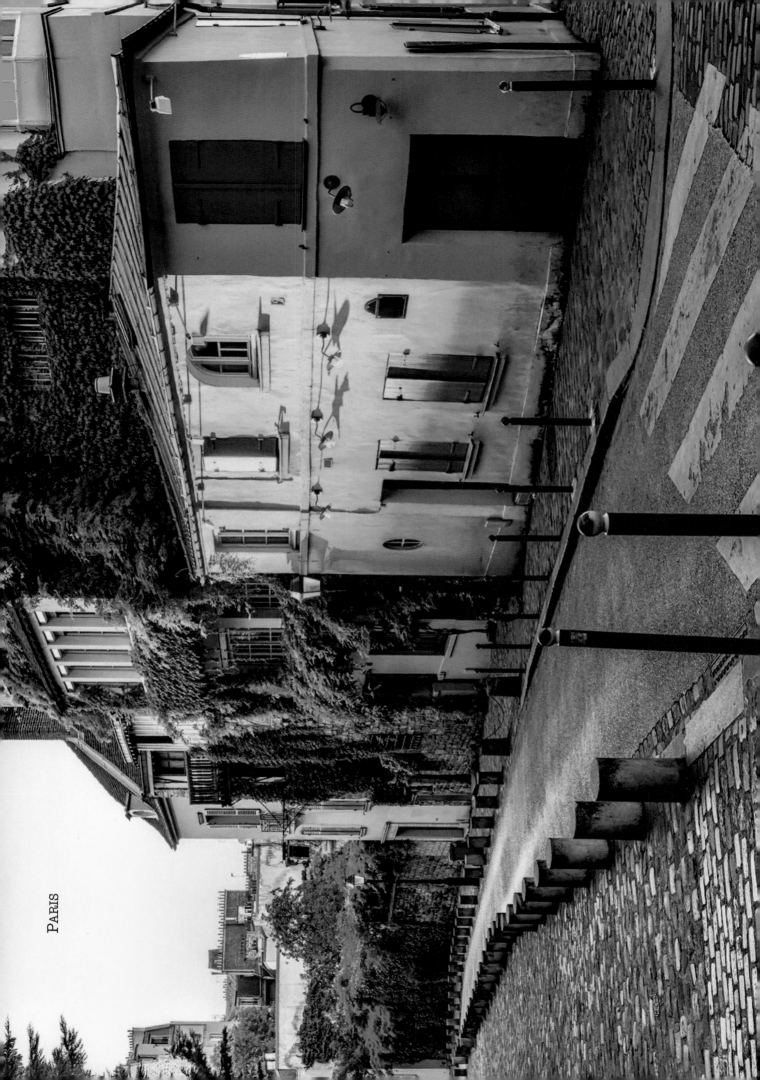

PARIS

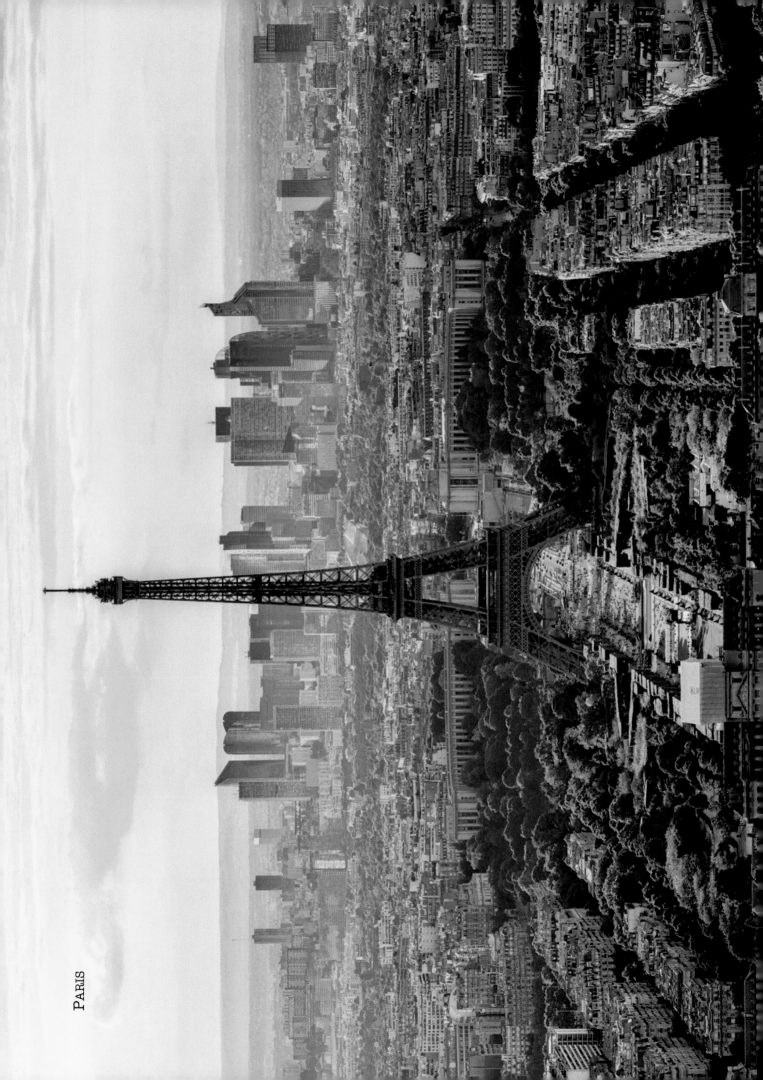

PARIS

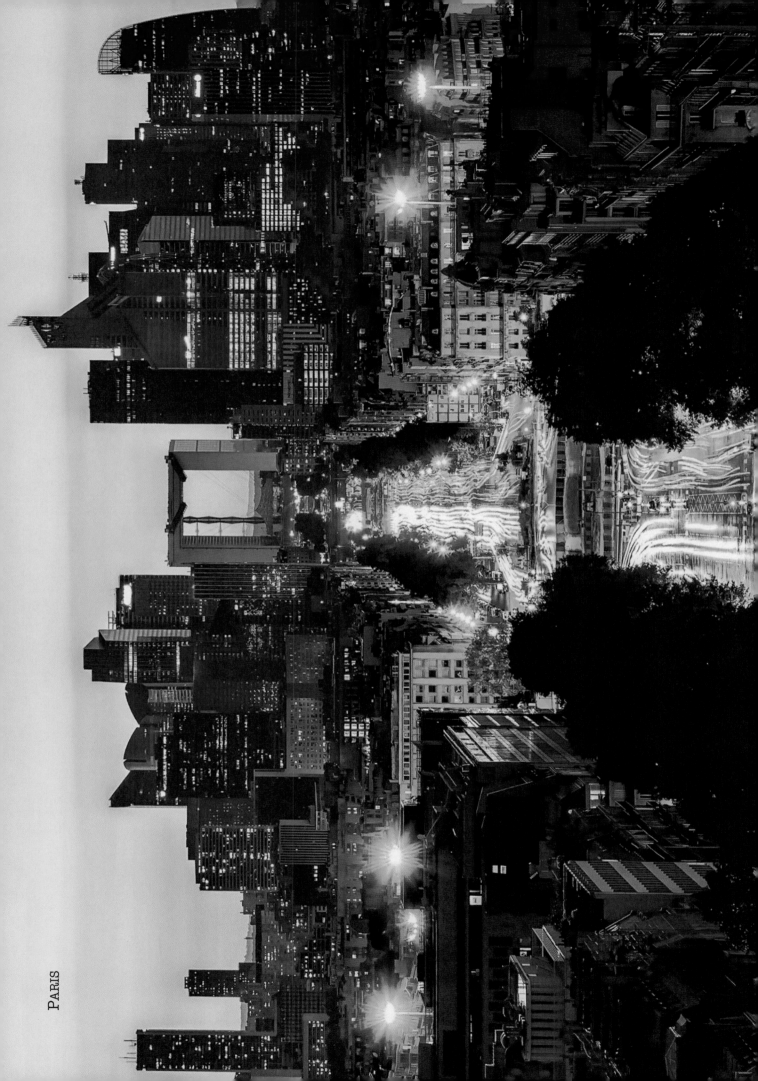

PARIS

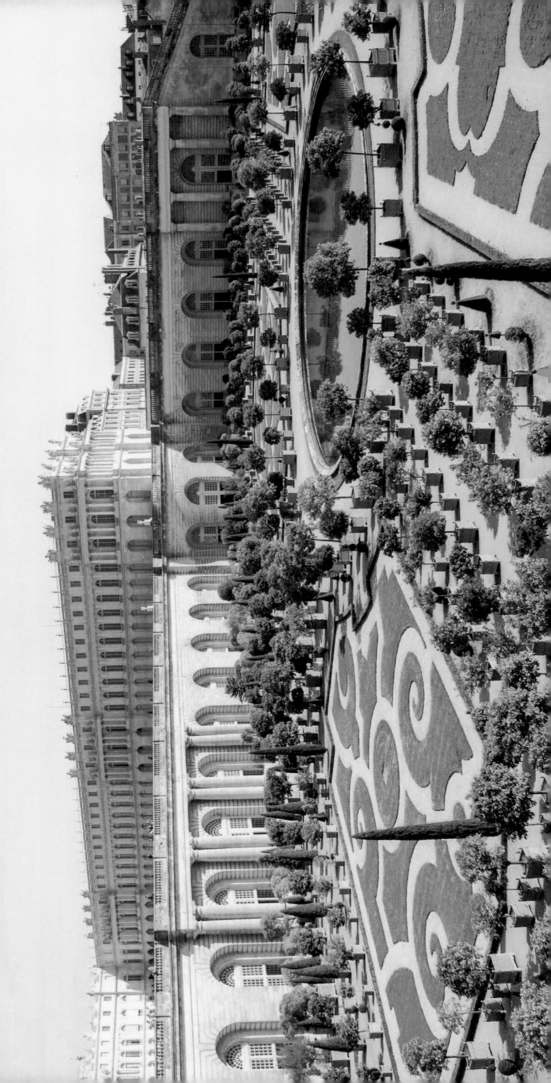

VERSAILLES

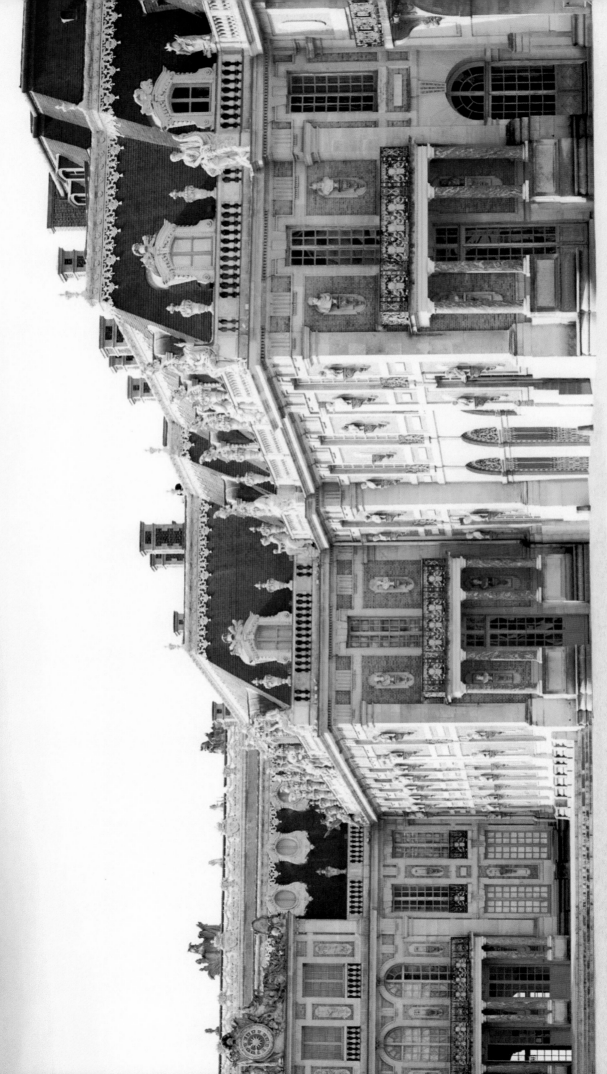

VERSAILLES

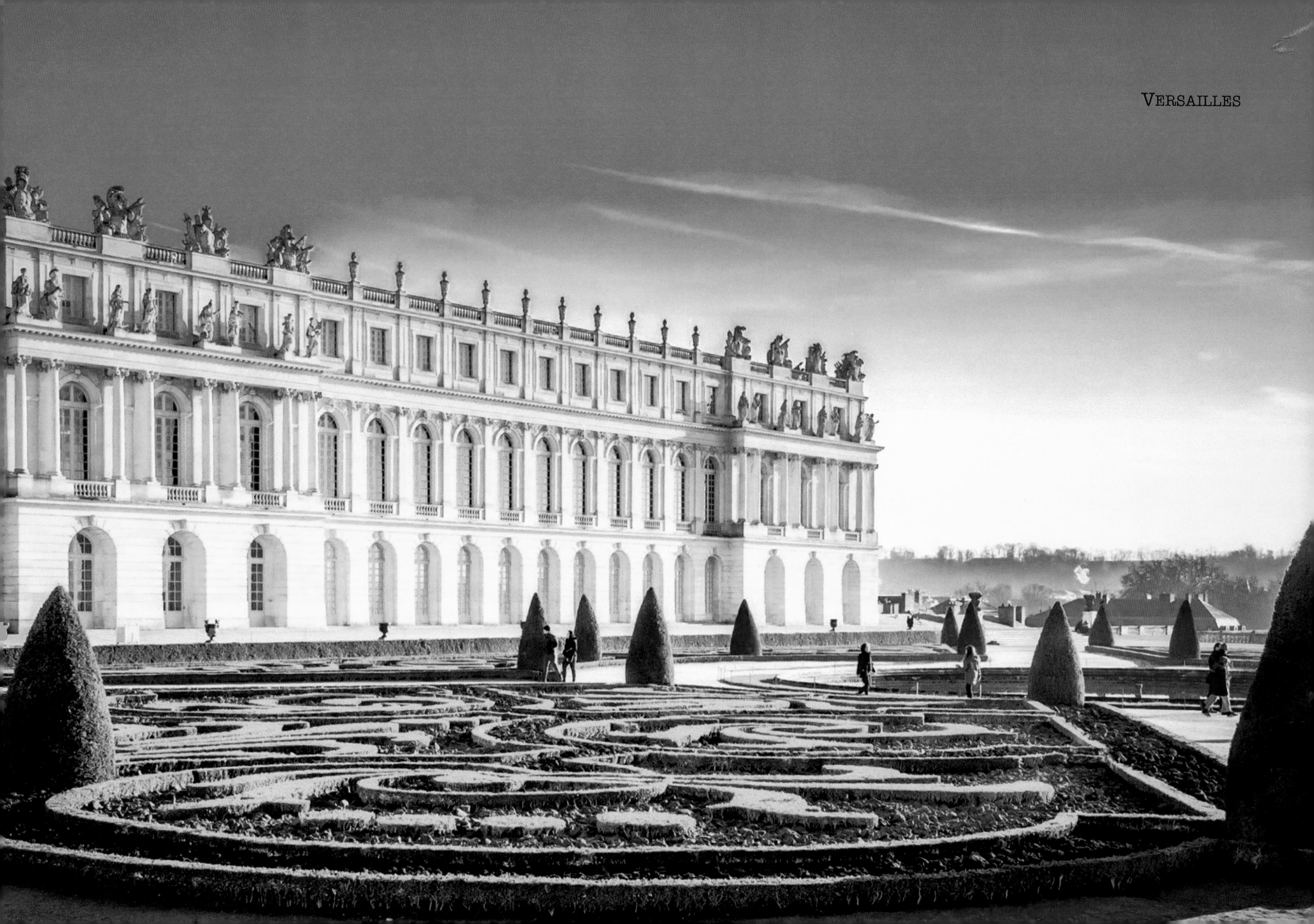

Versailles

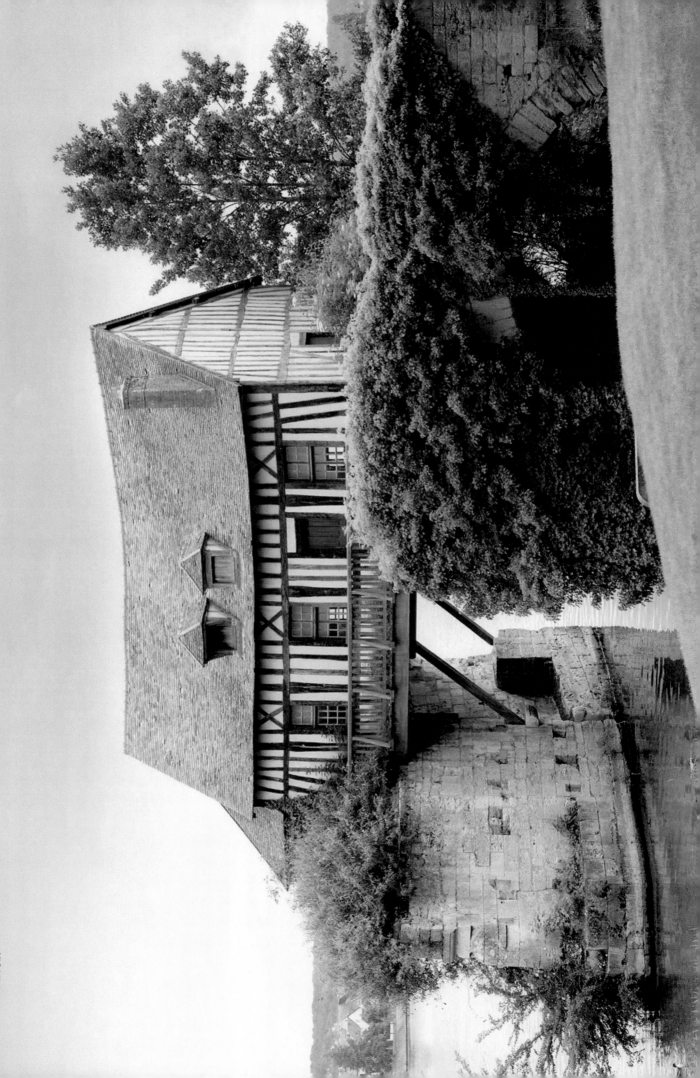

VERNON

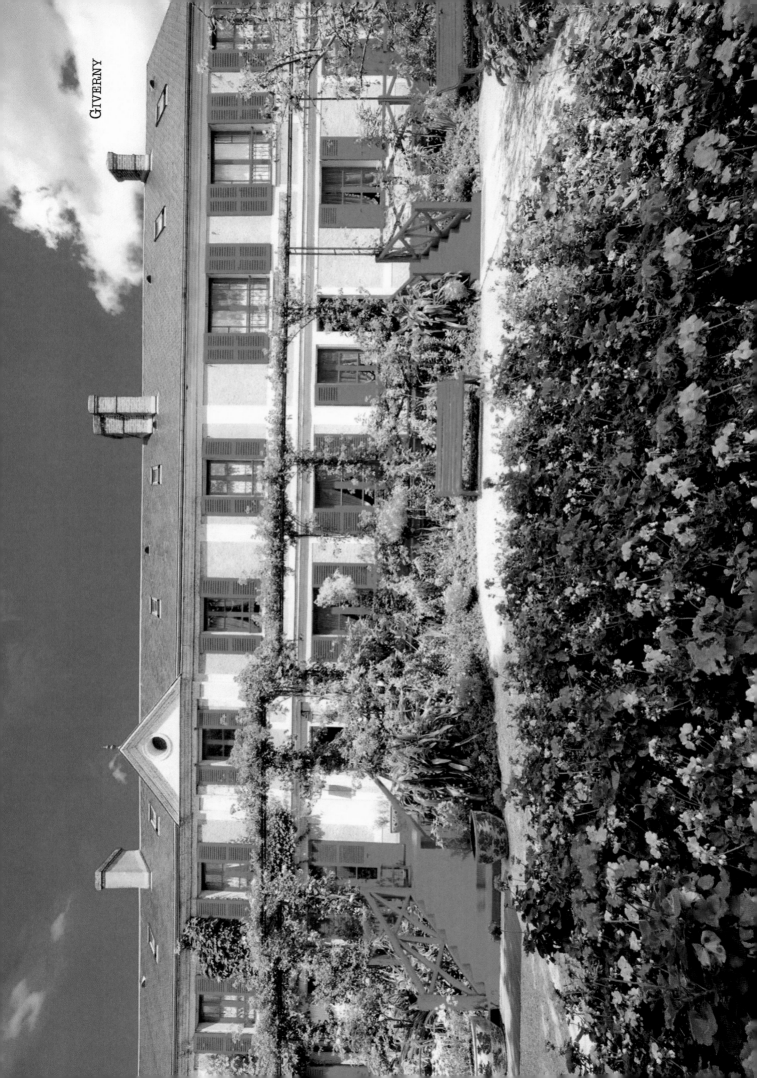

GIVERNY

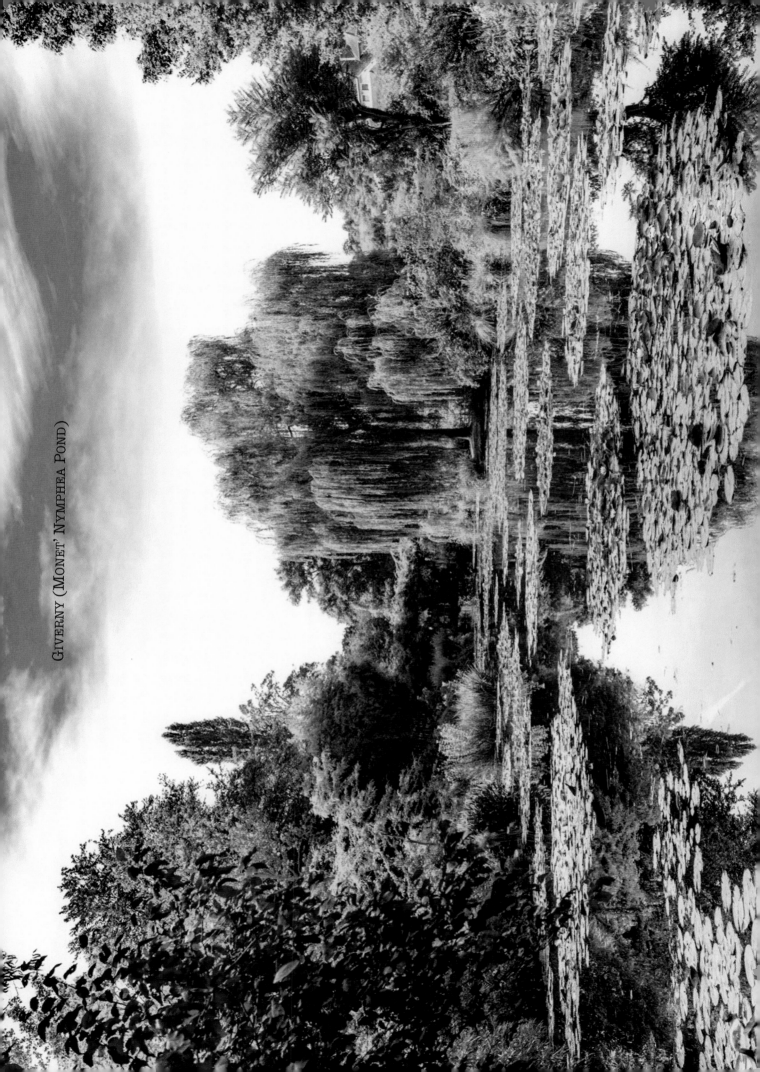

GIVERNY (MONET' NYMPHEA POND)

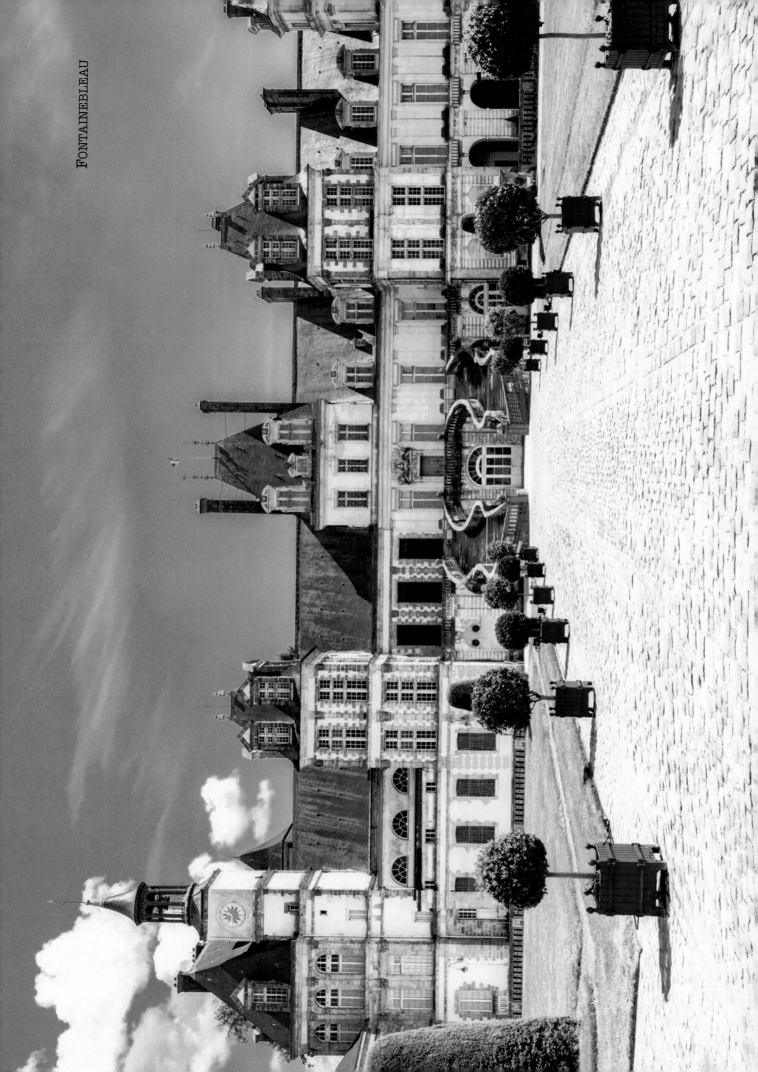

FONTAINEBLEAU

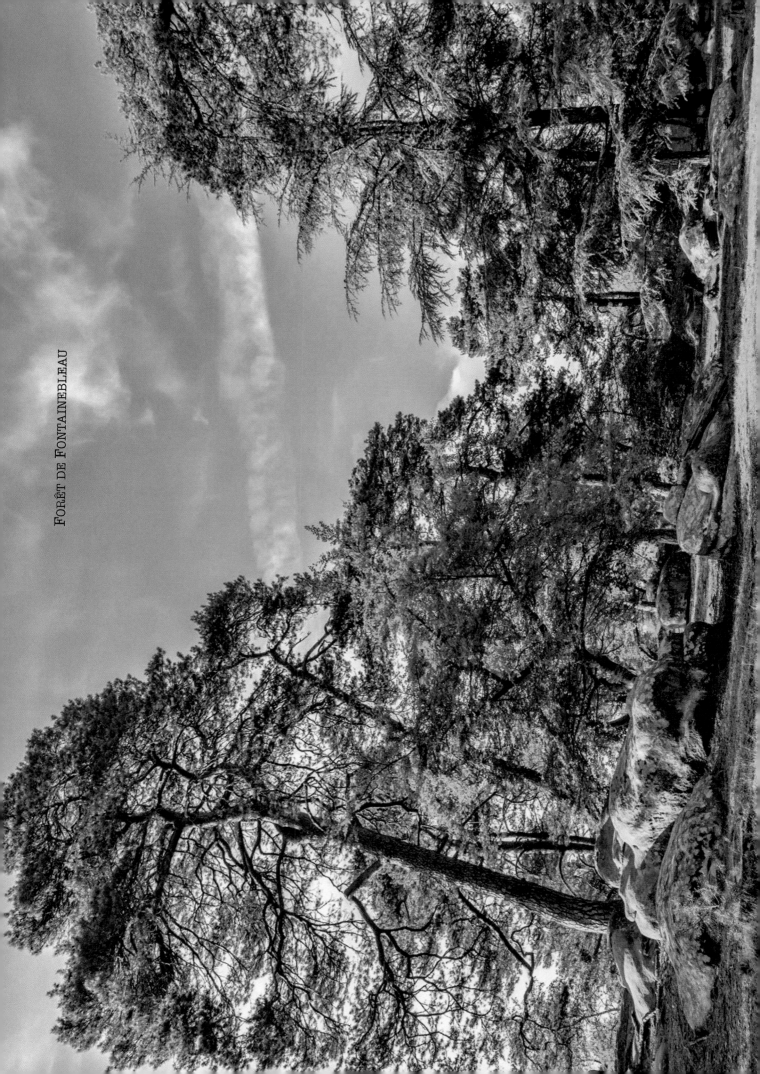

Forêt de Fontainebleau

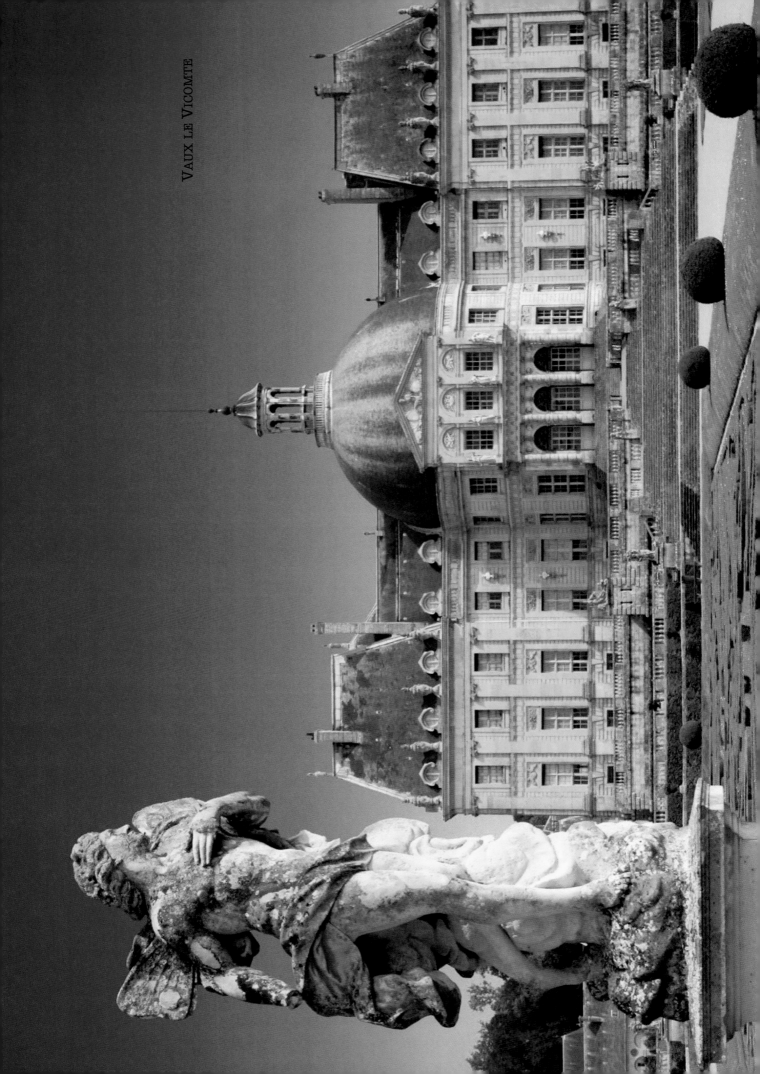

VAUX LE VICOMTE

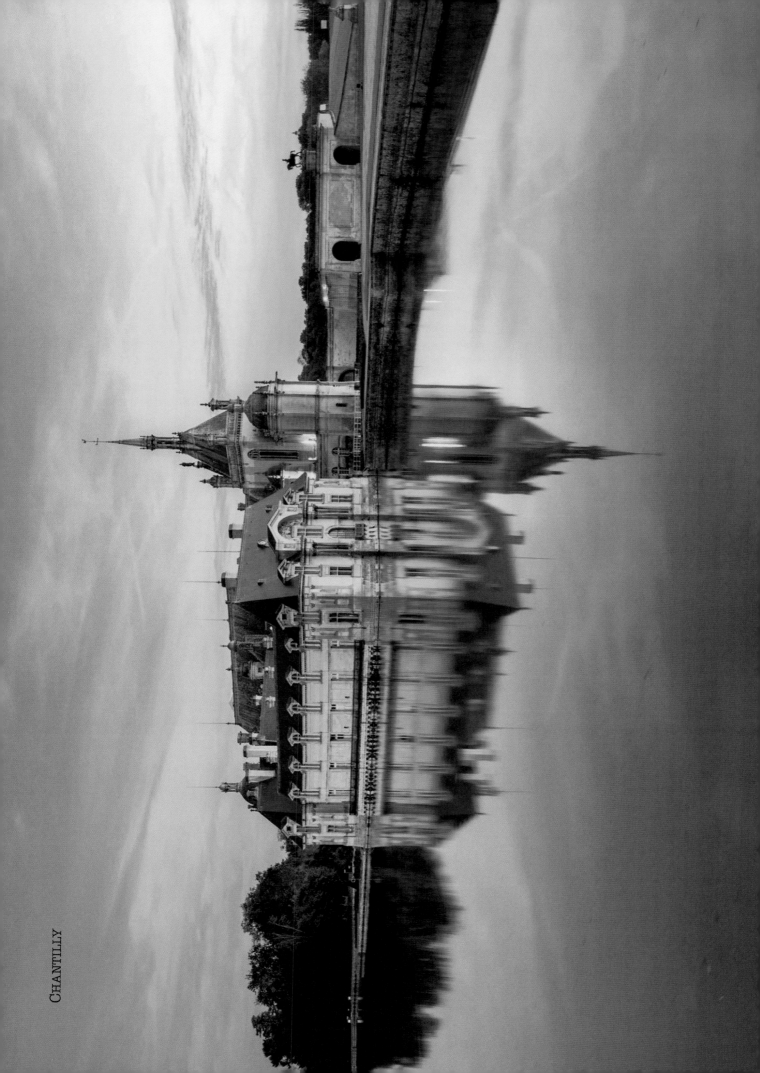

Chantilly

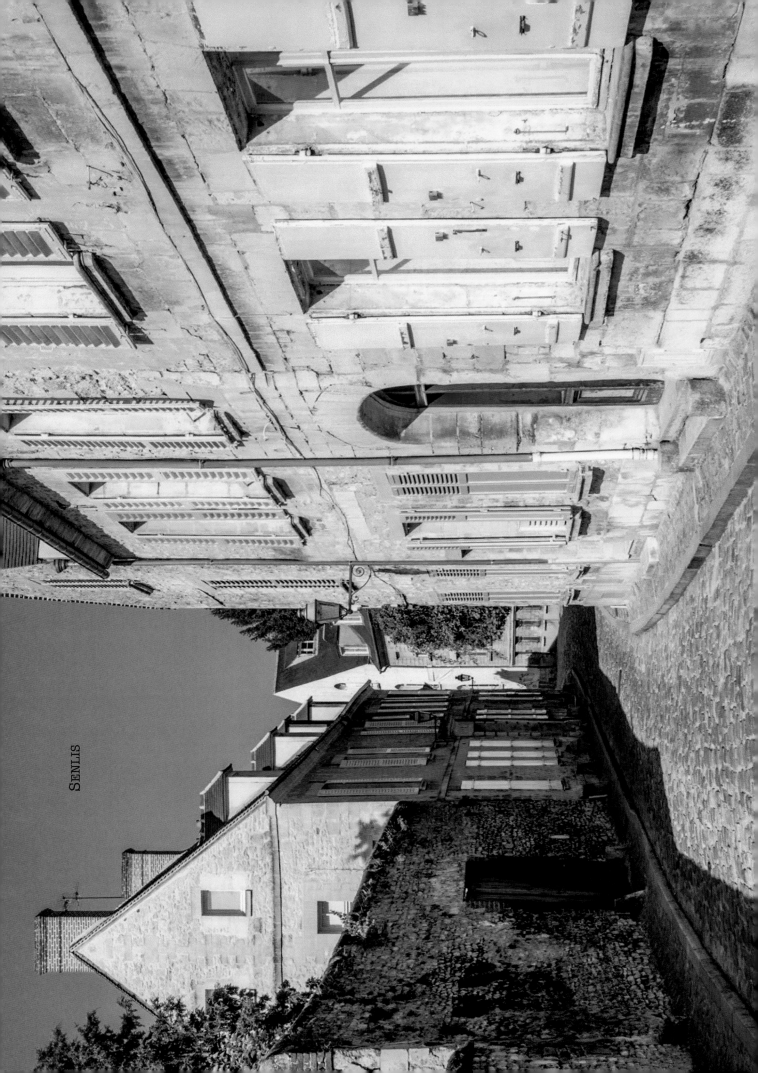

Senlis

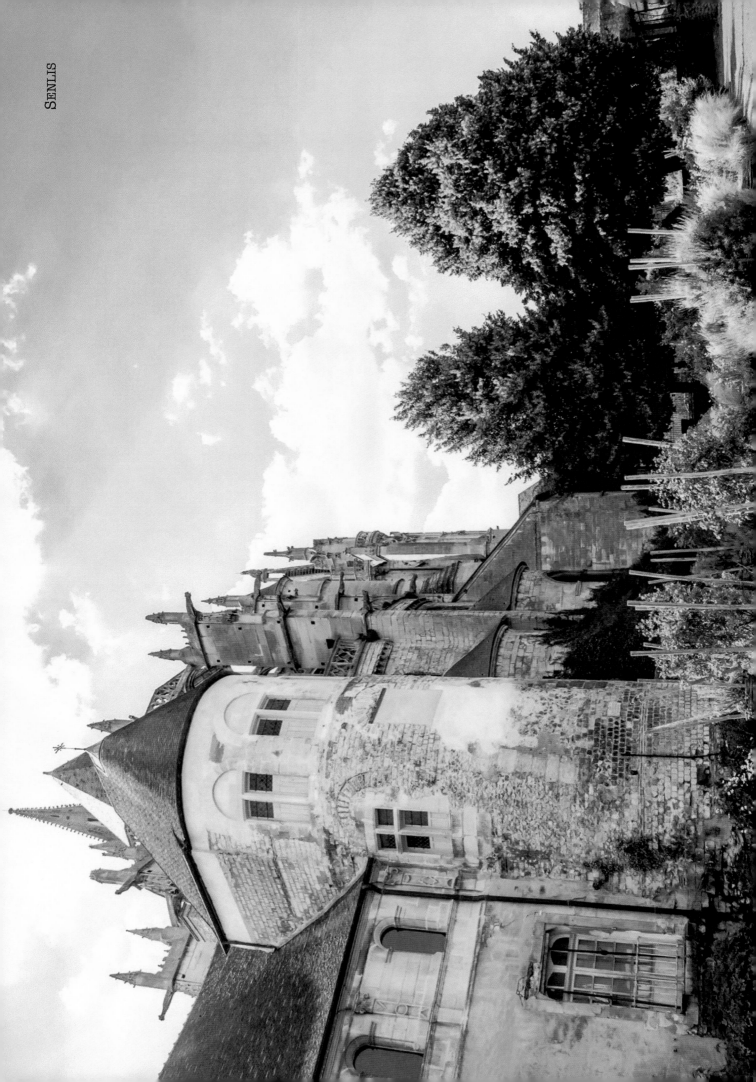

SENLIS

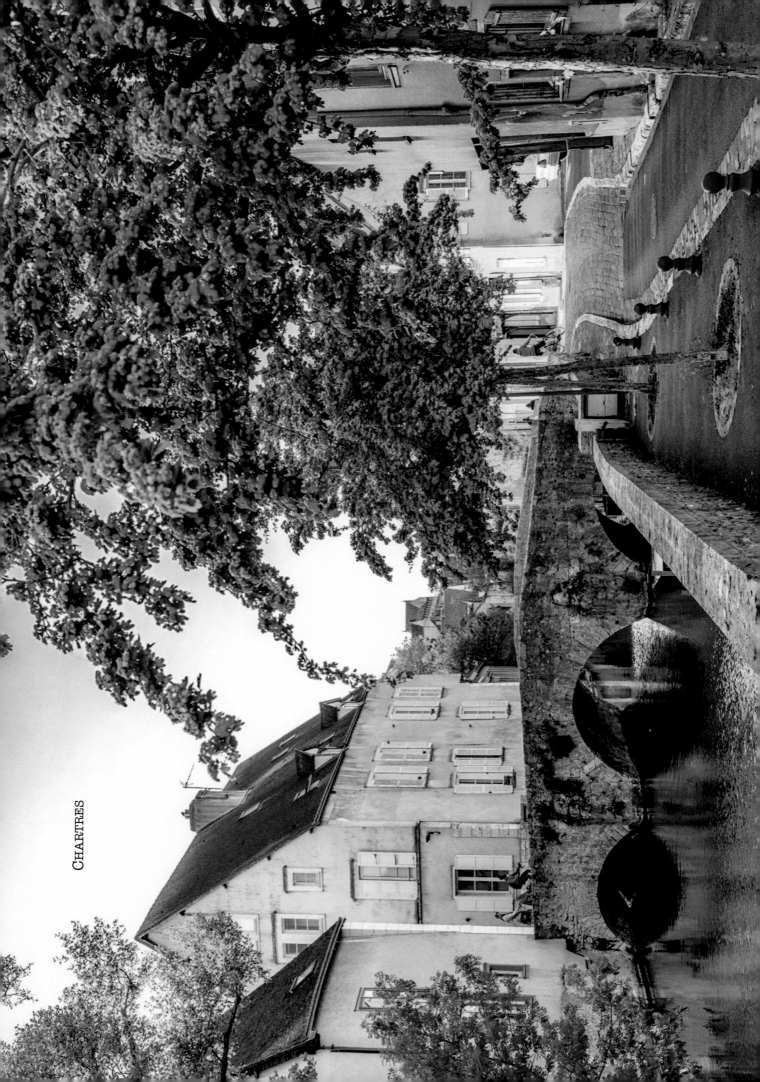

CHARTRES

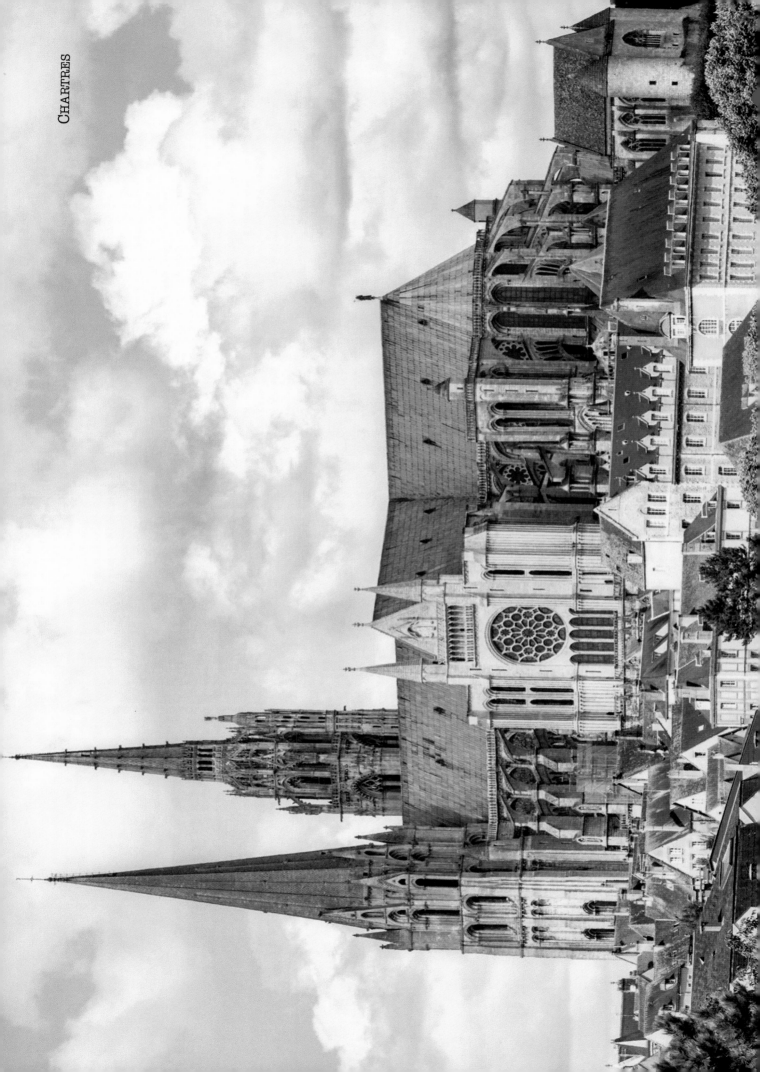

NORTH

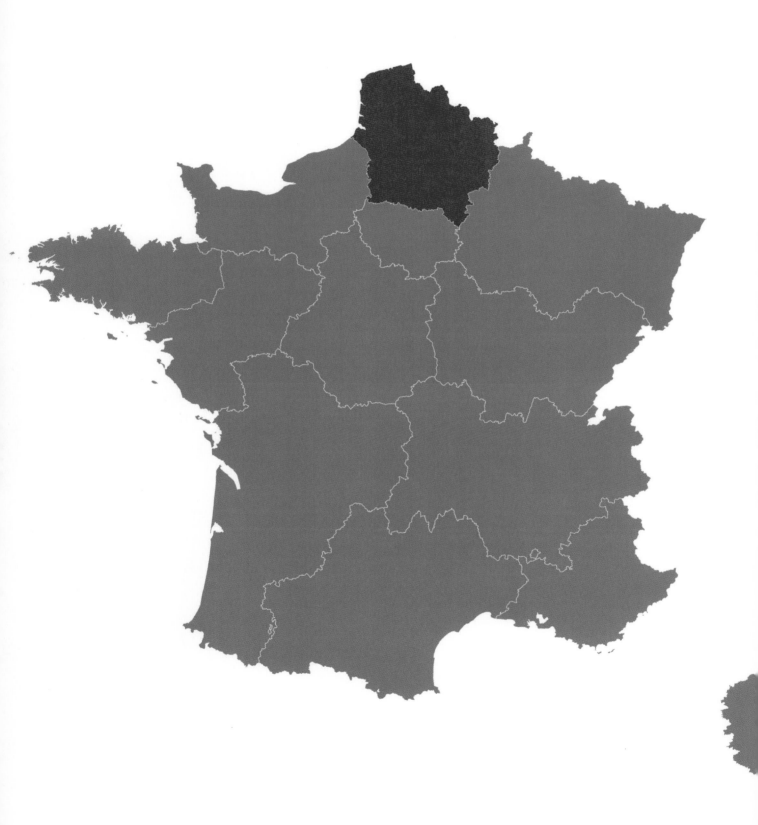

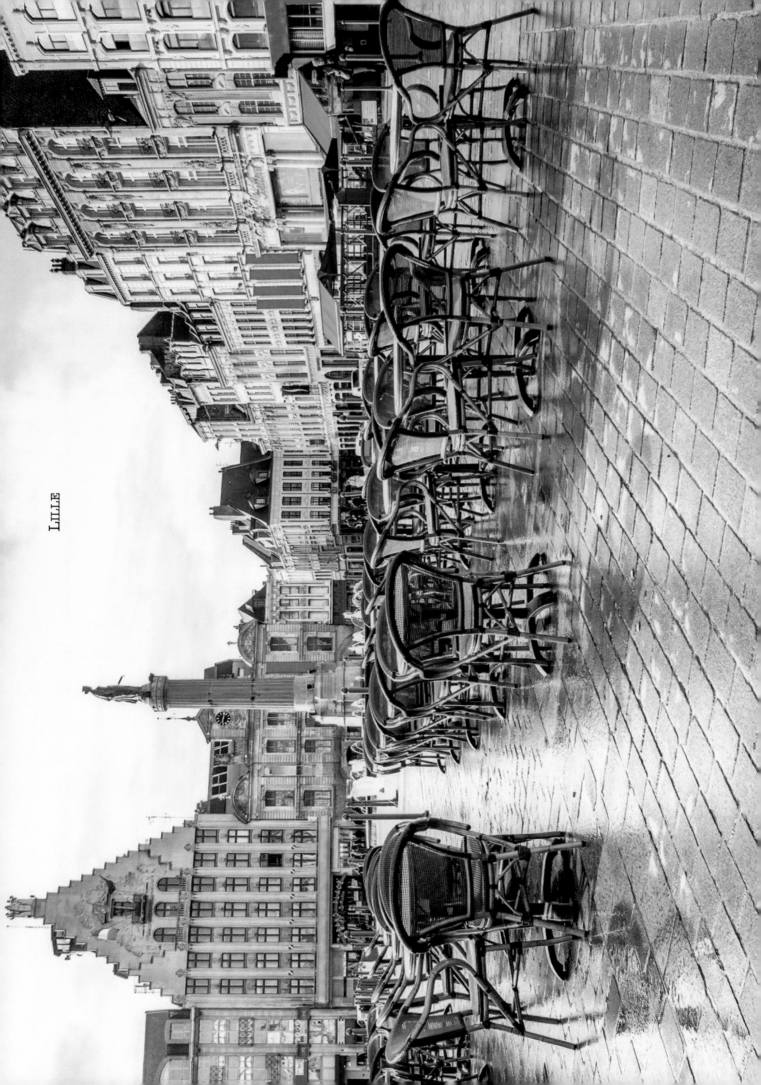

LILLE

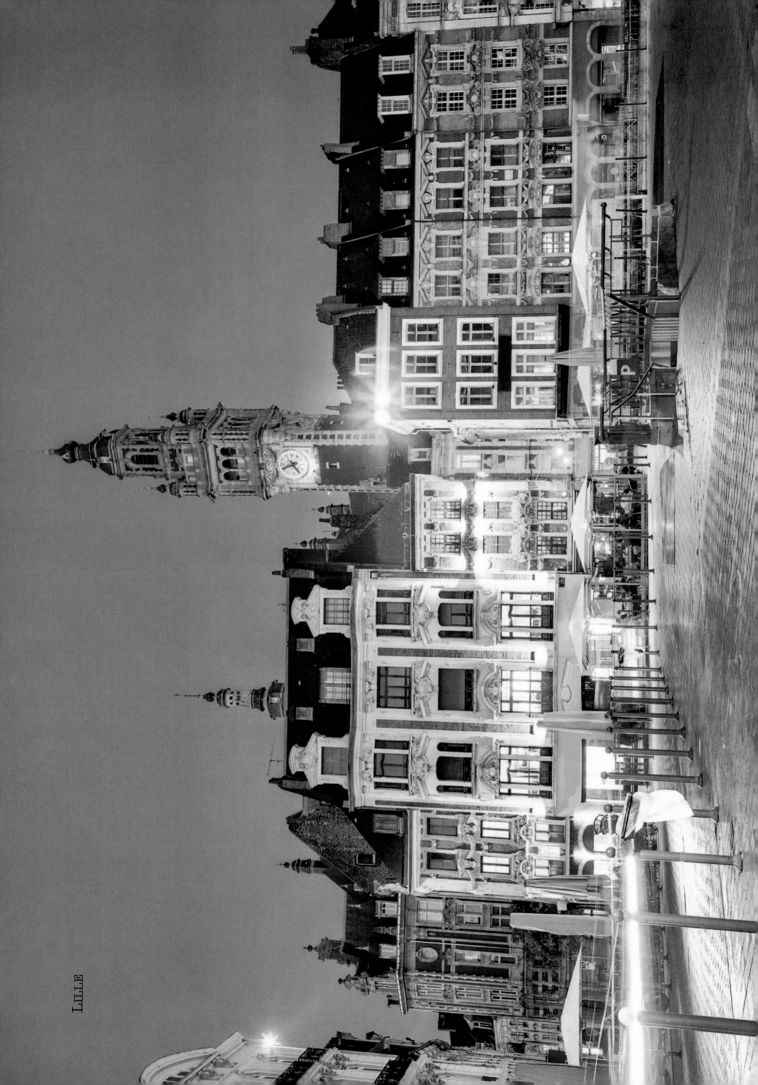

LILLE

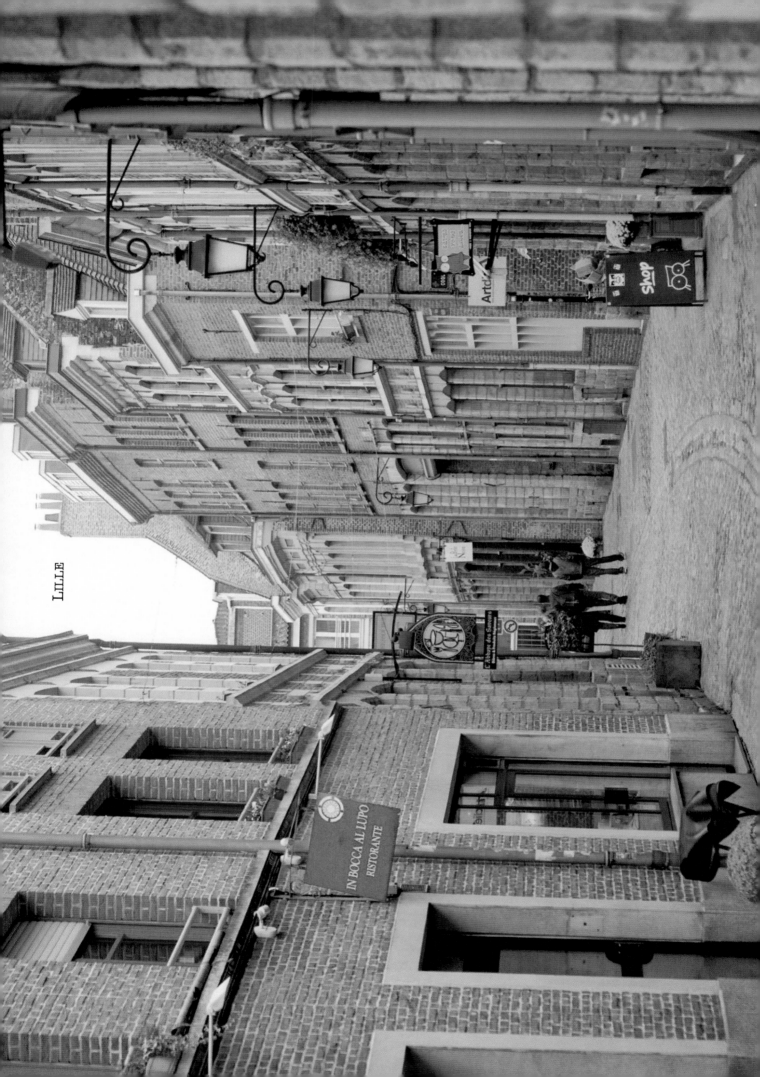

LILLE

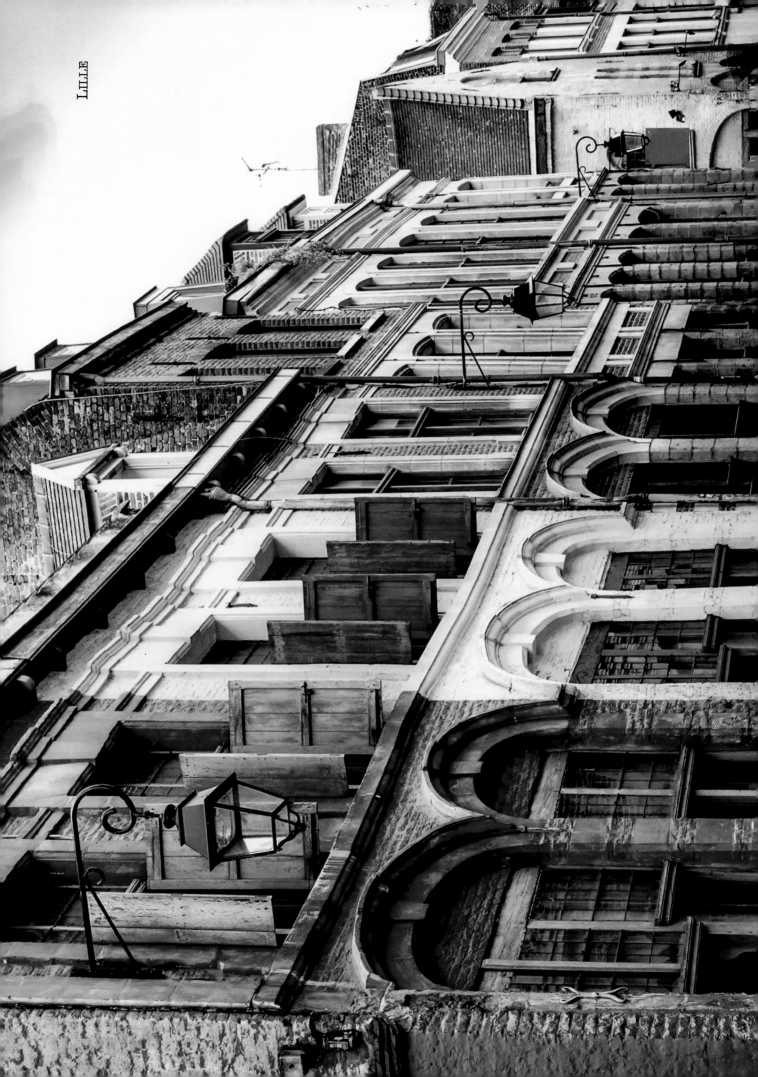

LILLE

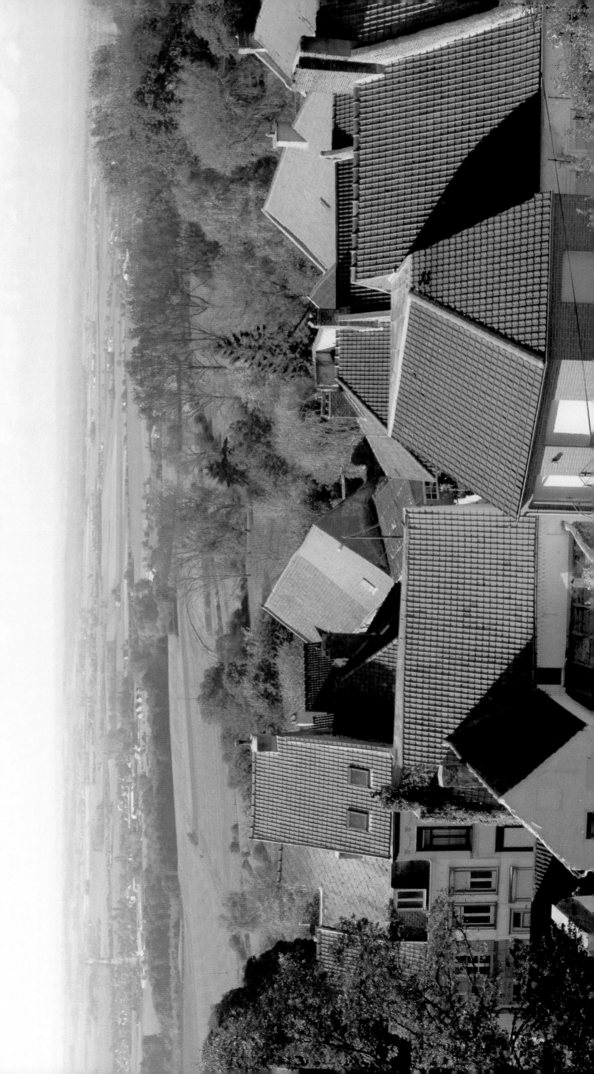

CASSEL

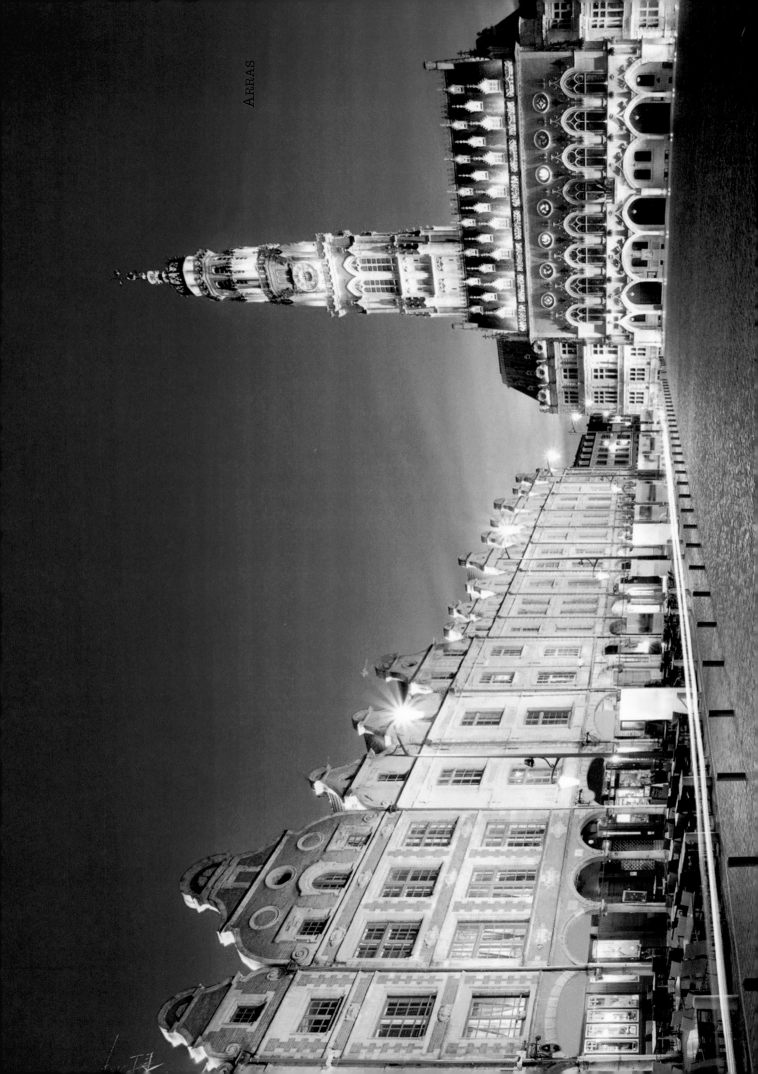

ARRAS

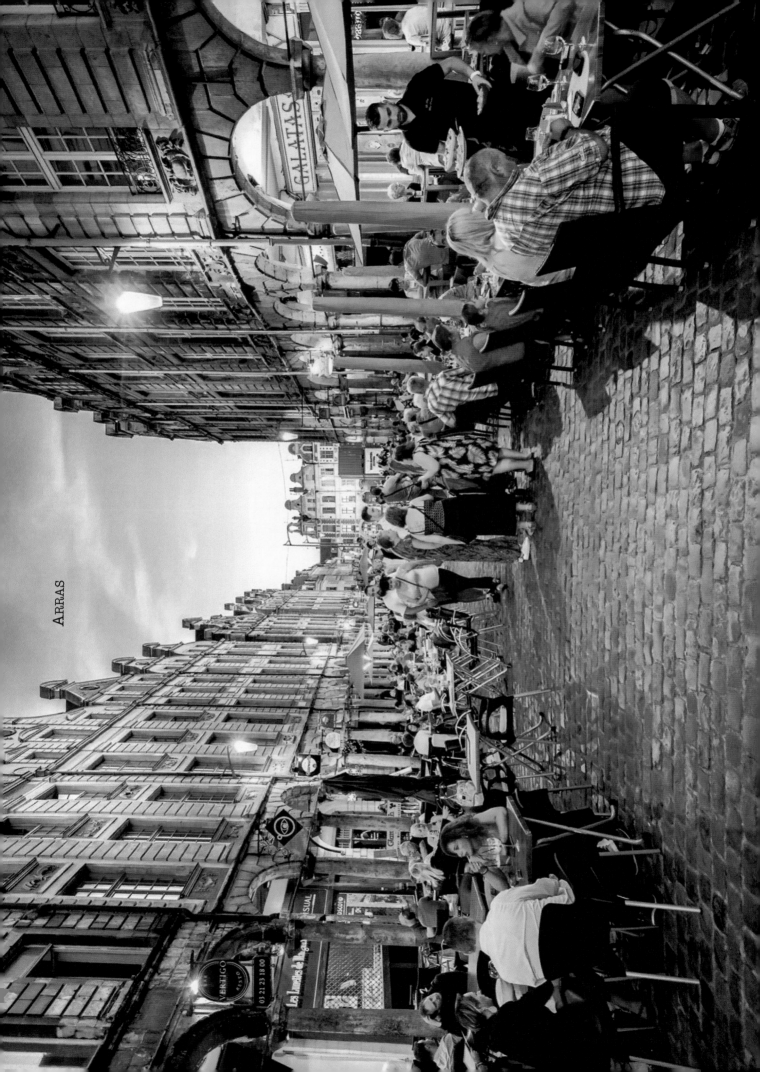

ARRAS

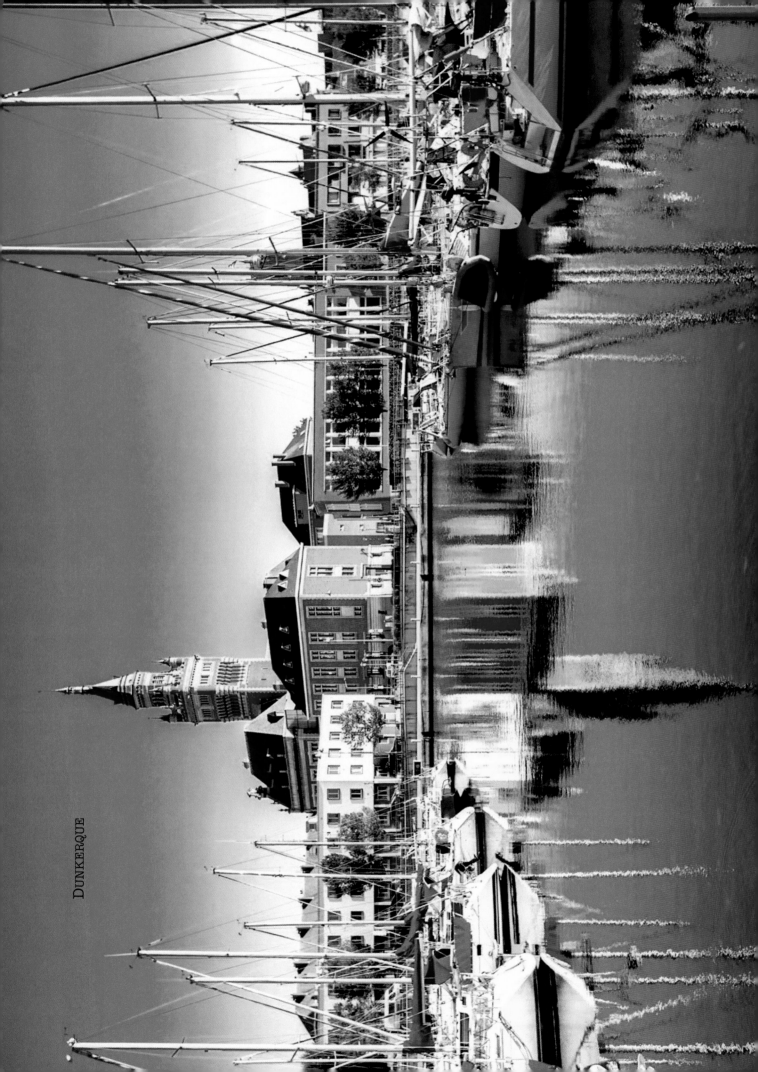

DUNKERQUE

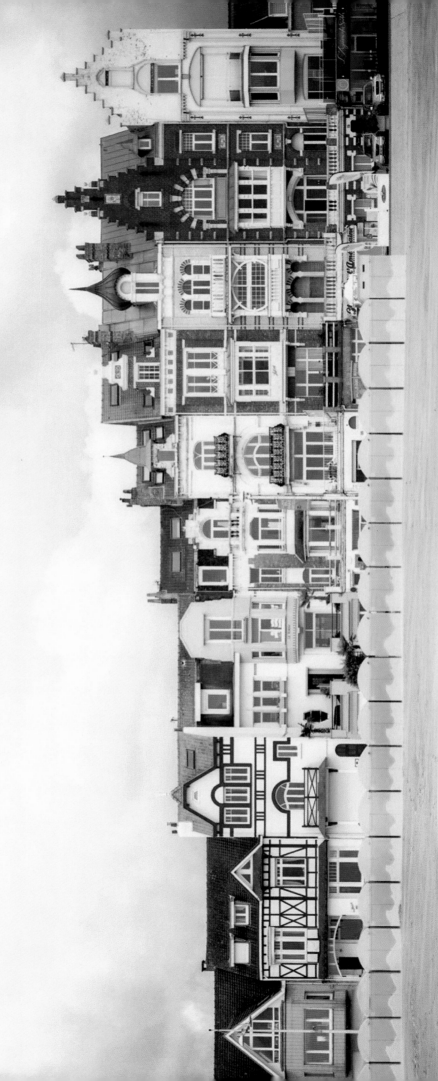

MALO LES BAINS

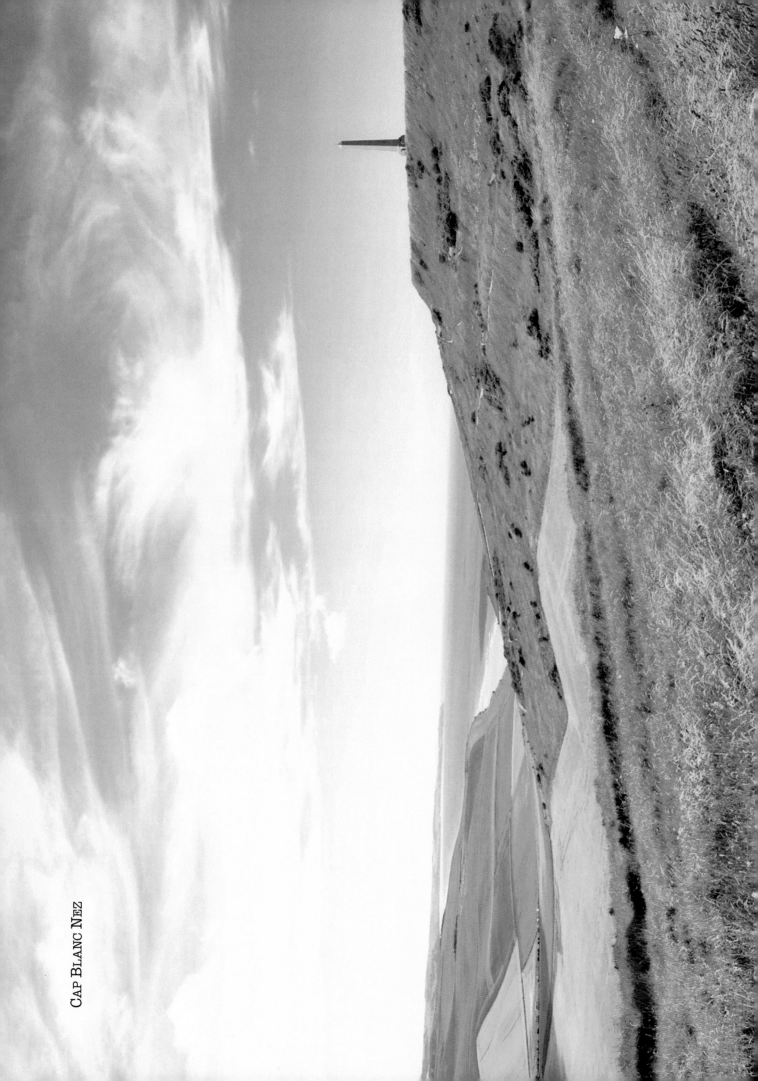

Cap Blanc Nez

Cap Gris Nez

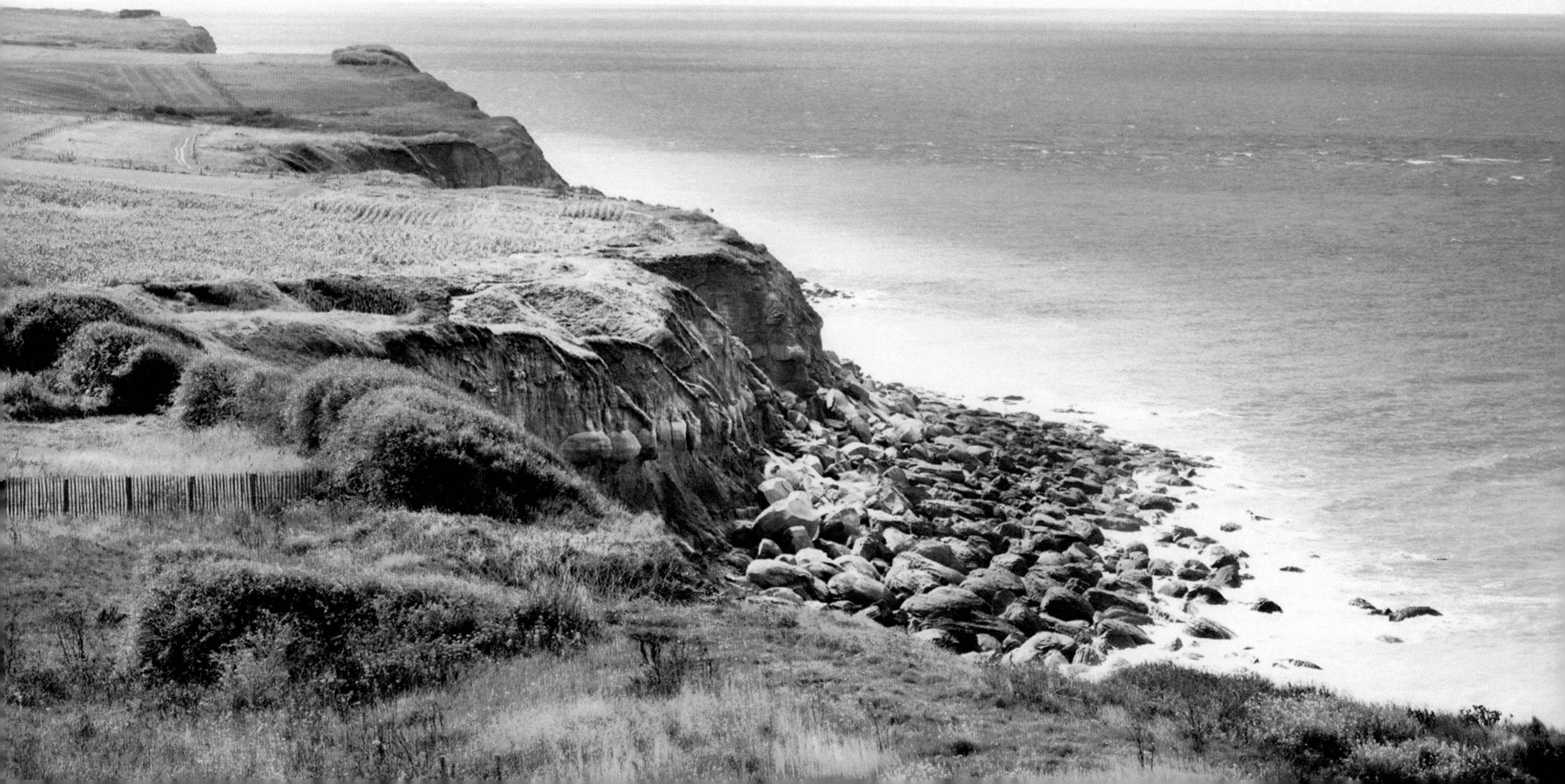

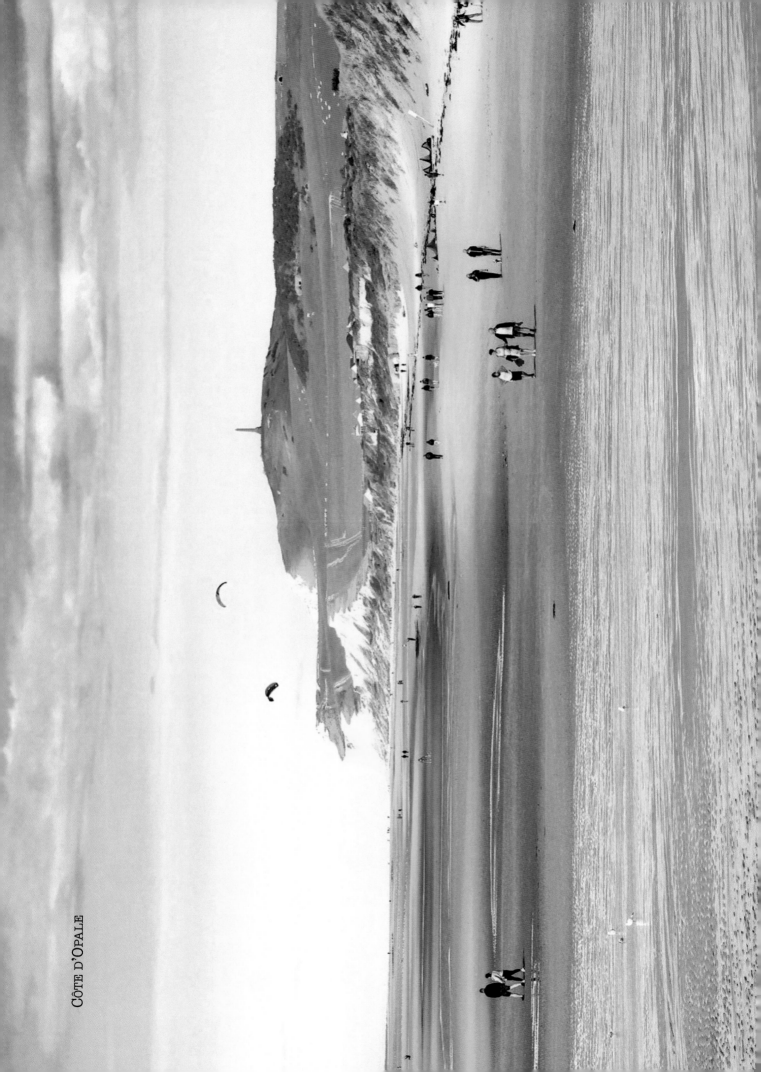

CÔTE D'OPALE

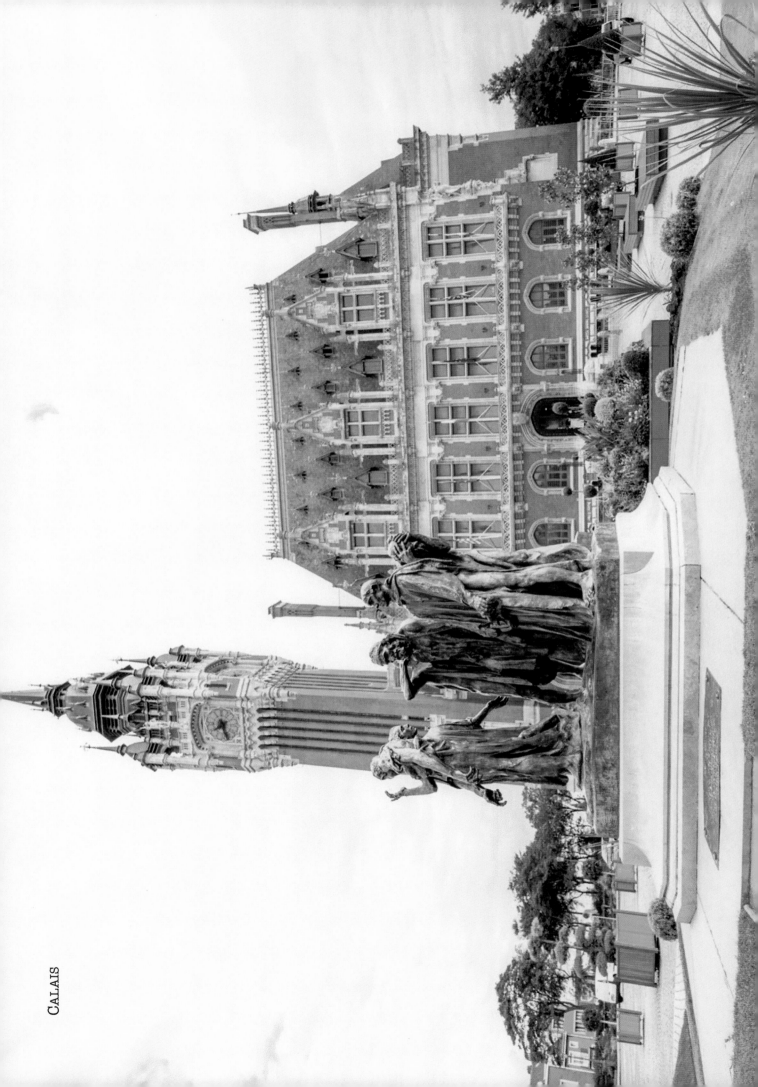

Calais

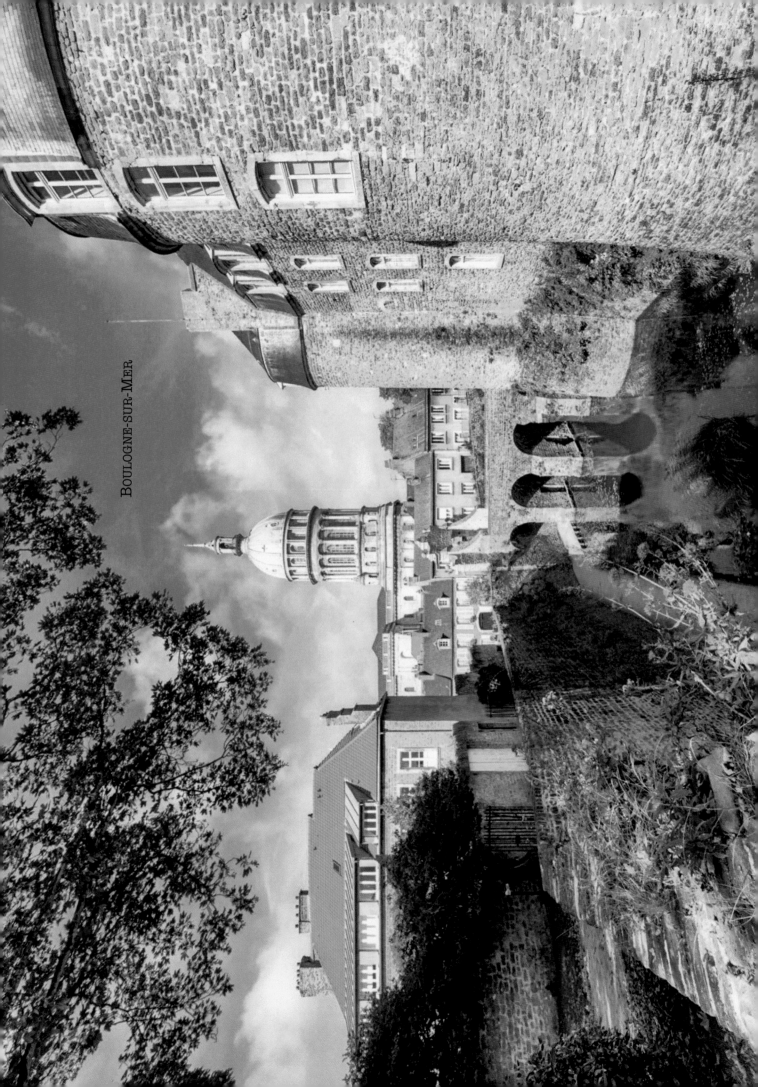

BOULOGNE-SUR-MER

BOULOGNE-SUR-MER

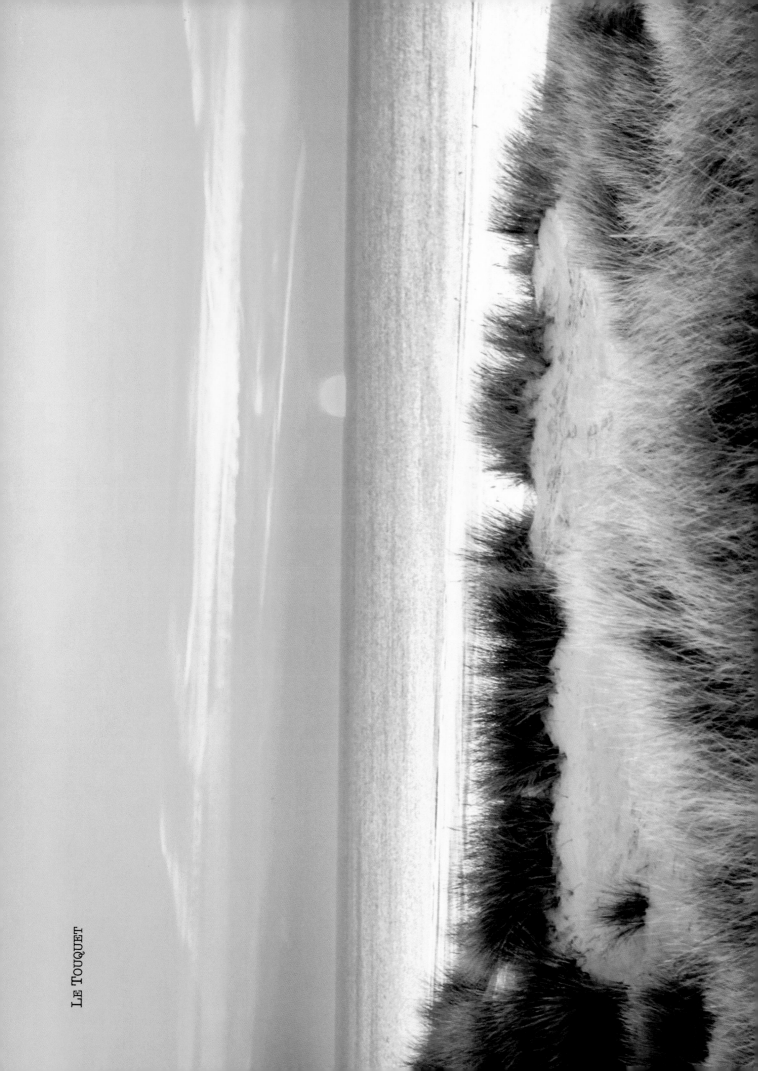

LE TOUQUET

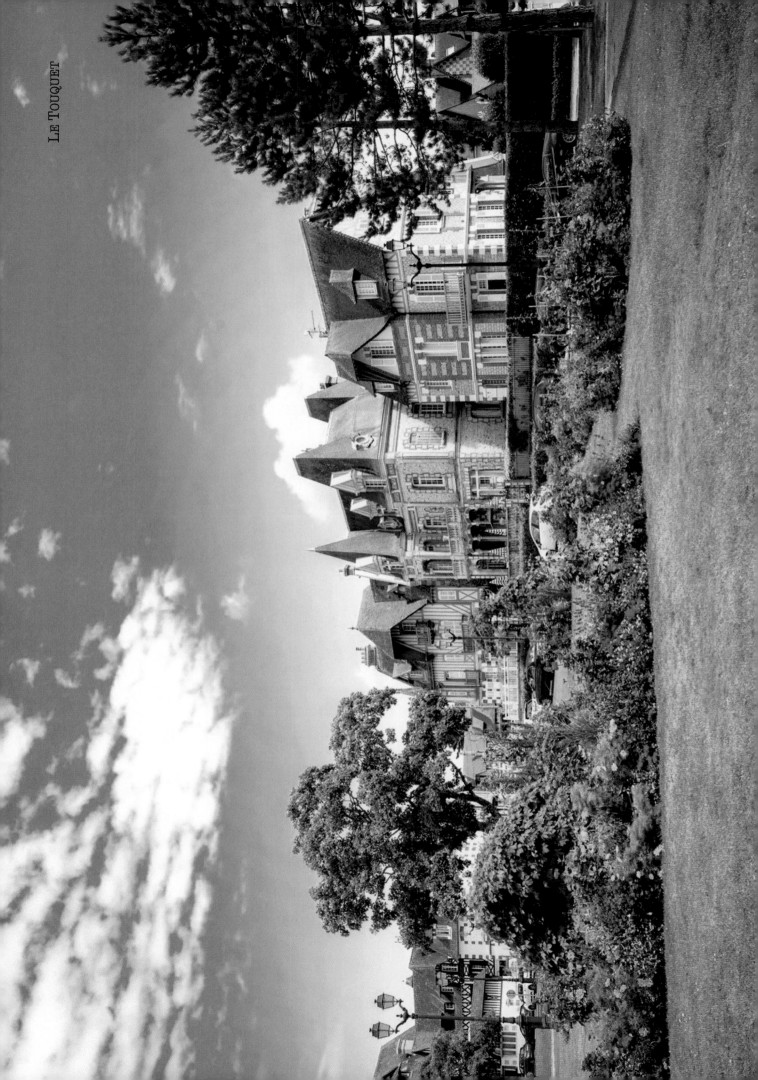

Le Touquet

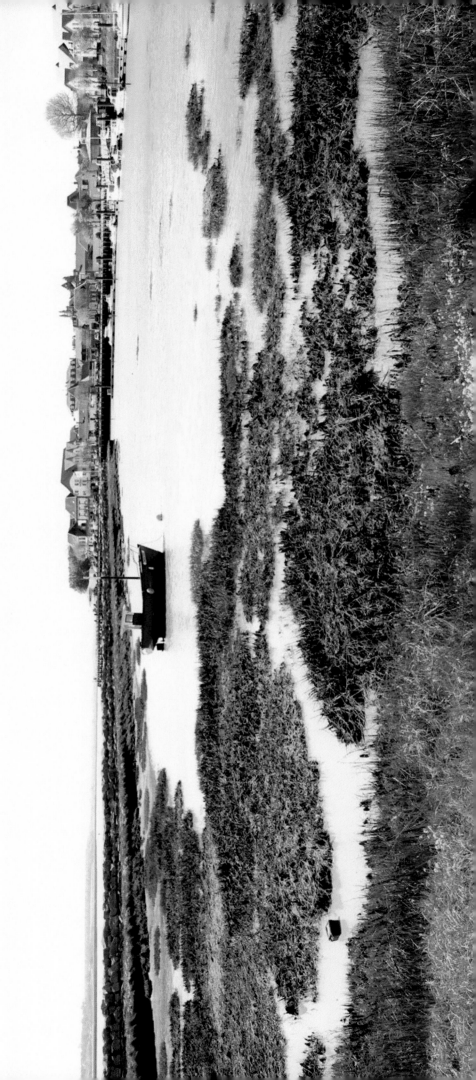

LE CROTOY

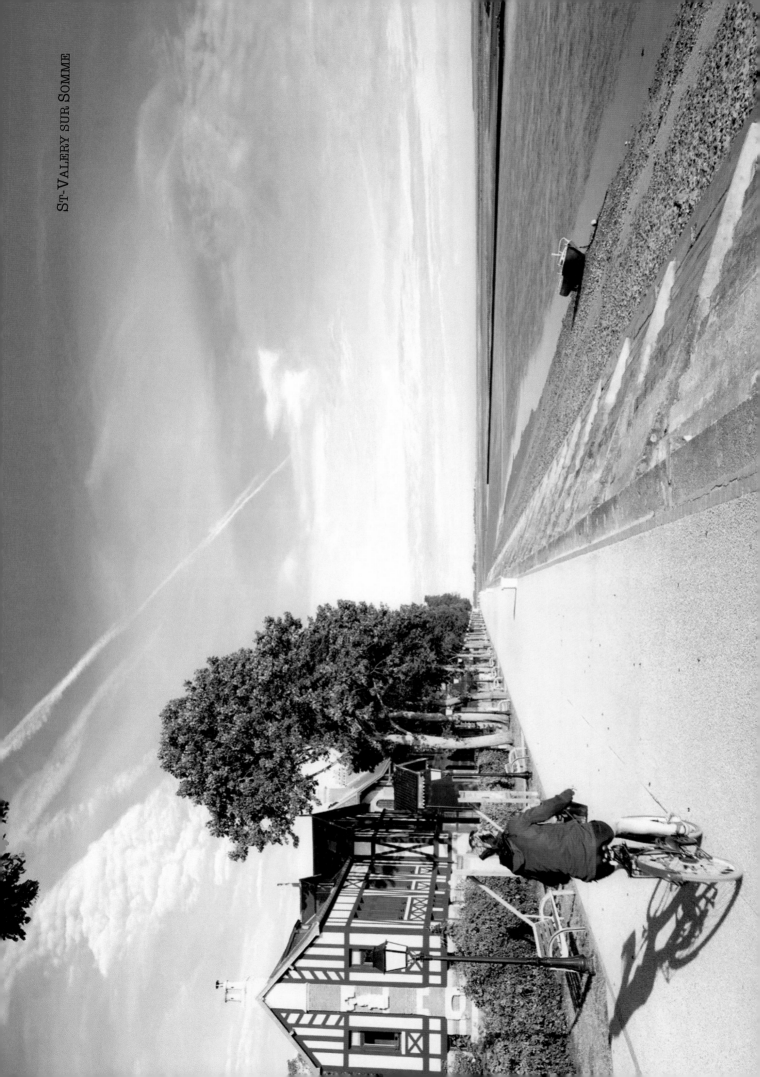

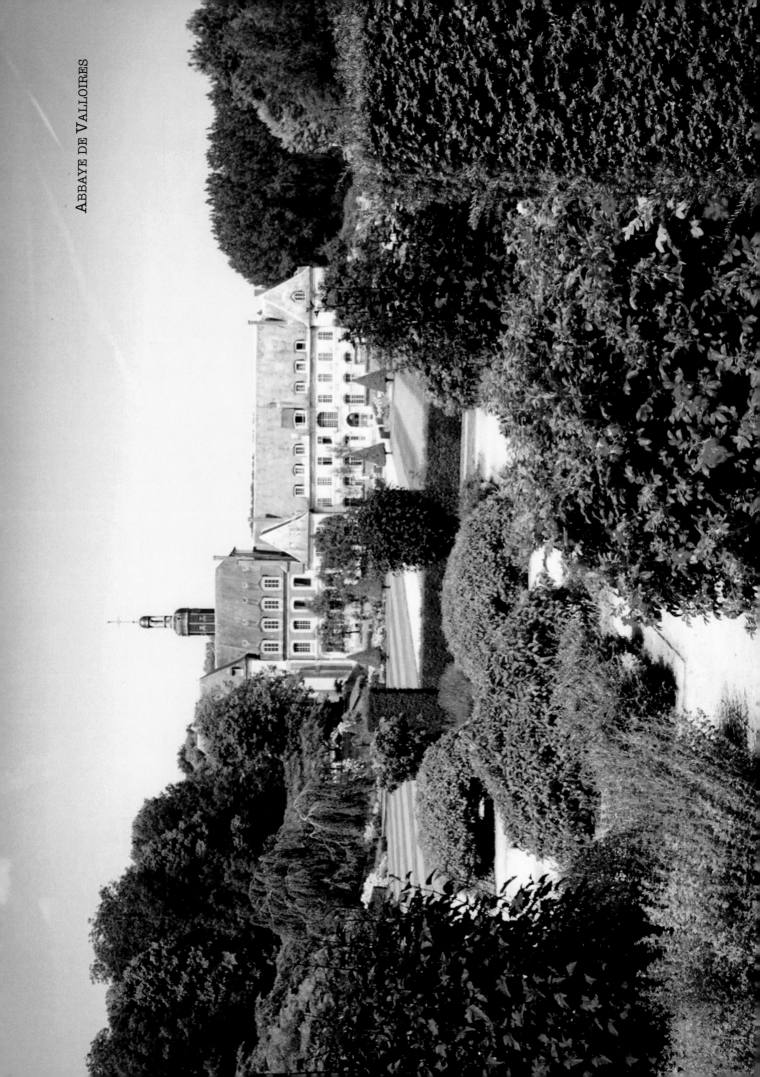

MARQUENTERRE

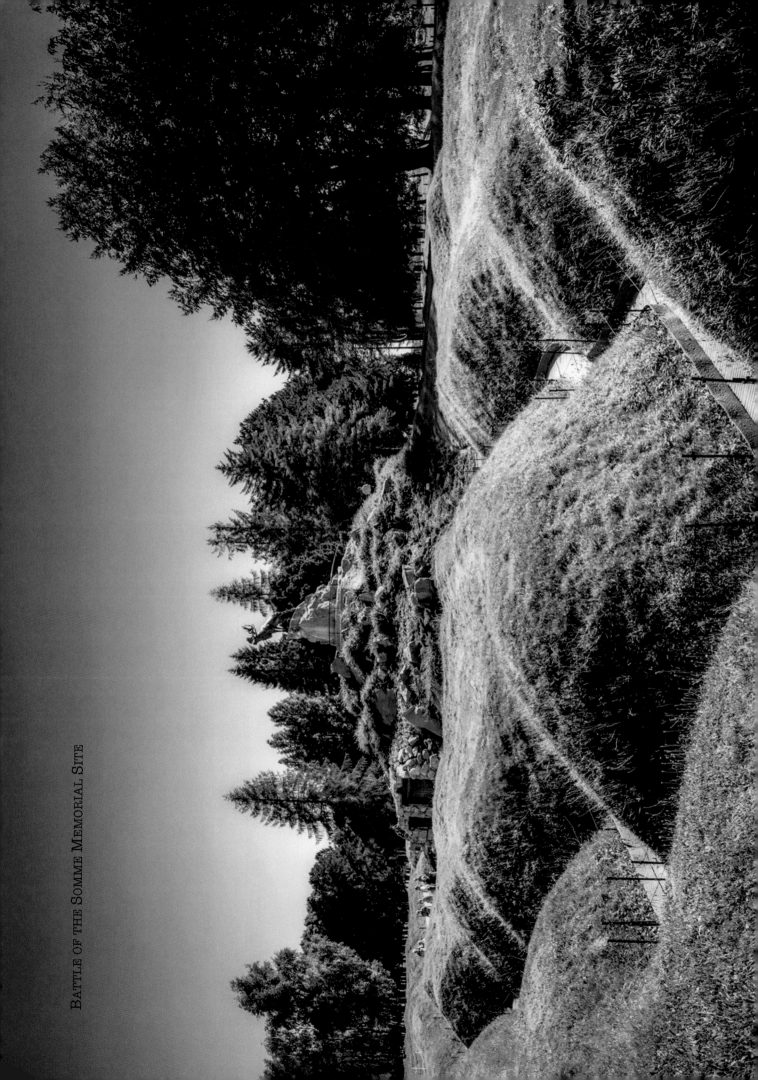

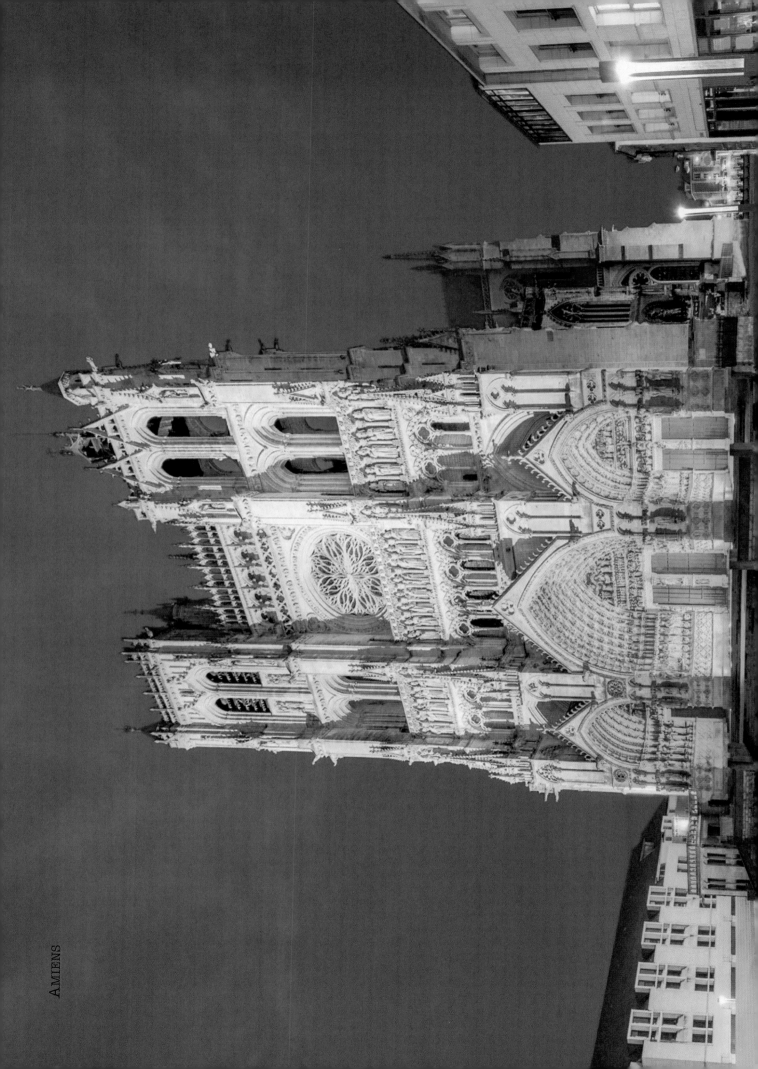

AMIENS

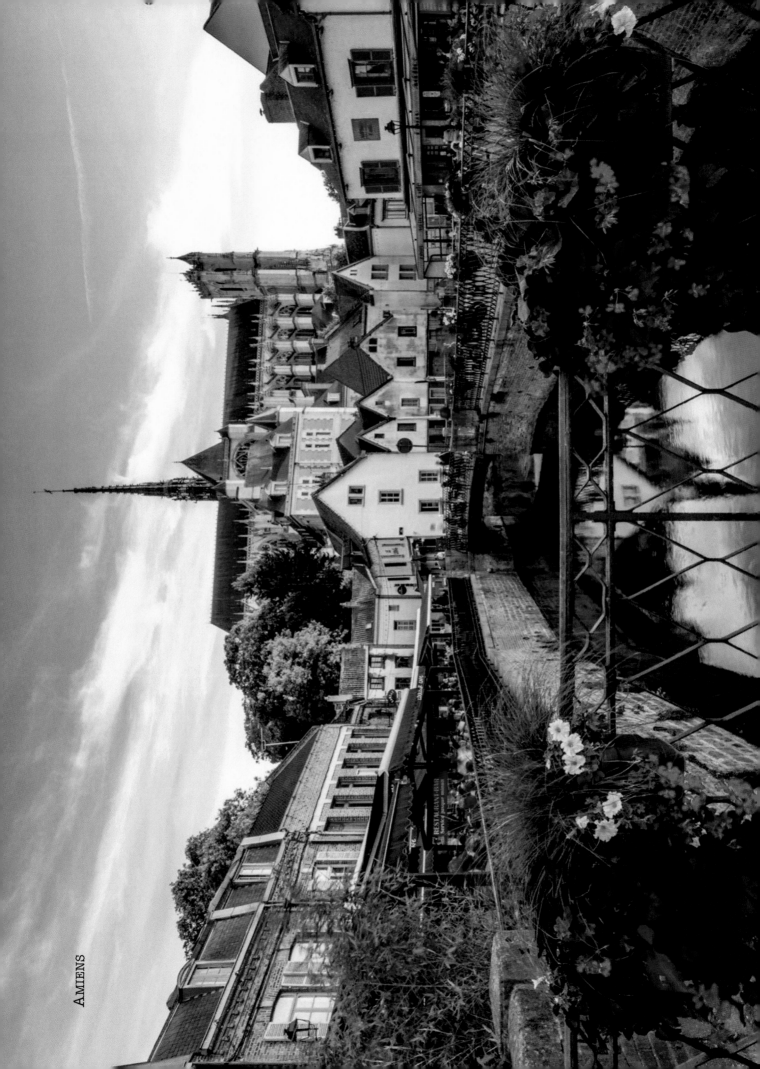

AMIENS

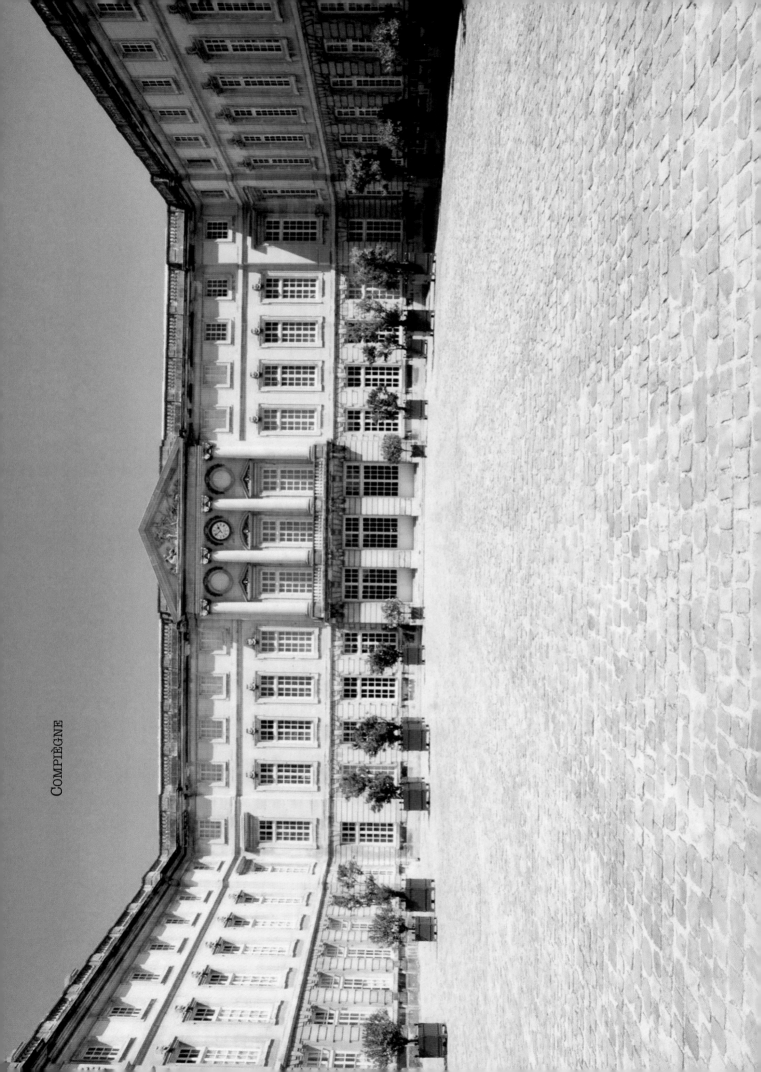

COMPIÈGNE

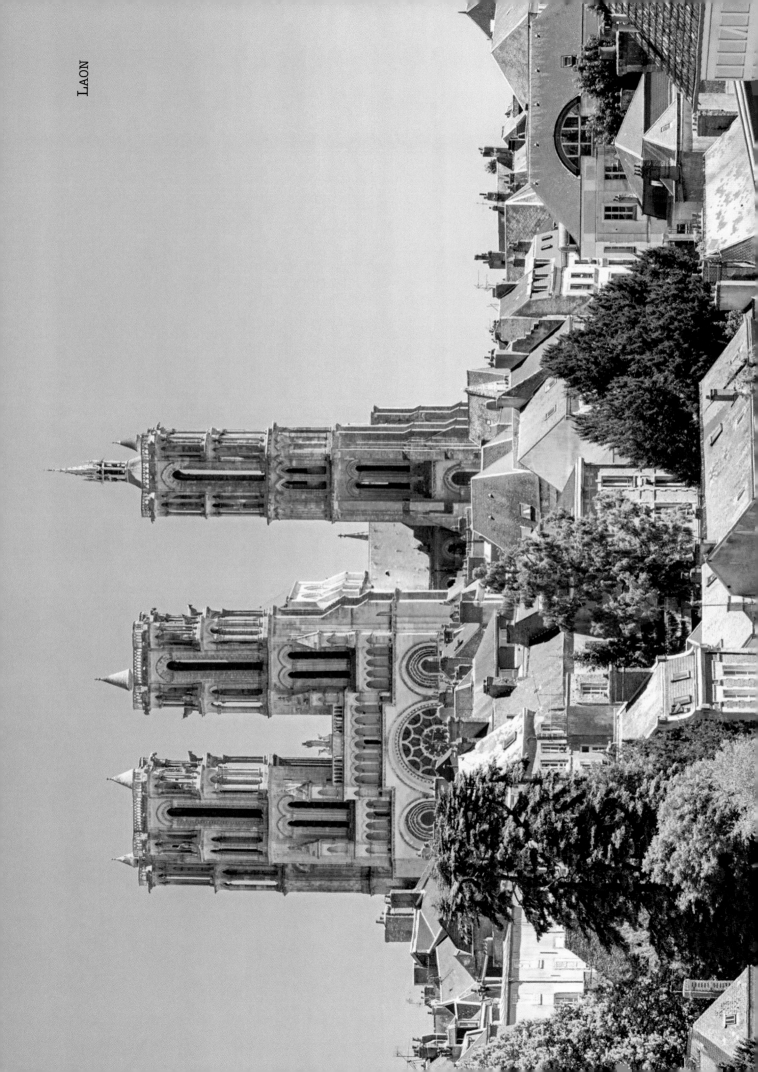

LAON

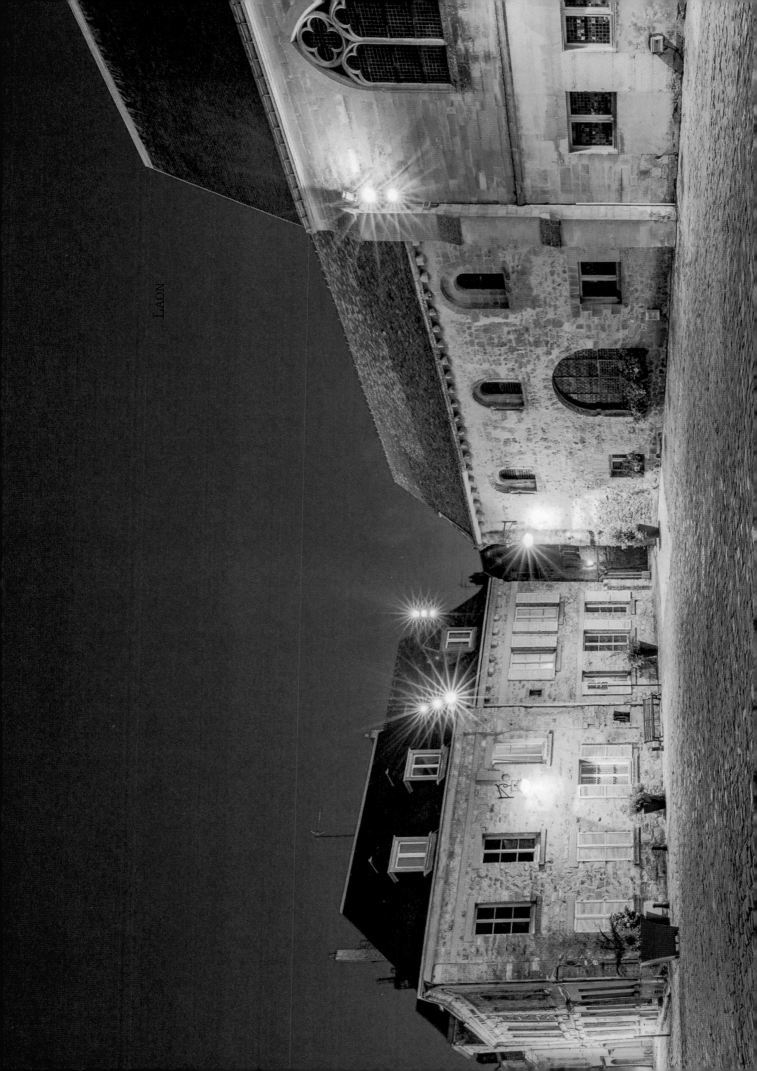

LAON

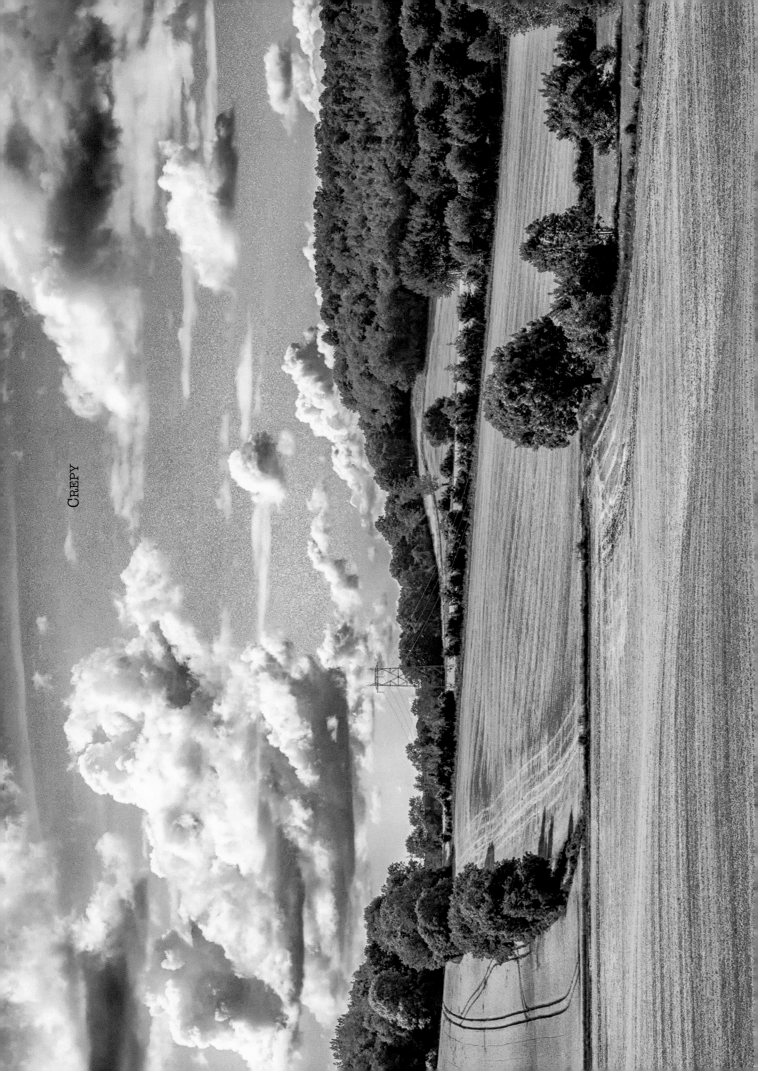

CREPY

NORMANDY

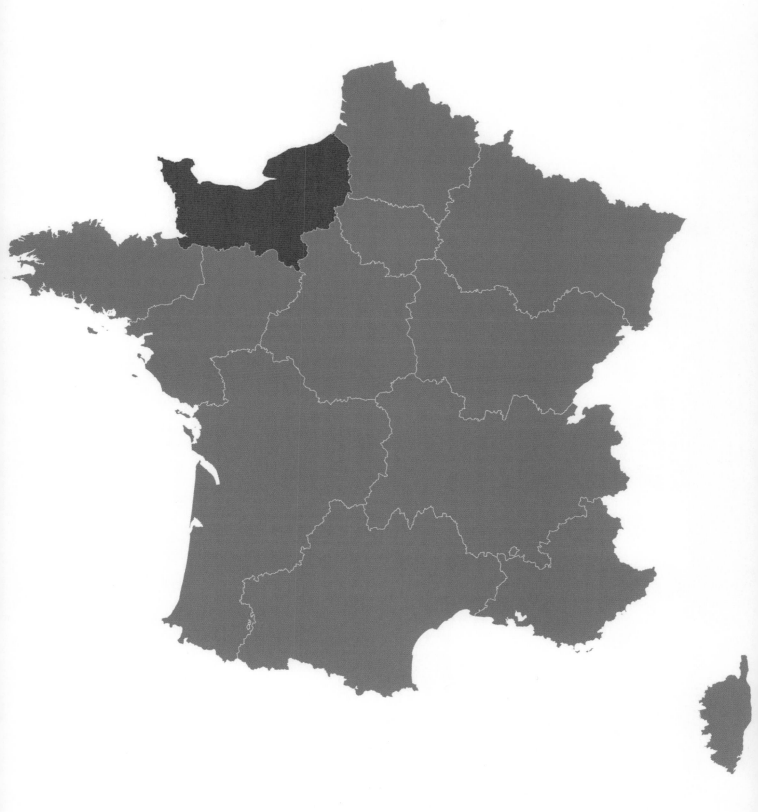

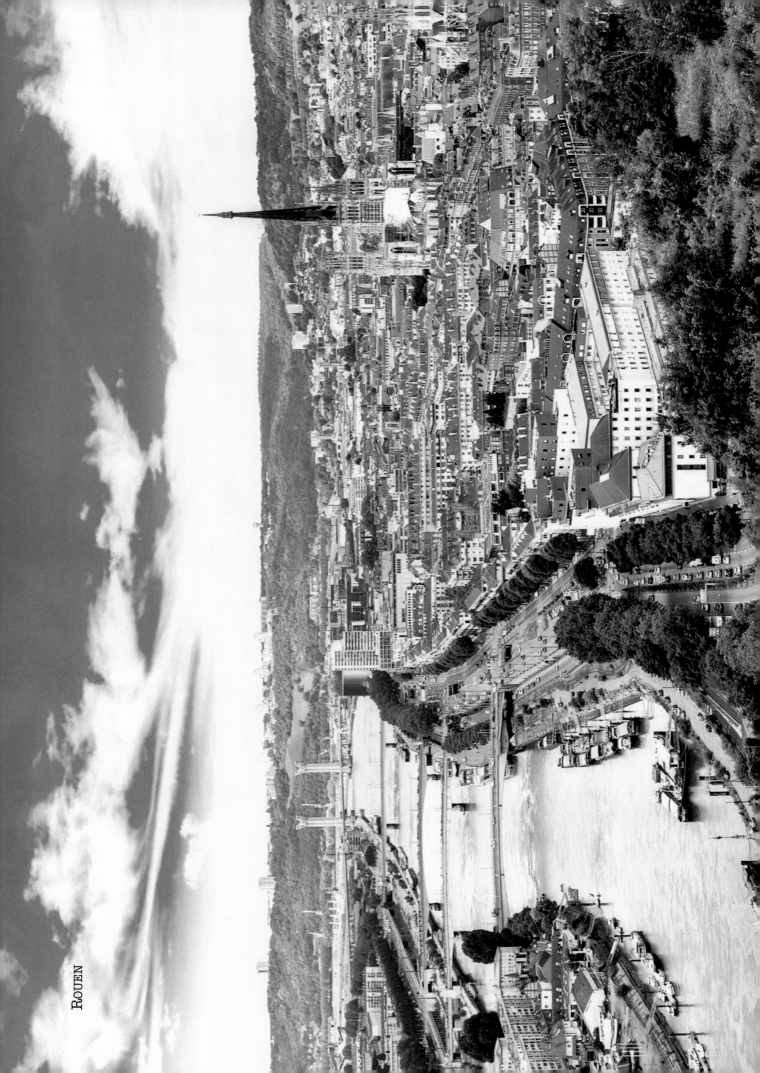

ROUEN

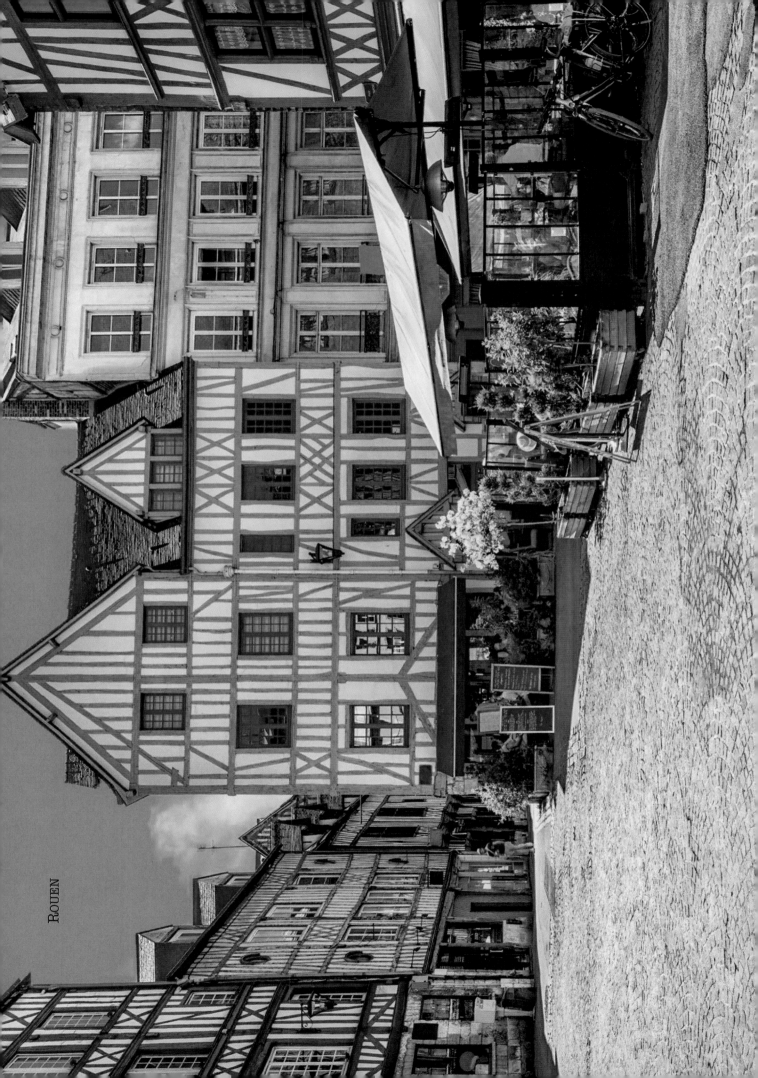

ROUEN

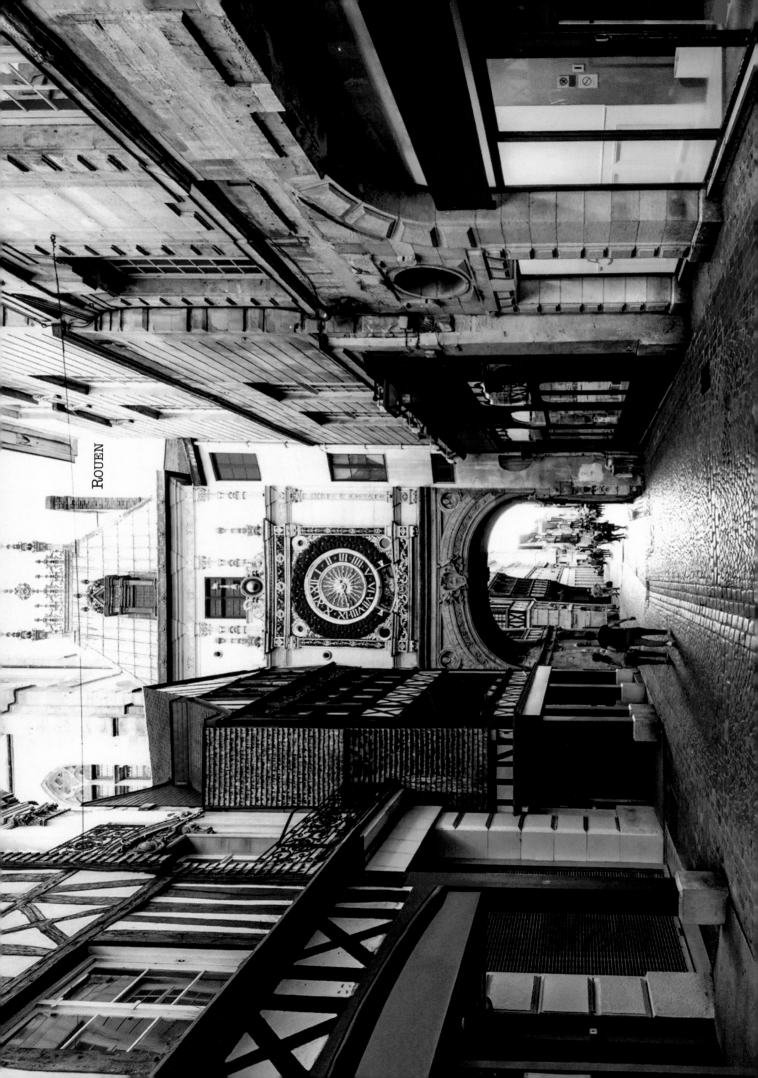

ROUEN

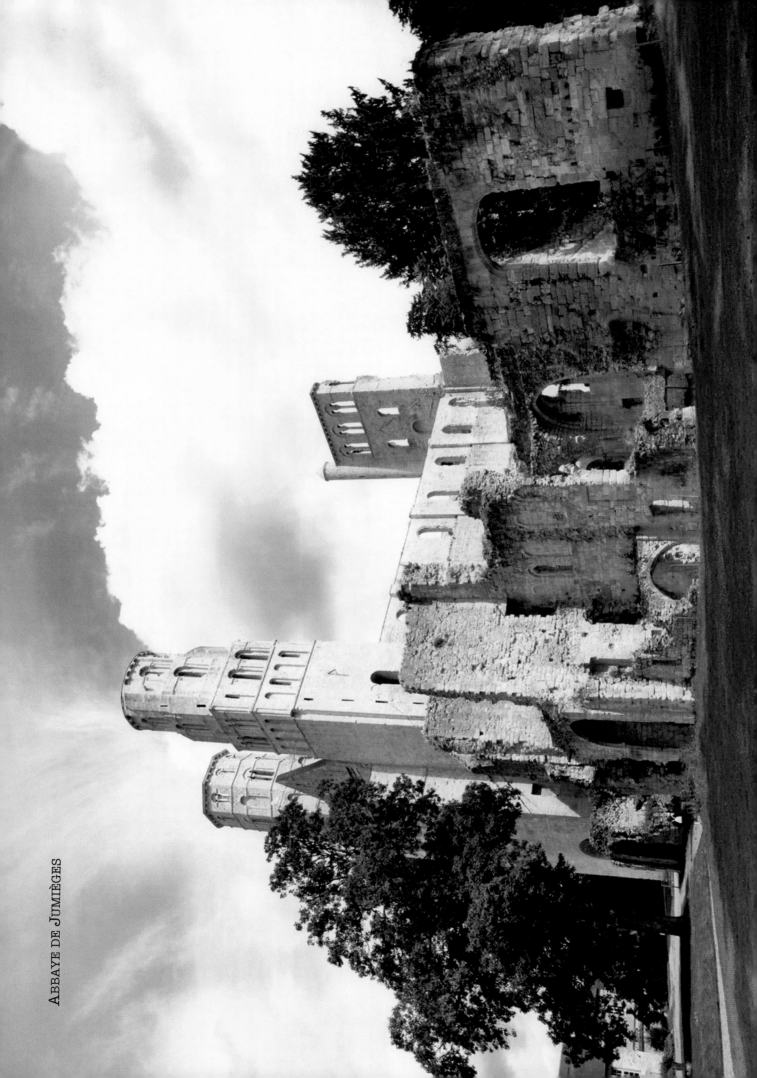

ABBAYE DE JUMIÈGES

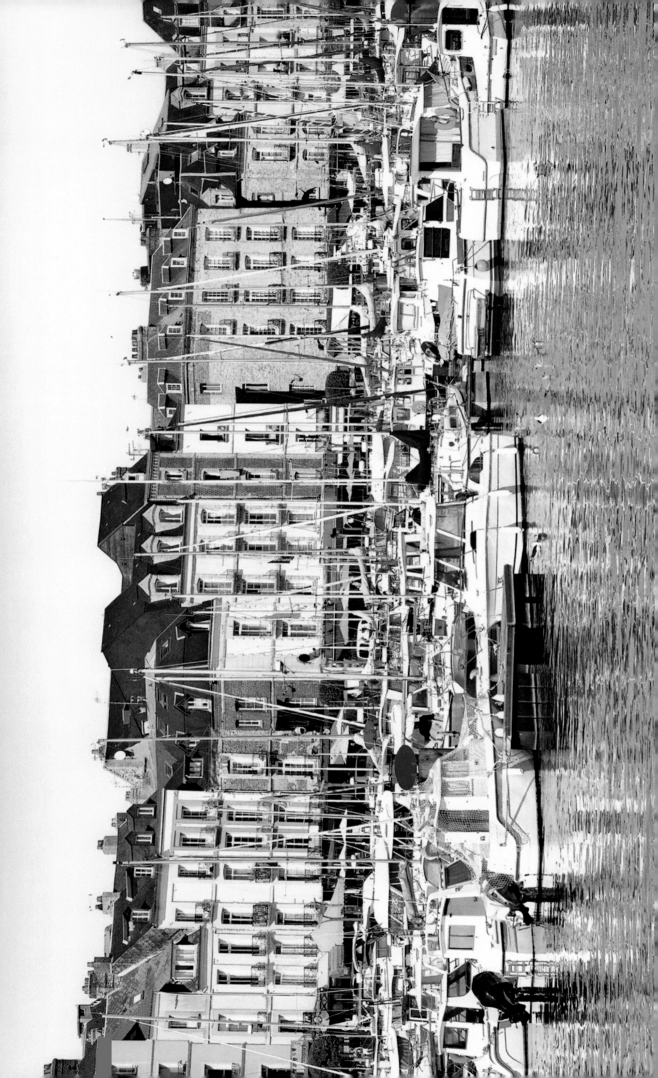

DIEPPE

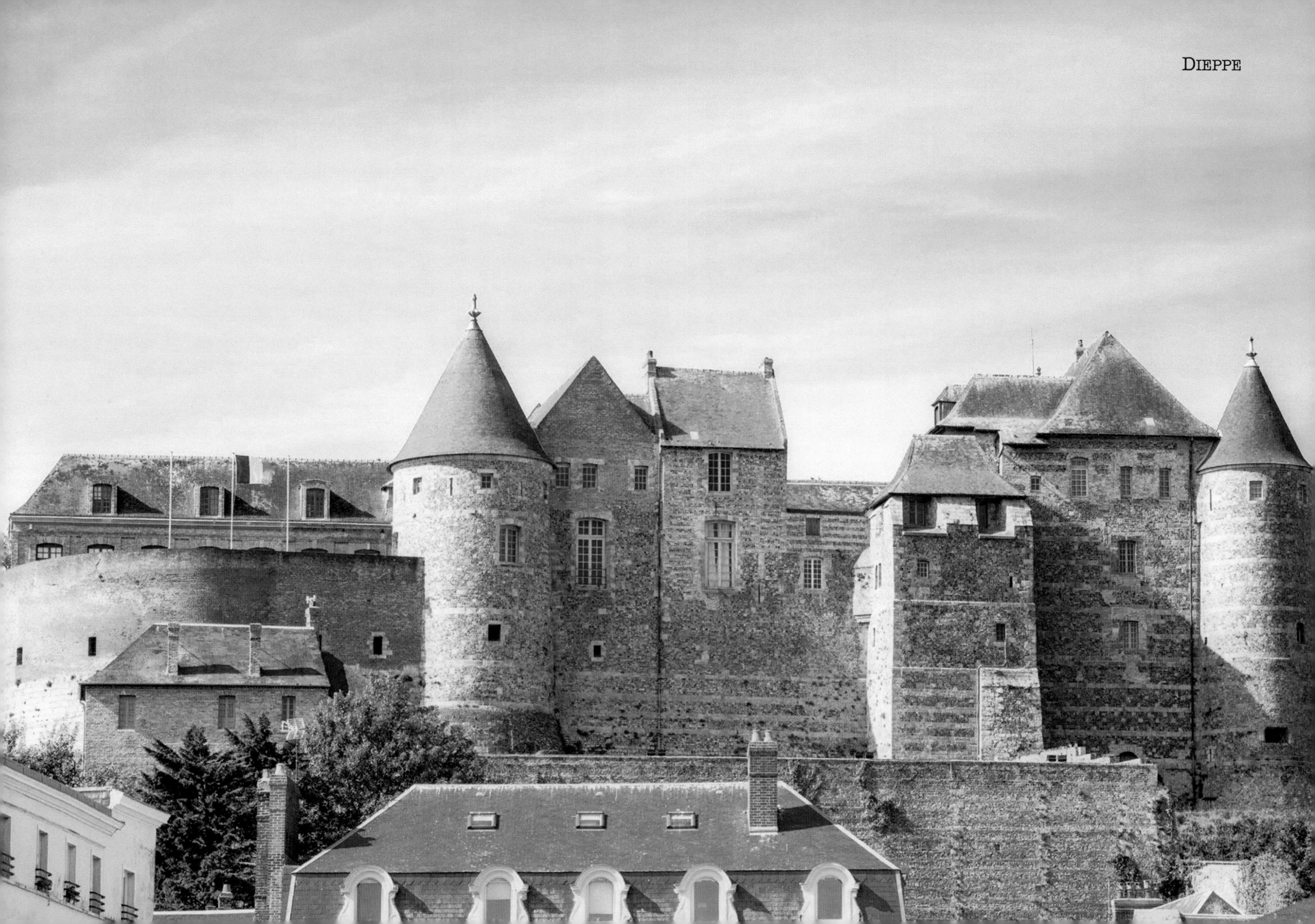

DIEPPE

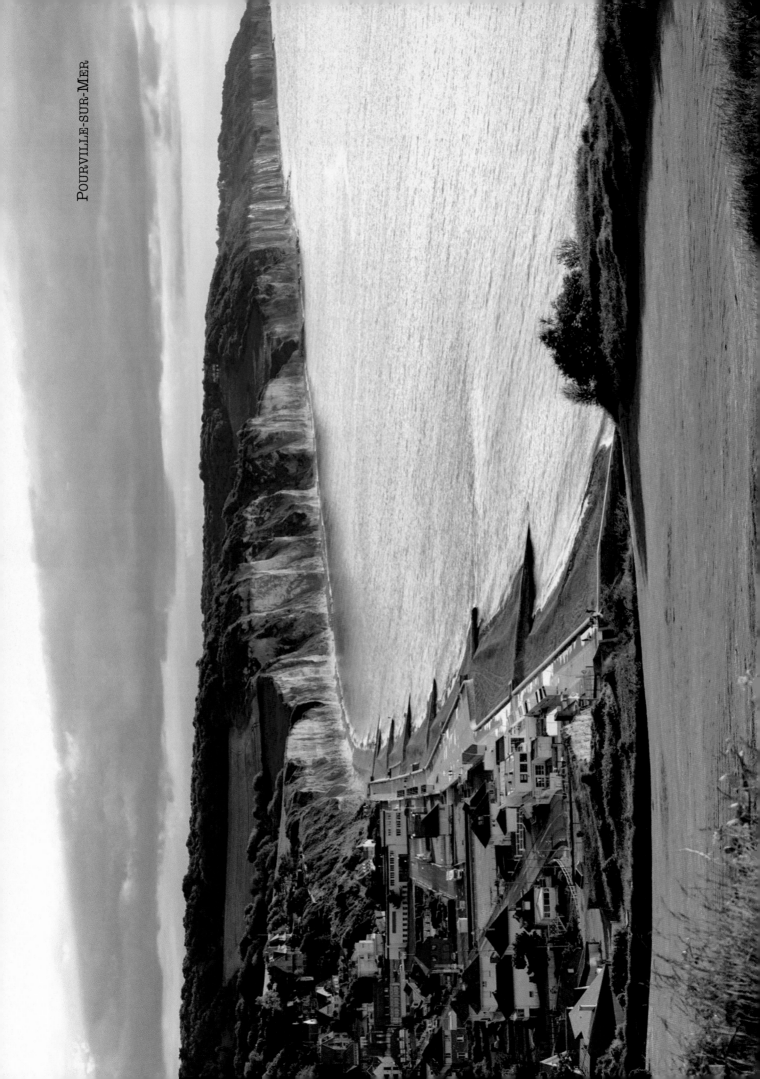

POURVILLE-SUR-MER

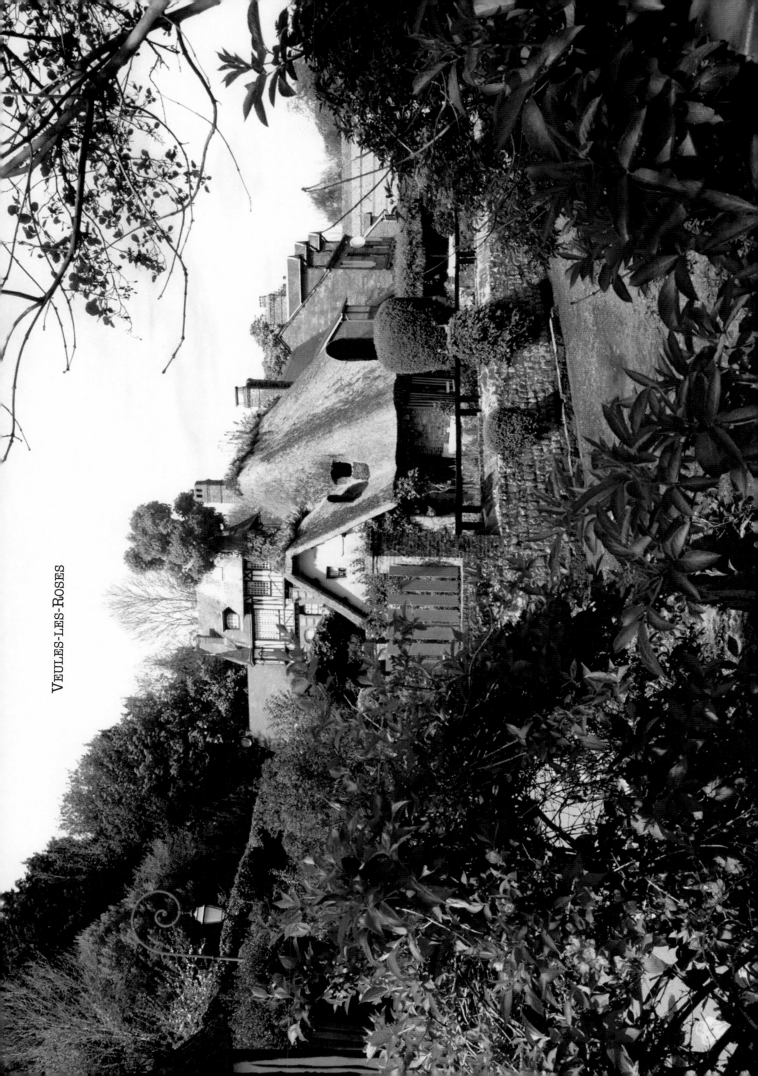

VEULES-LES-ROSES

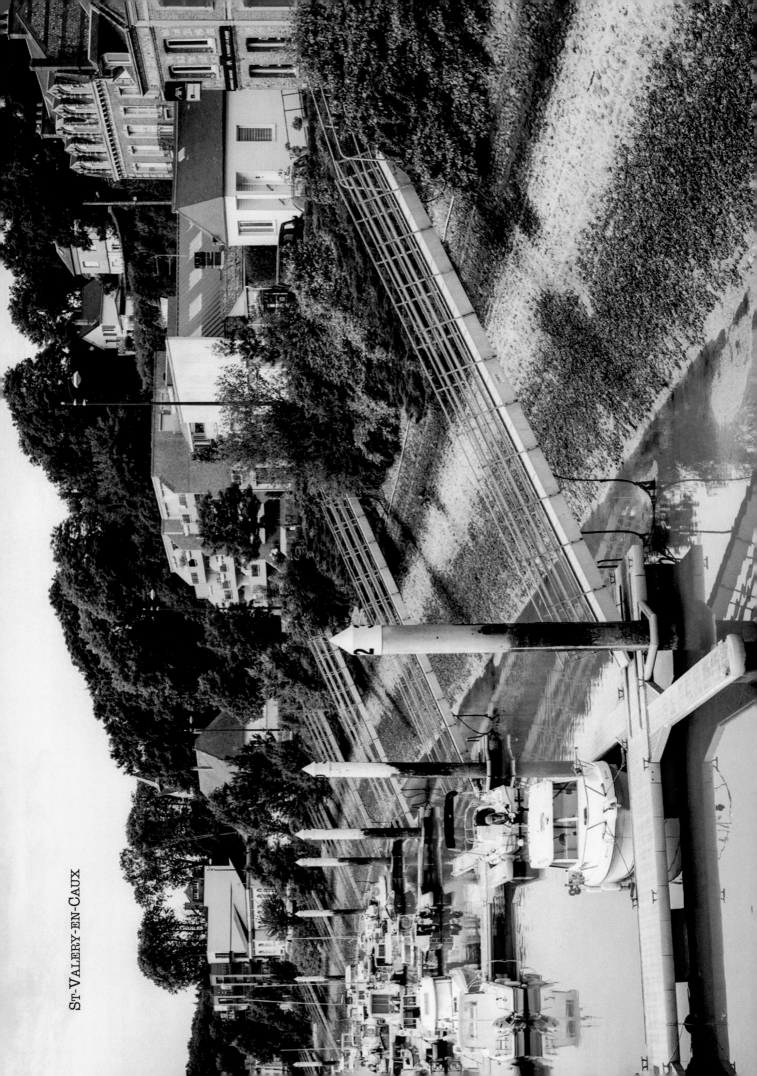

St-Valery-en-Caux

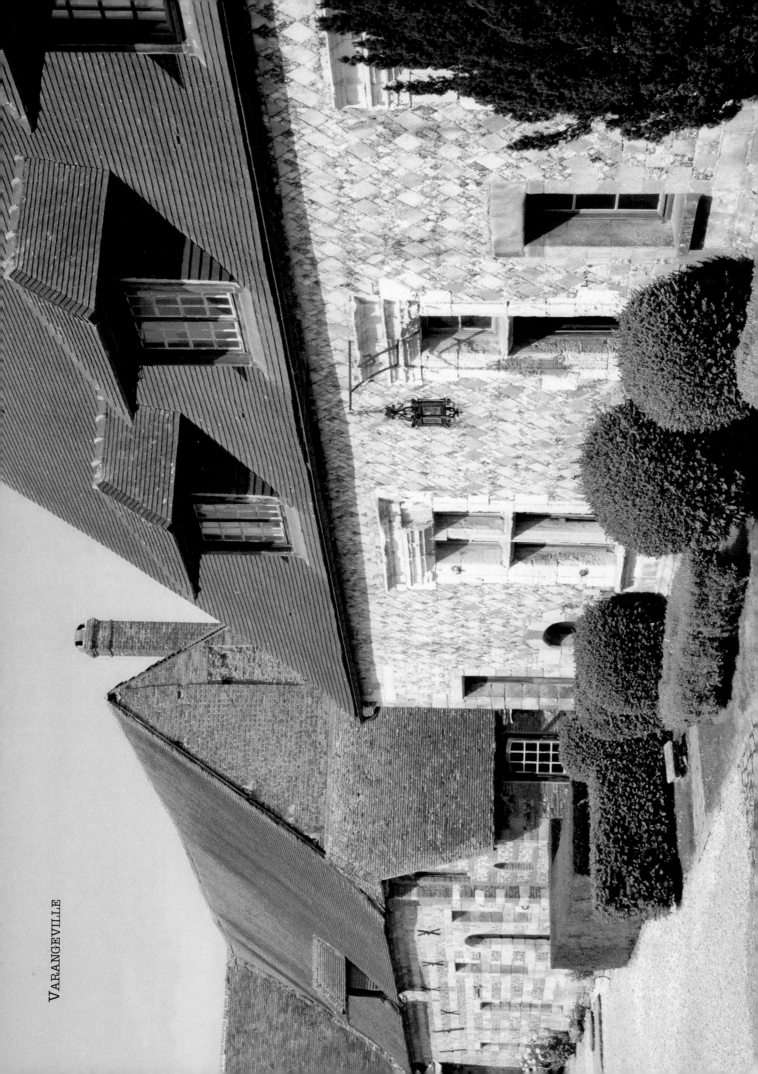

VARANGEVILLE

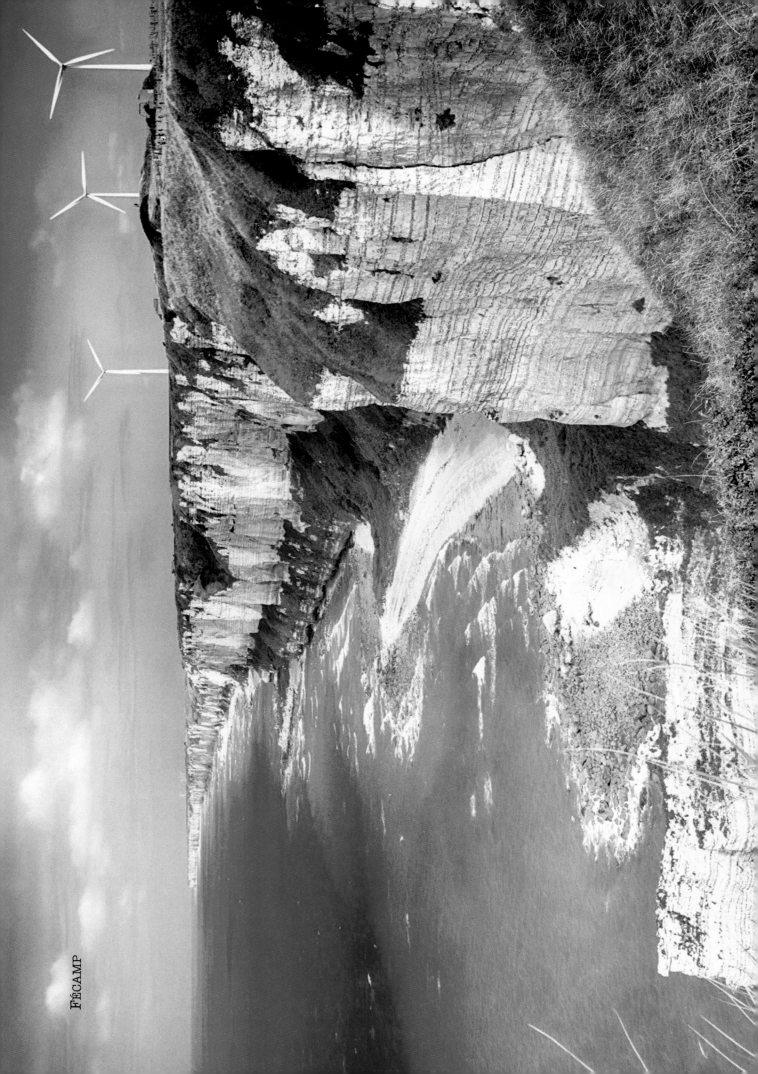

FÉCAMP

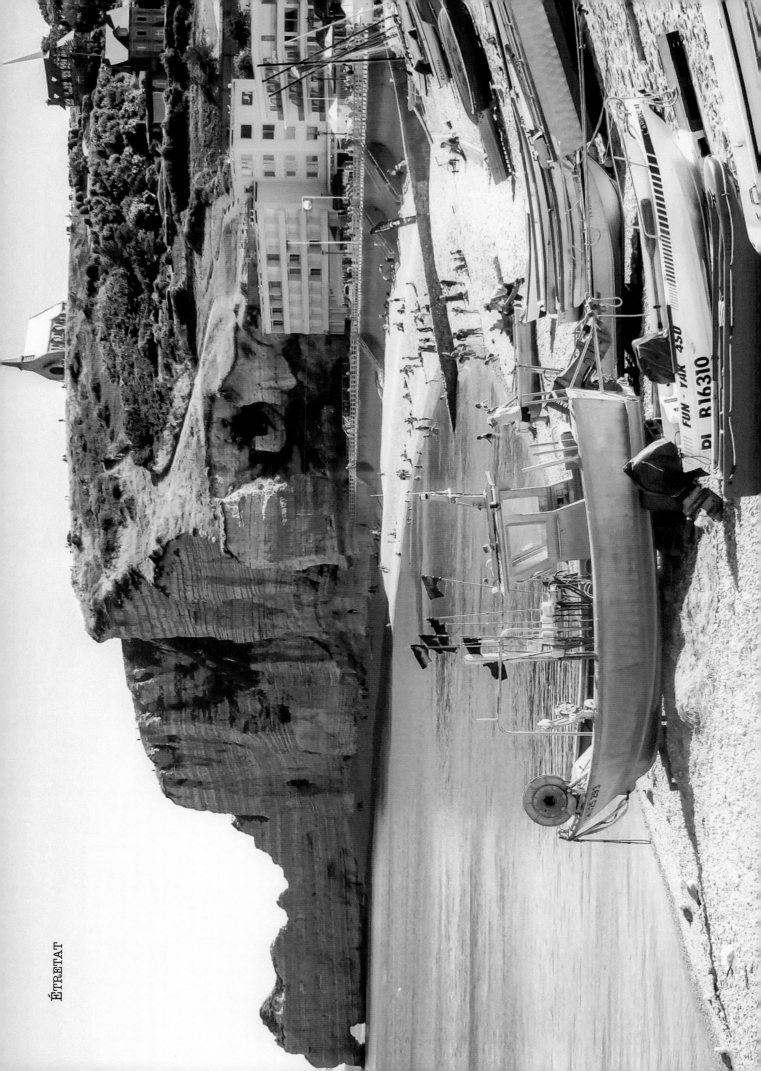

ÉTRETAT

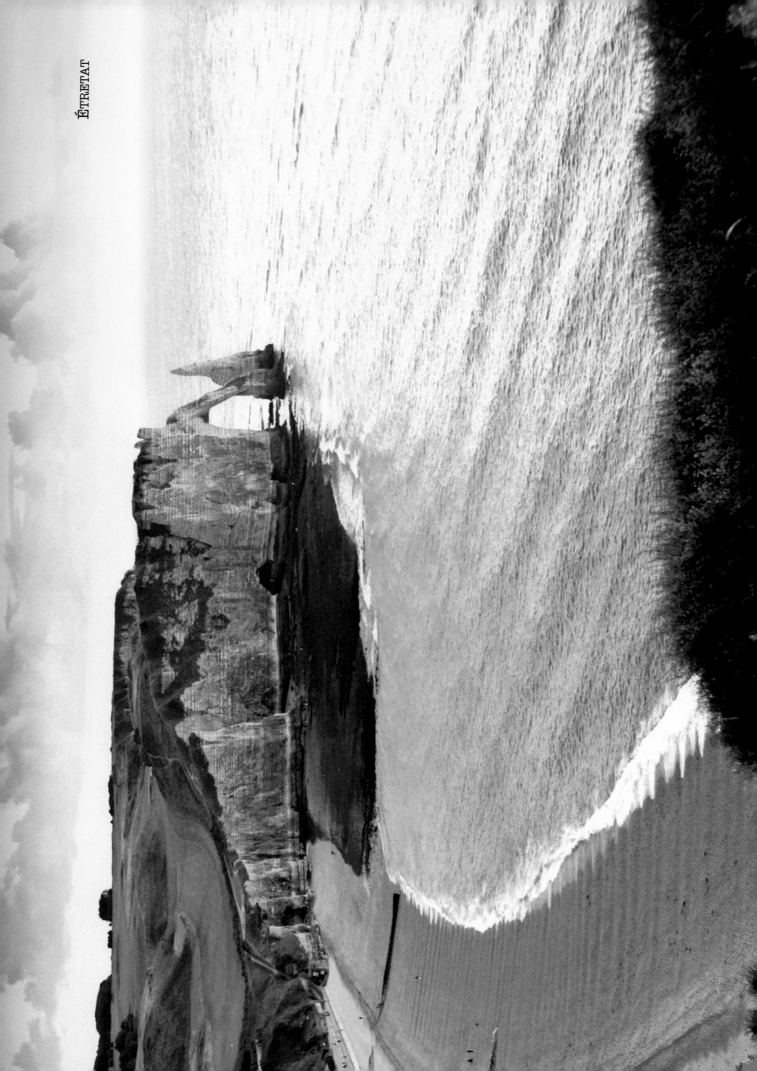

ÉTRETAT

LE HAVRE

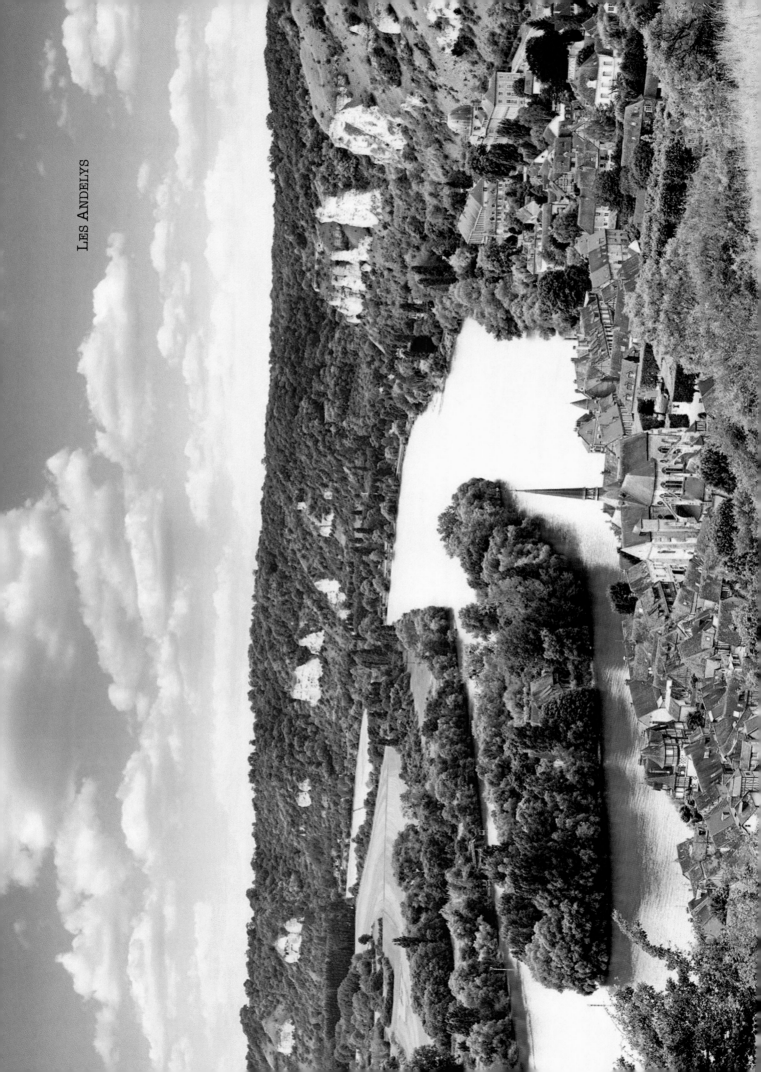

LES ANDELYS

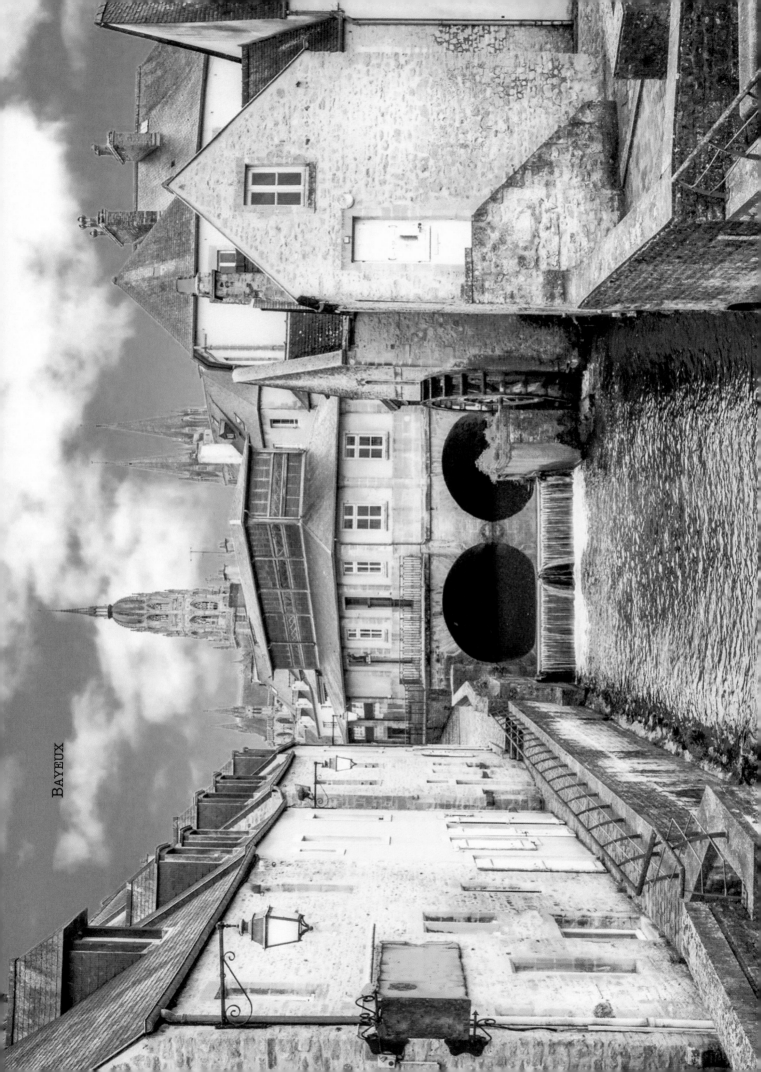

BAYEUX

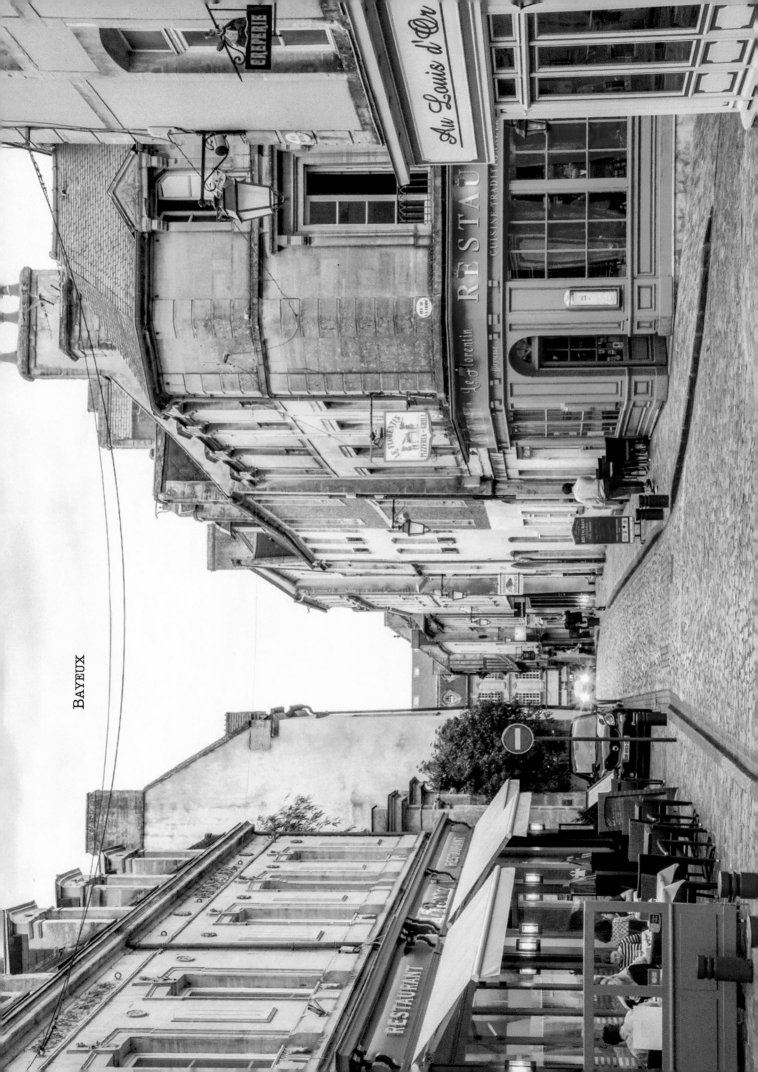

BAYEUX

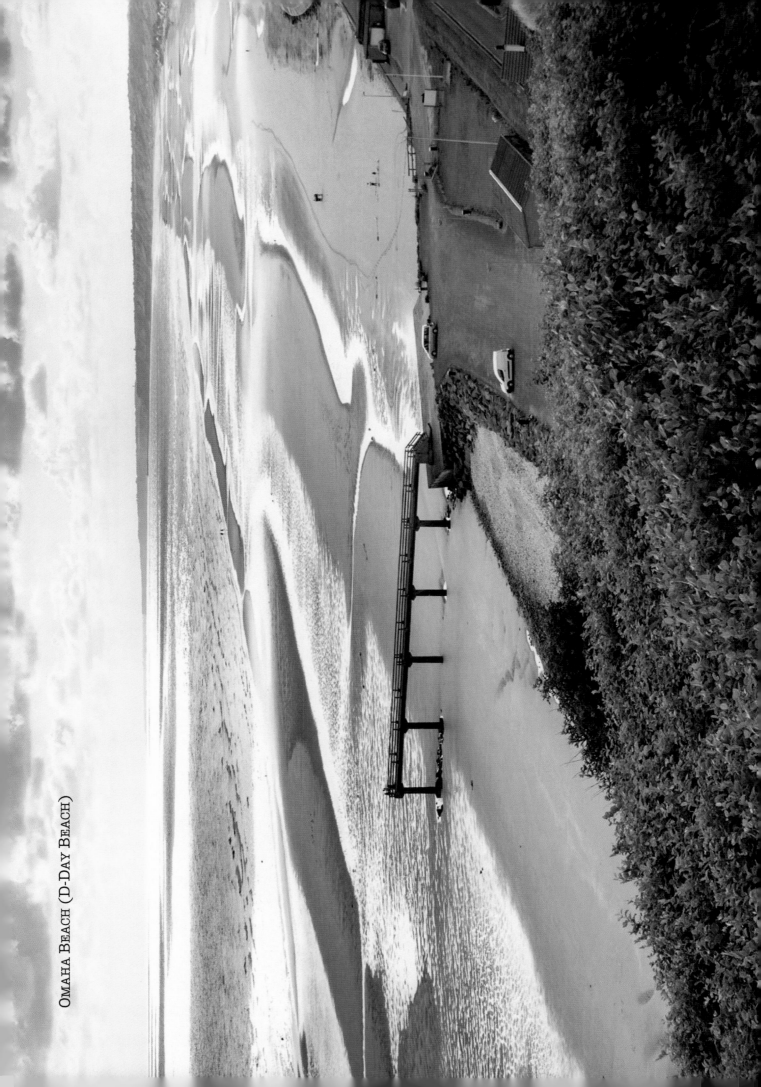

Omaha Beach (D-Day Beach)

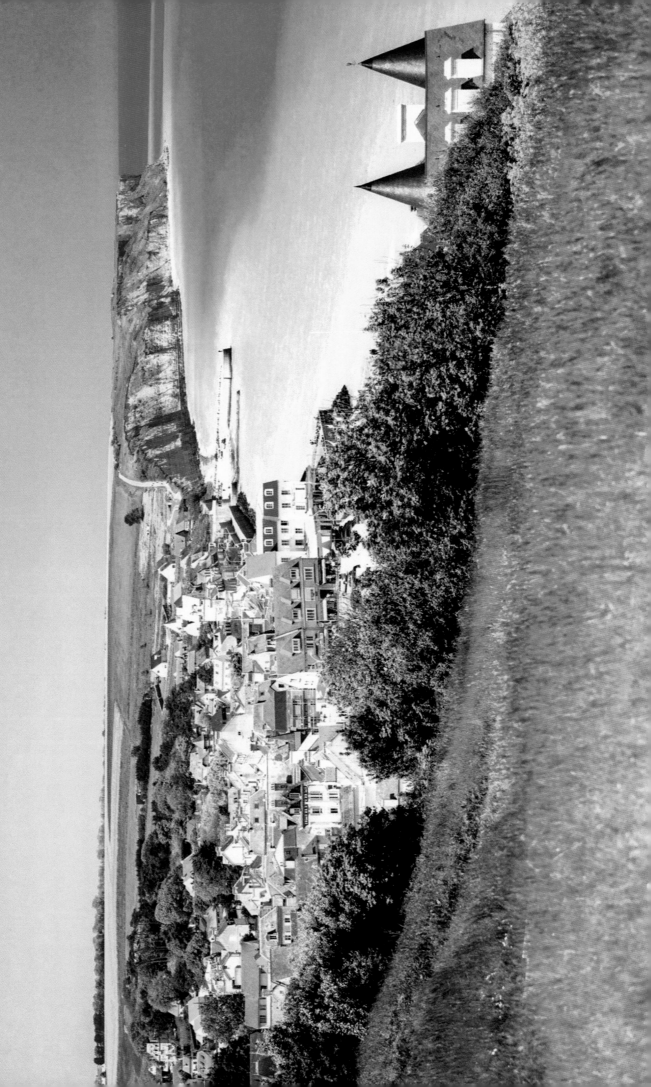

ARROMANCHES-LES-BAINS

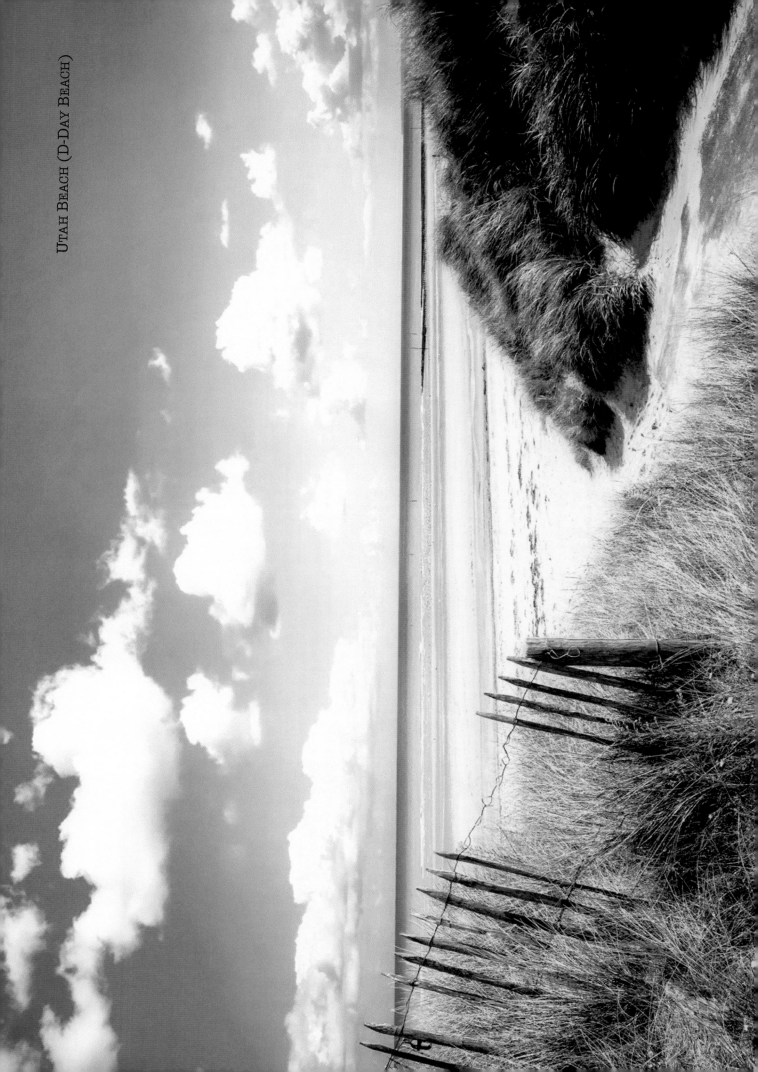

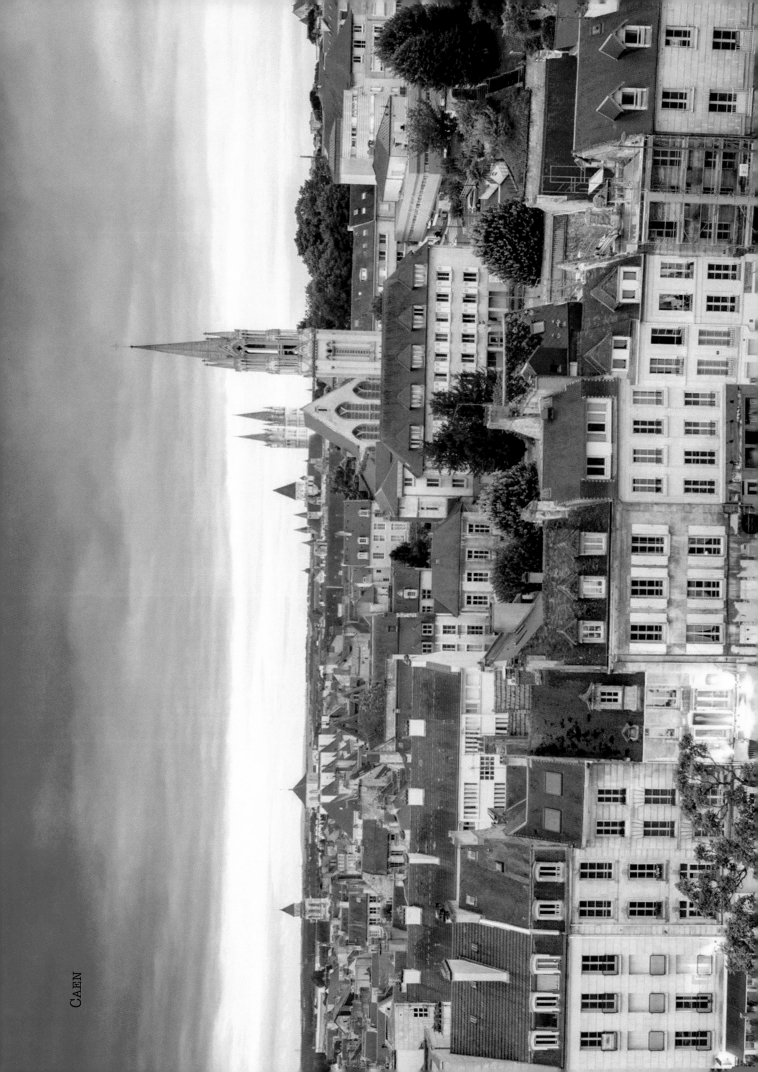

CAEN

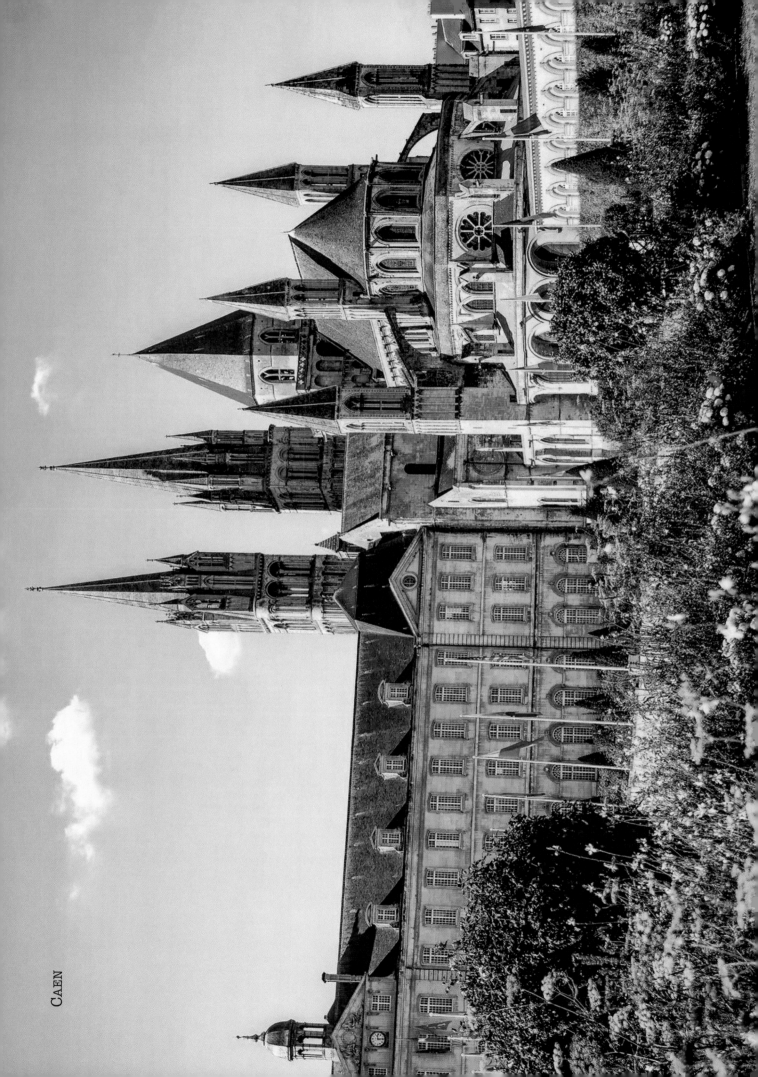

CAEN

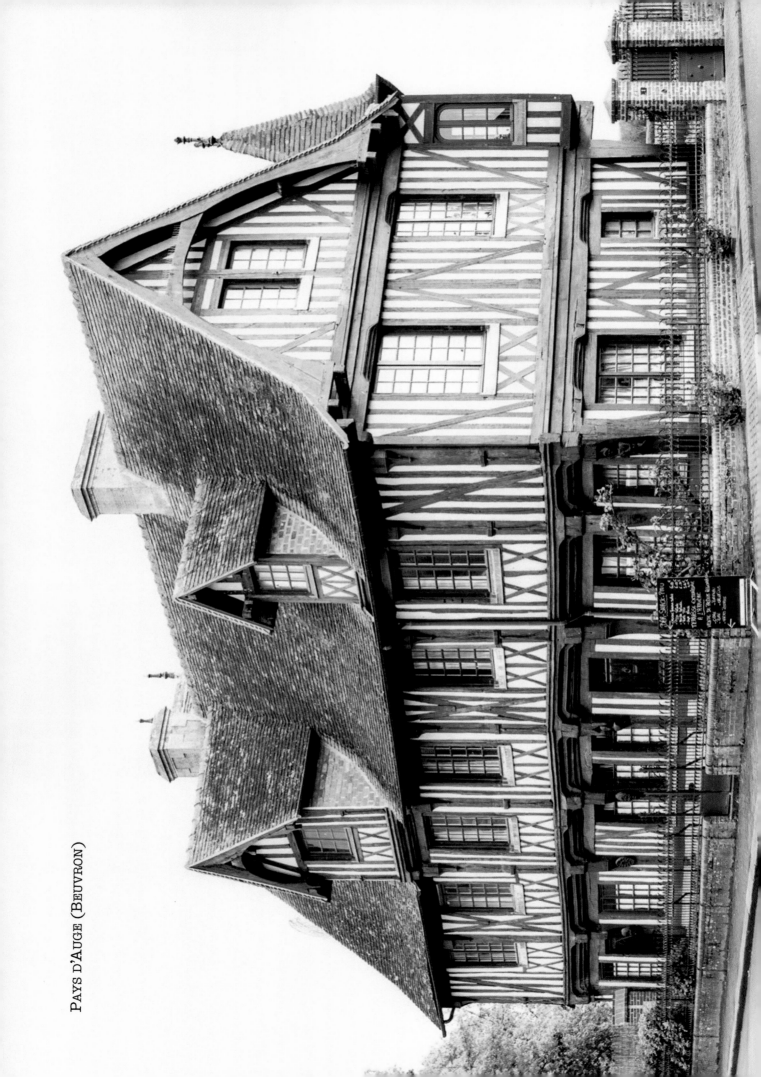

PAYS D'AUGE (BEUVRON)

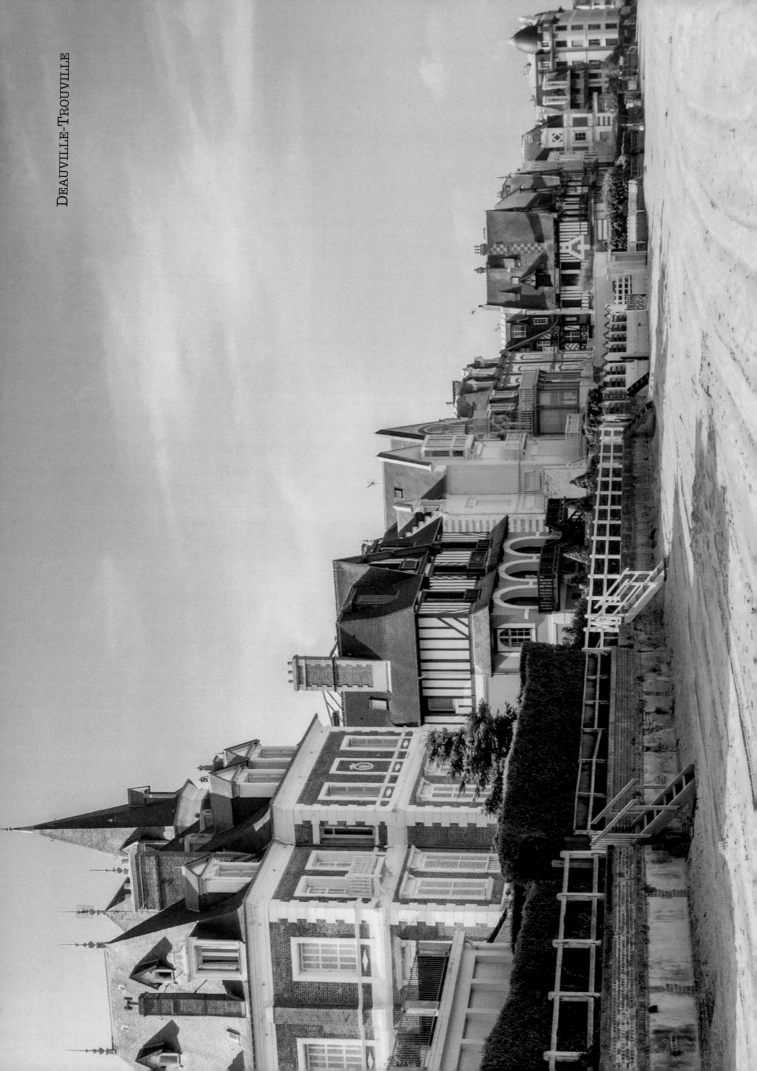

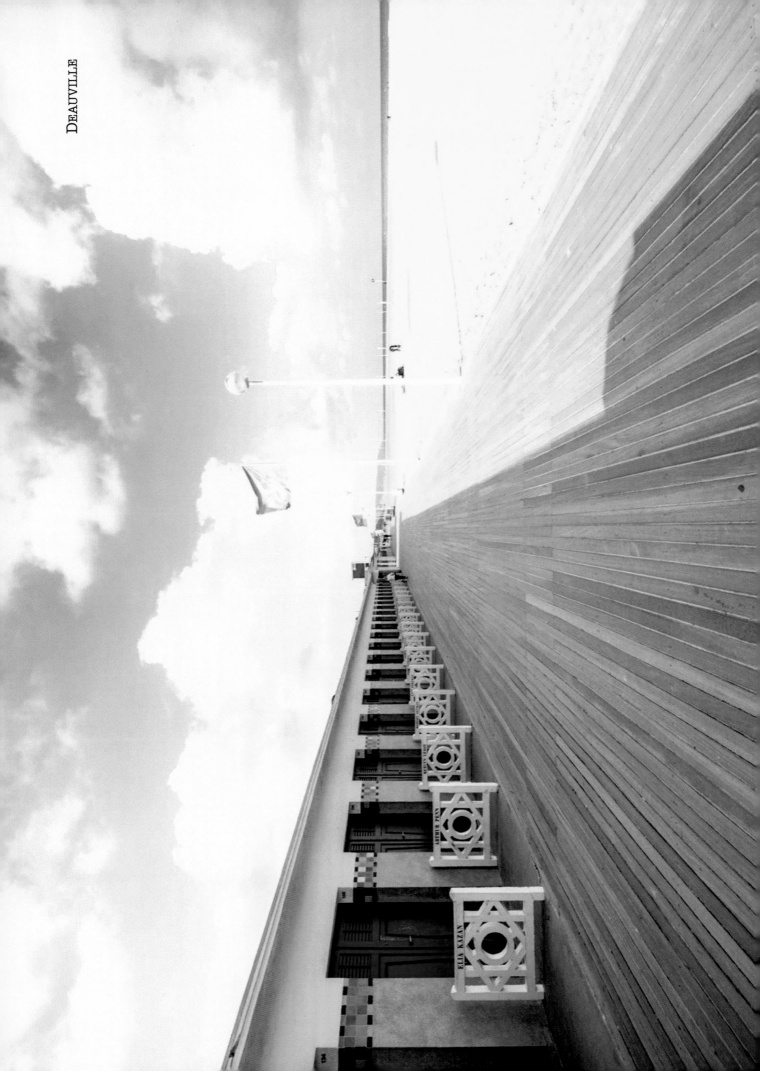

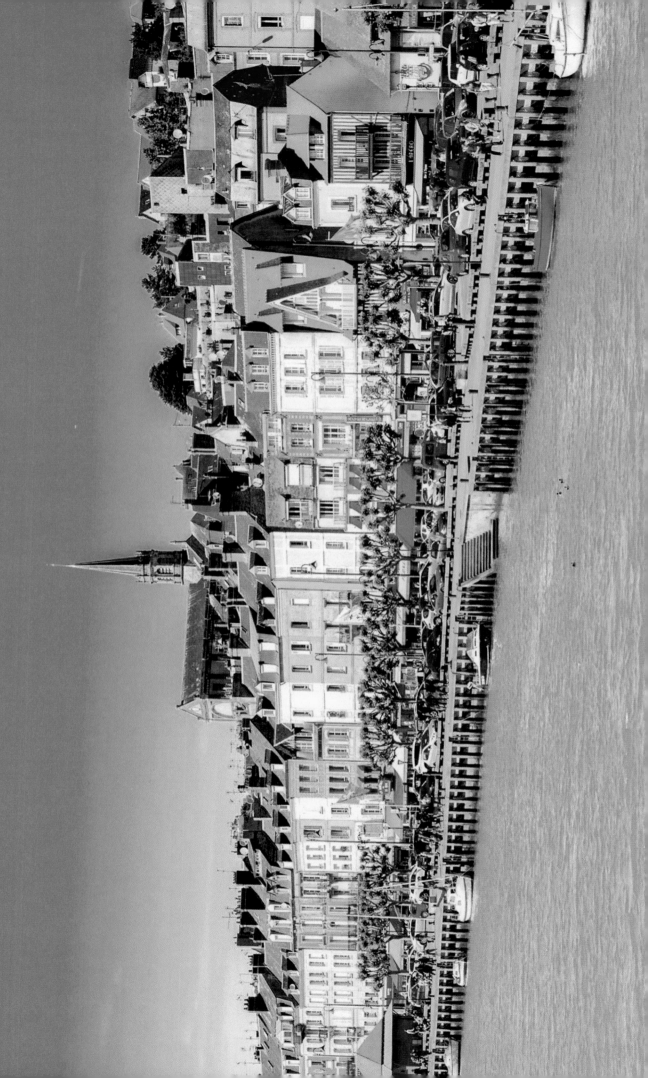

TROUVILLE

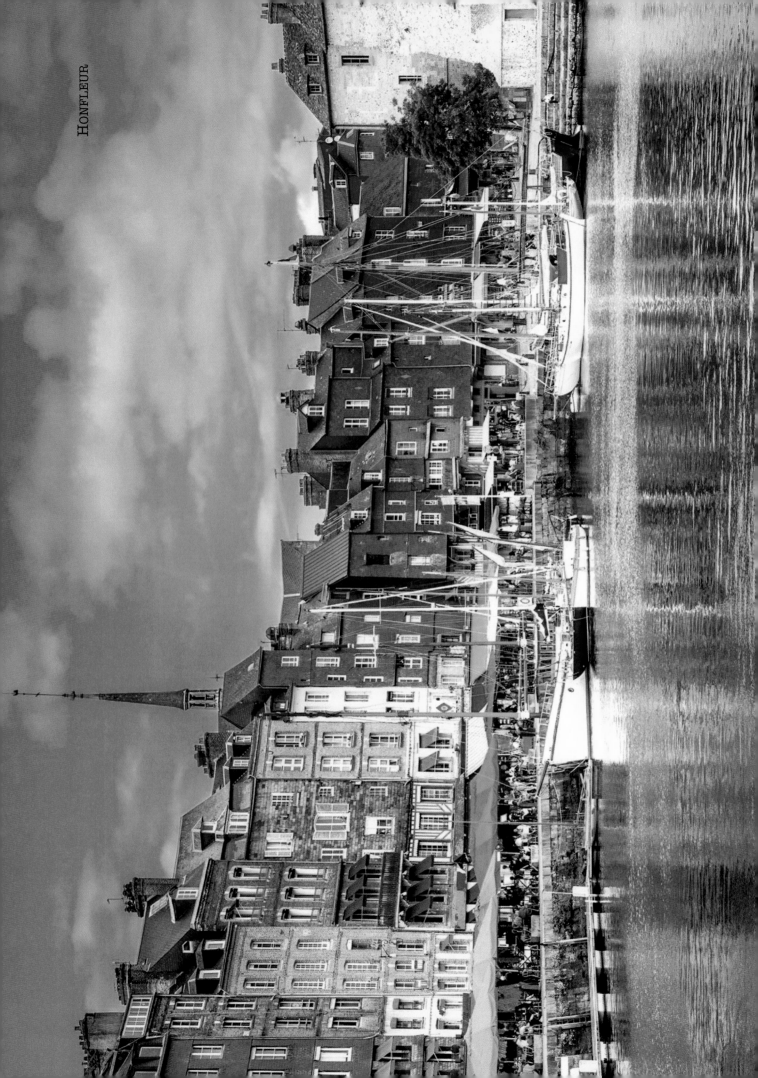

HONFLEUR.

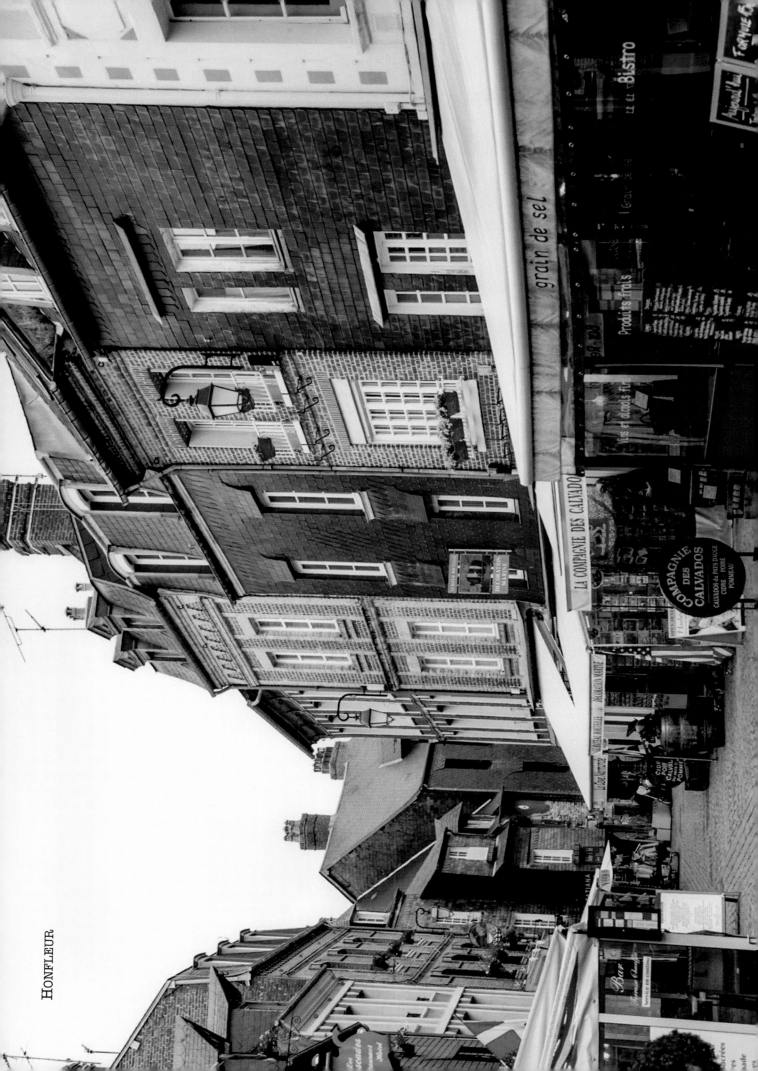

HONFLEUR

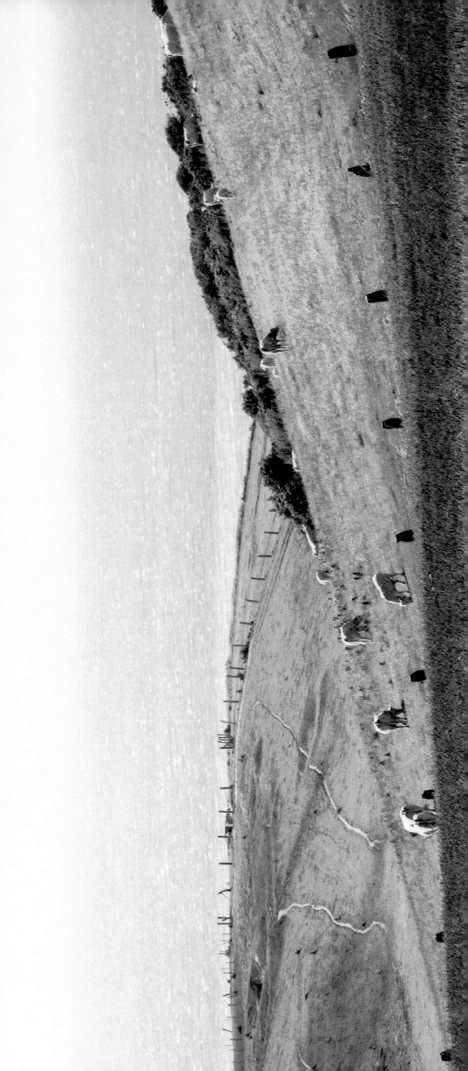

NORMANDY COUNTRYSDE

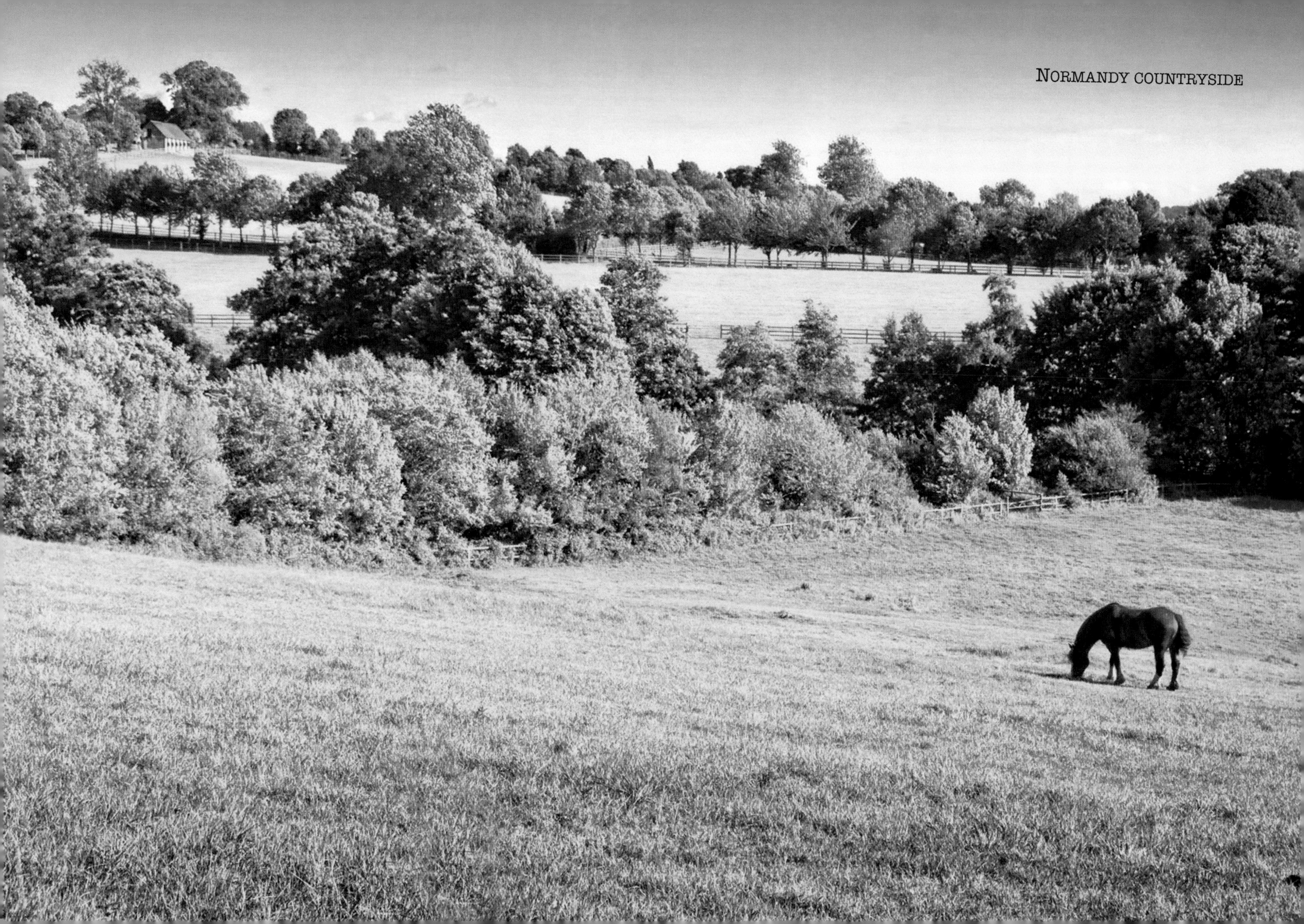

Normandy countryside

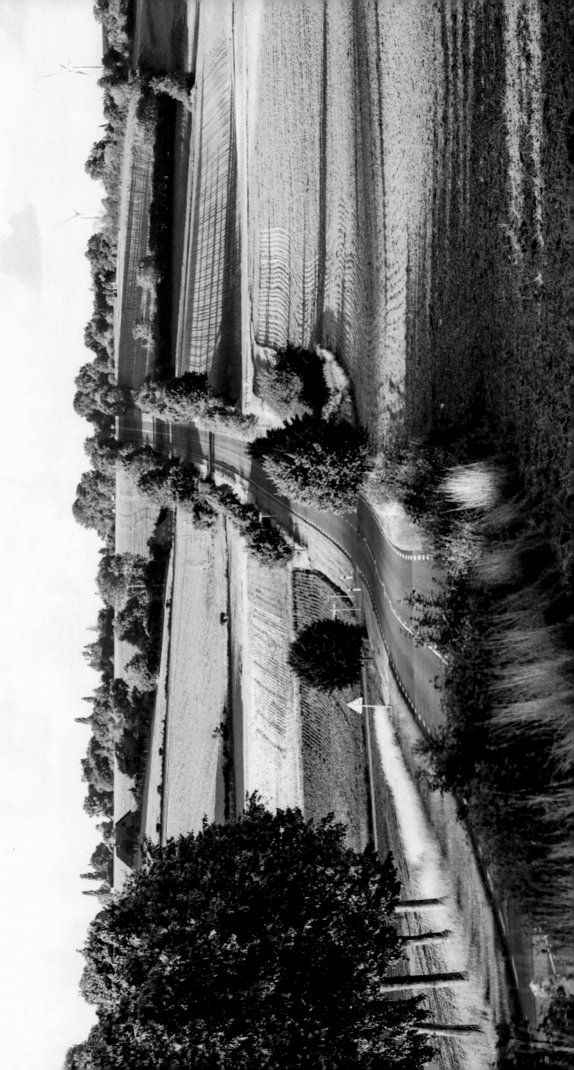

NORMANDY COUNTRYSIDE

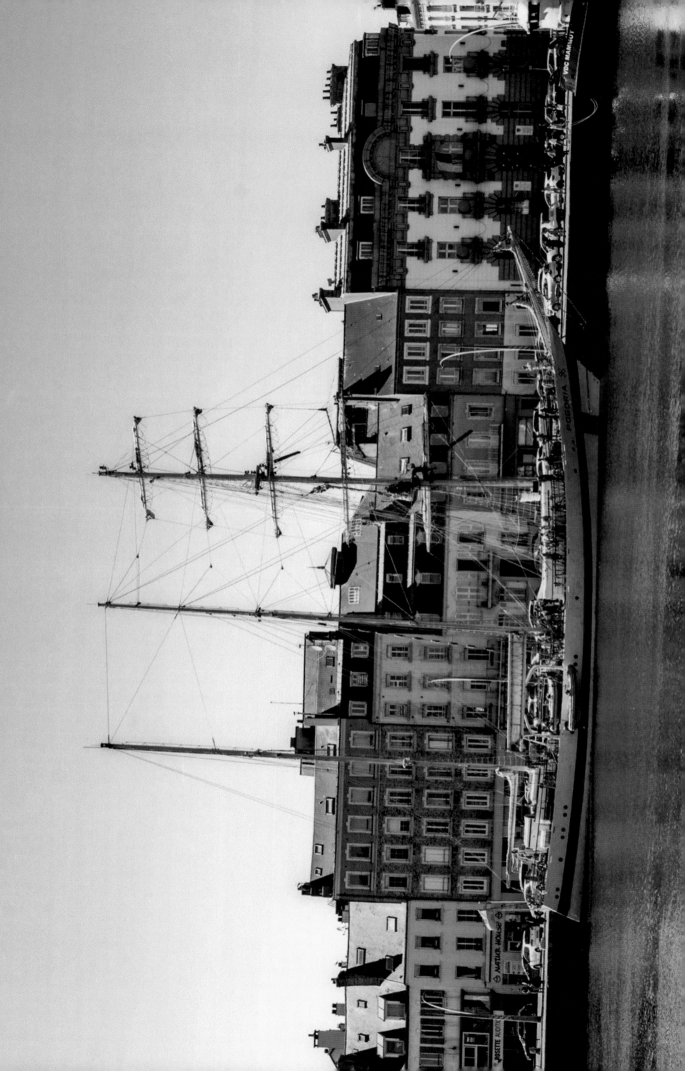

CHERBOURG

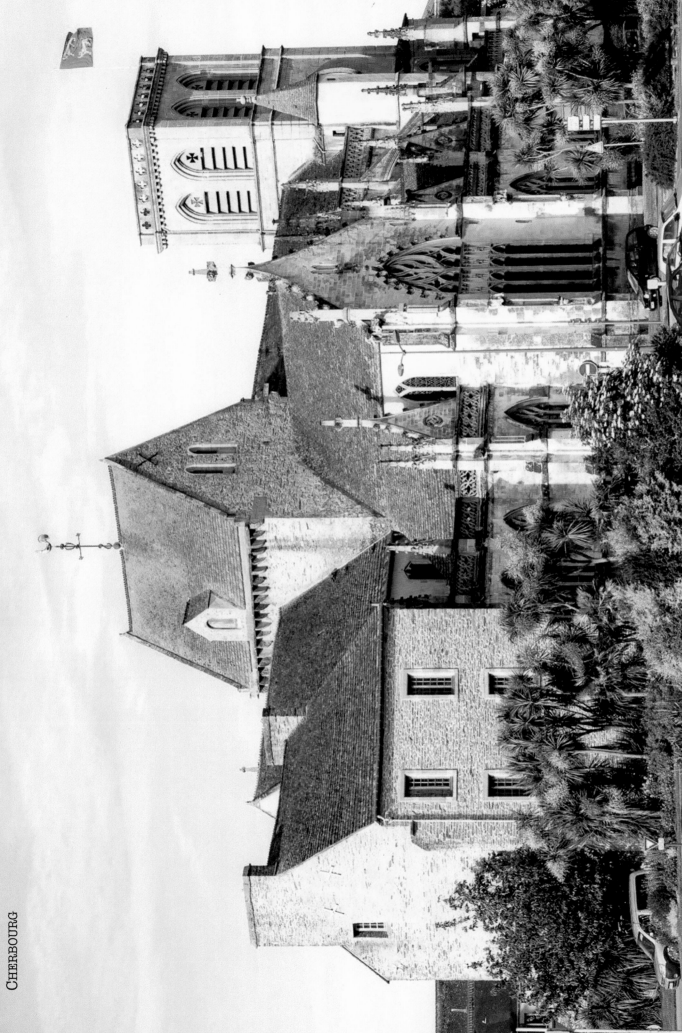

CHERBOURG

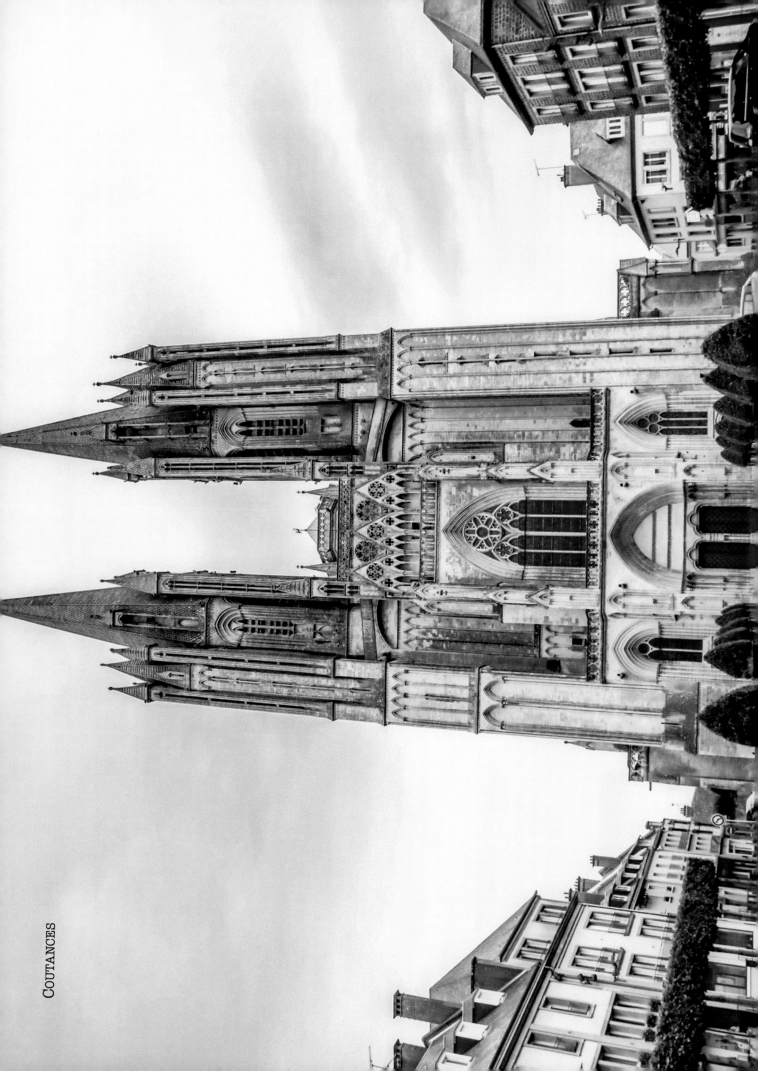

COUTANCES

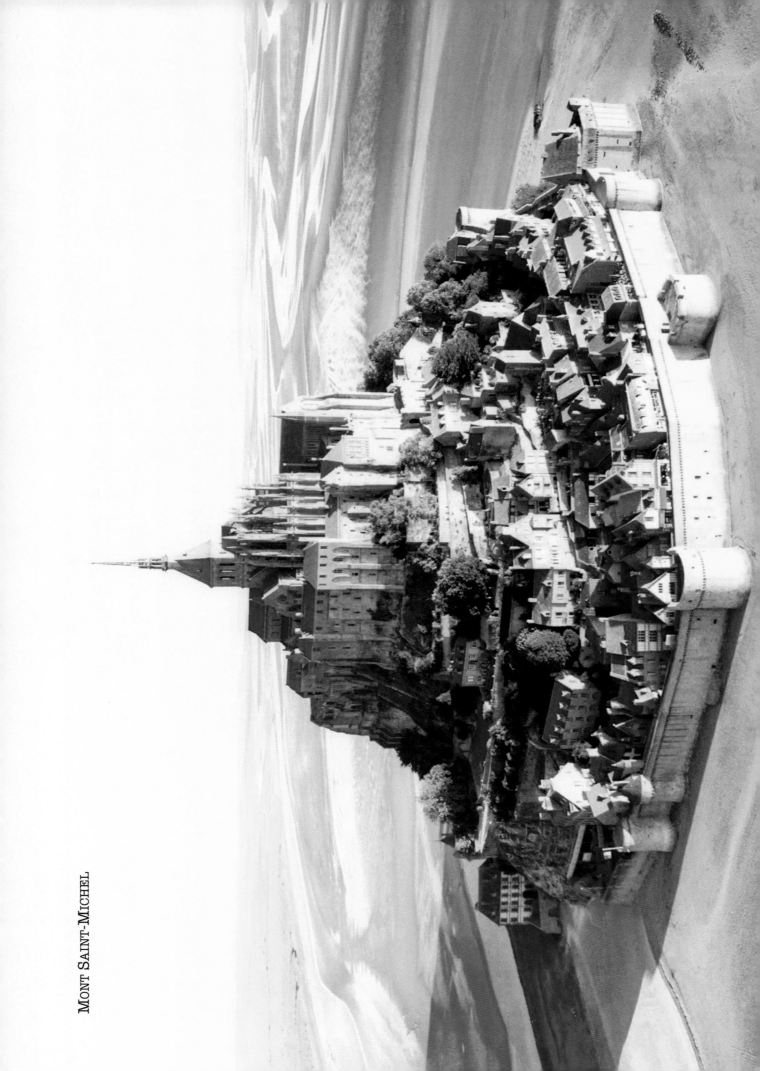

Mont Saint-Michel

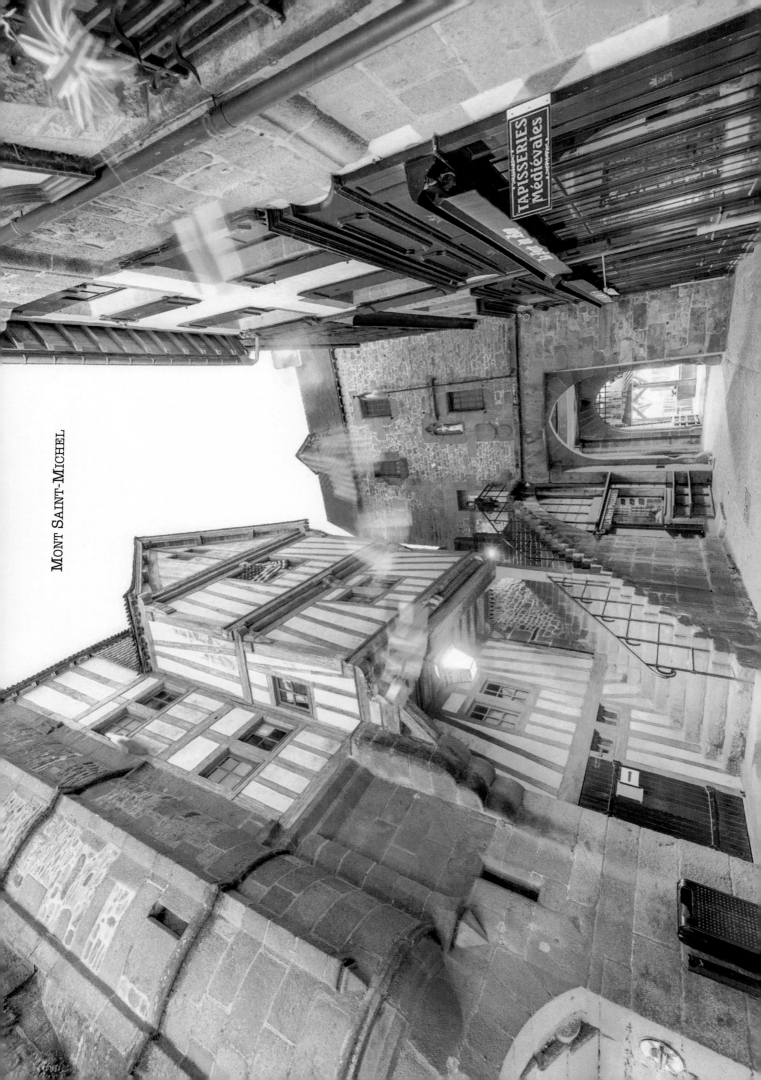

MONT SAINT-MICHEL

TAPISSERIES
Médiévales

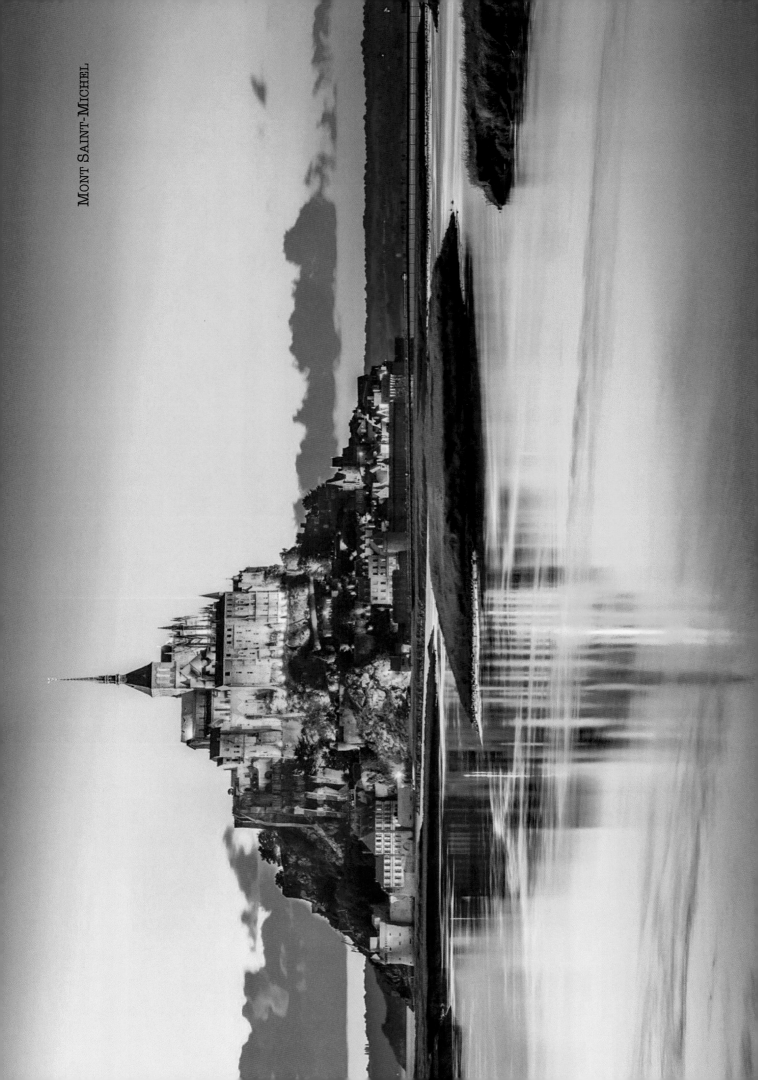

MONT SAINT-MICHEL

BRITTANY

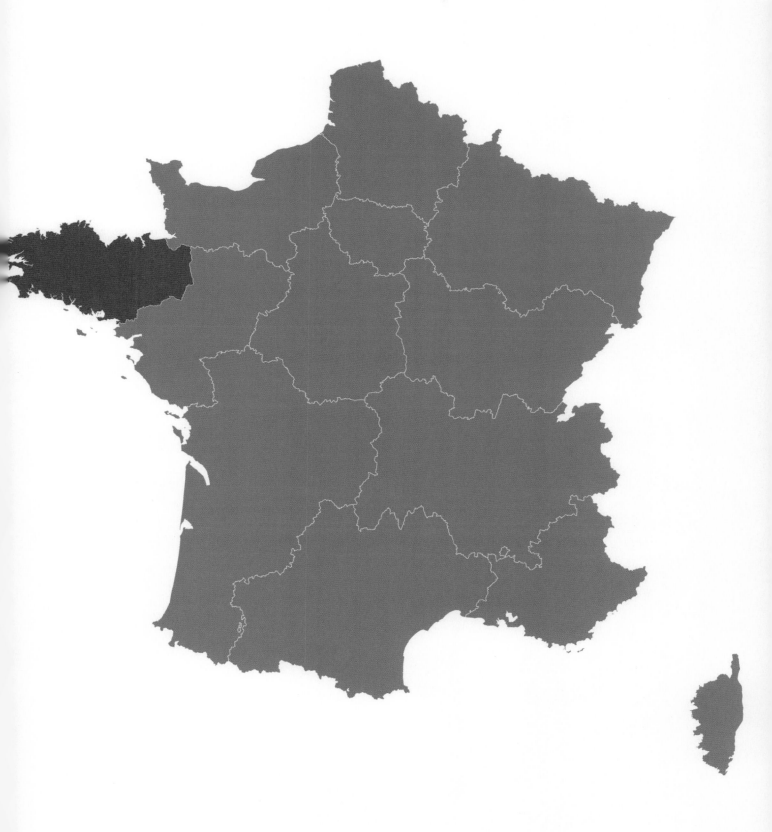

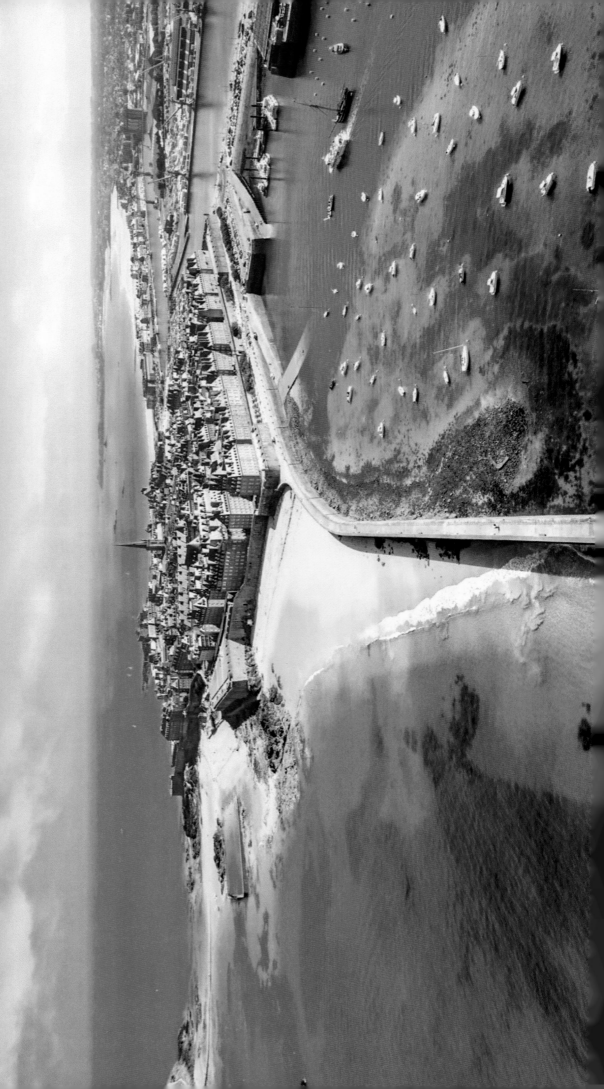

SAINT MALO

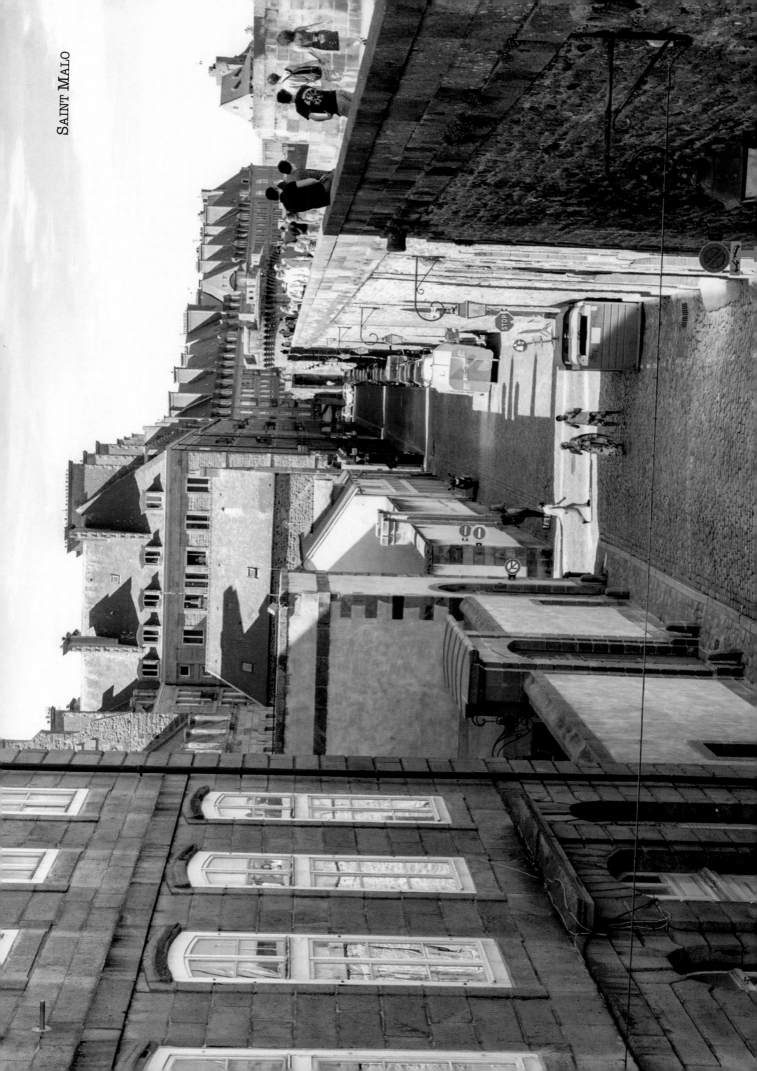

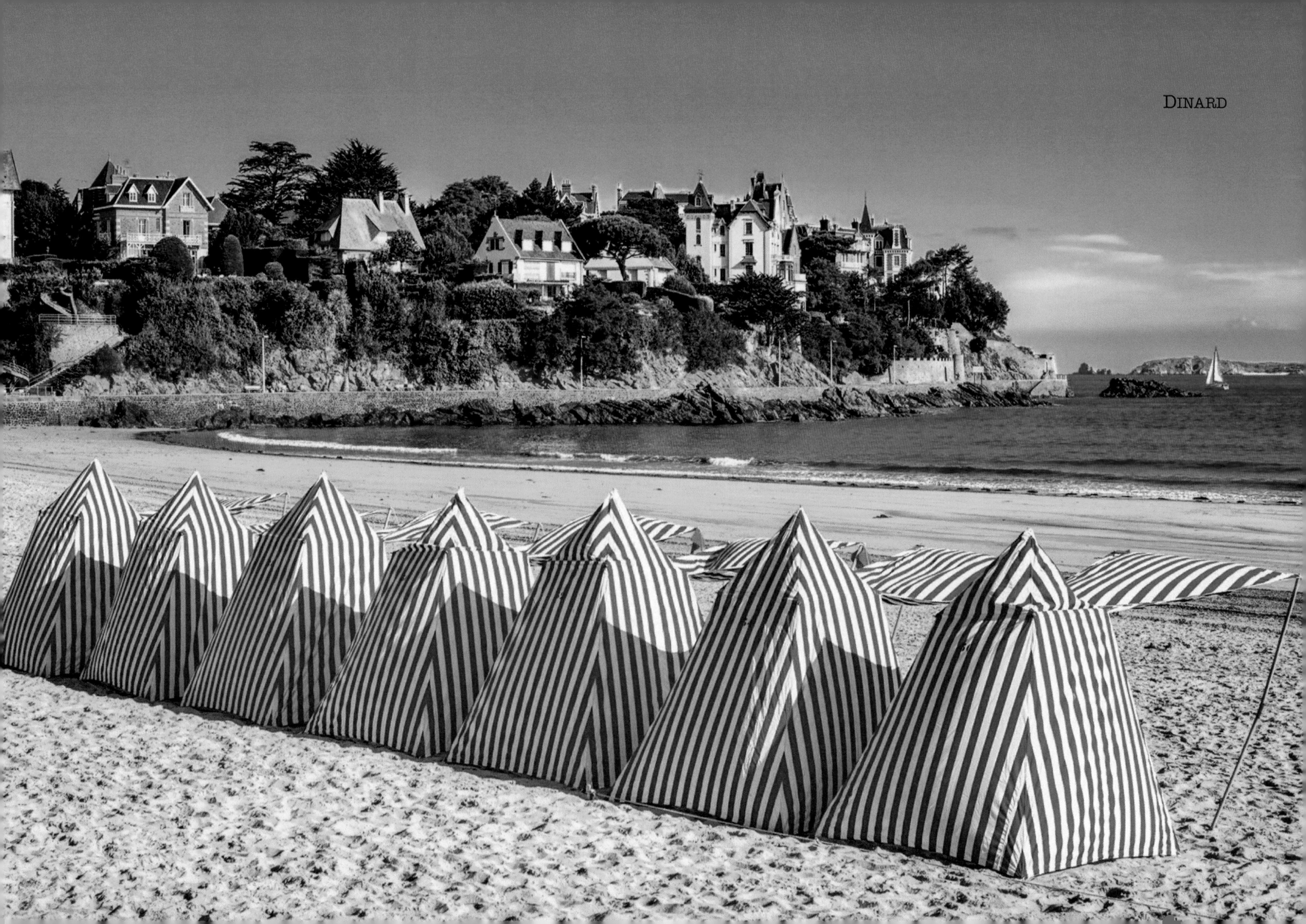

Dinard

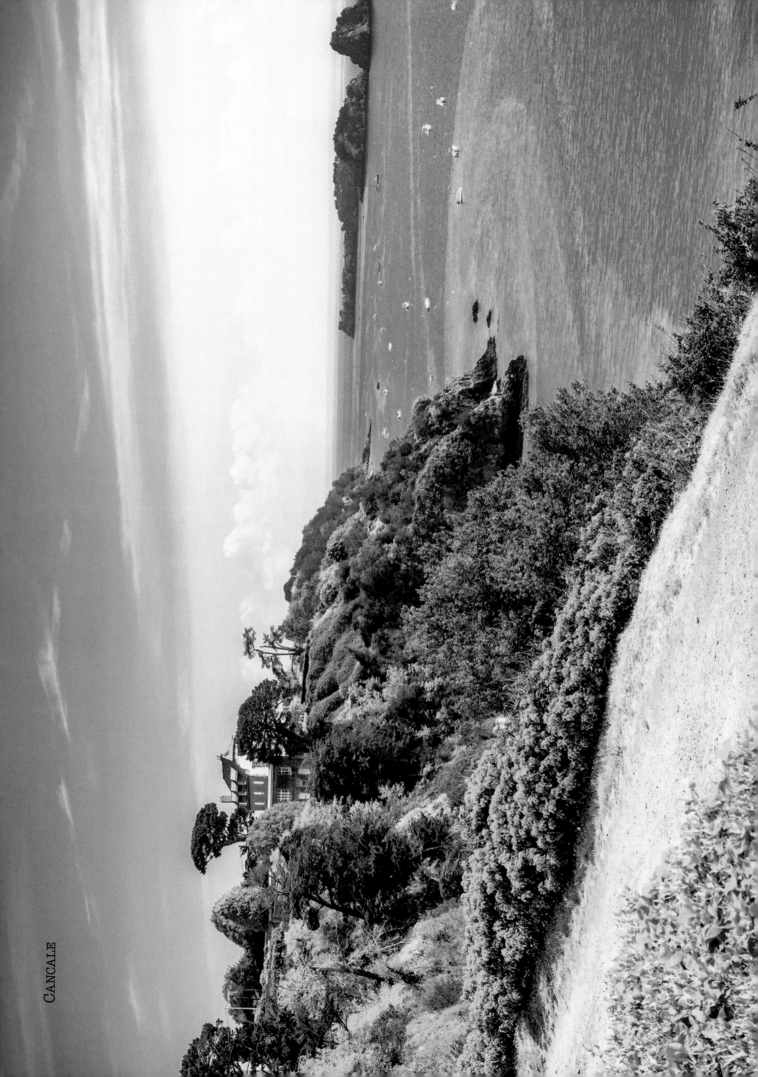

CANCALE

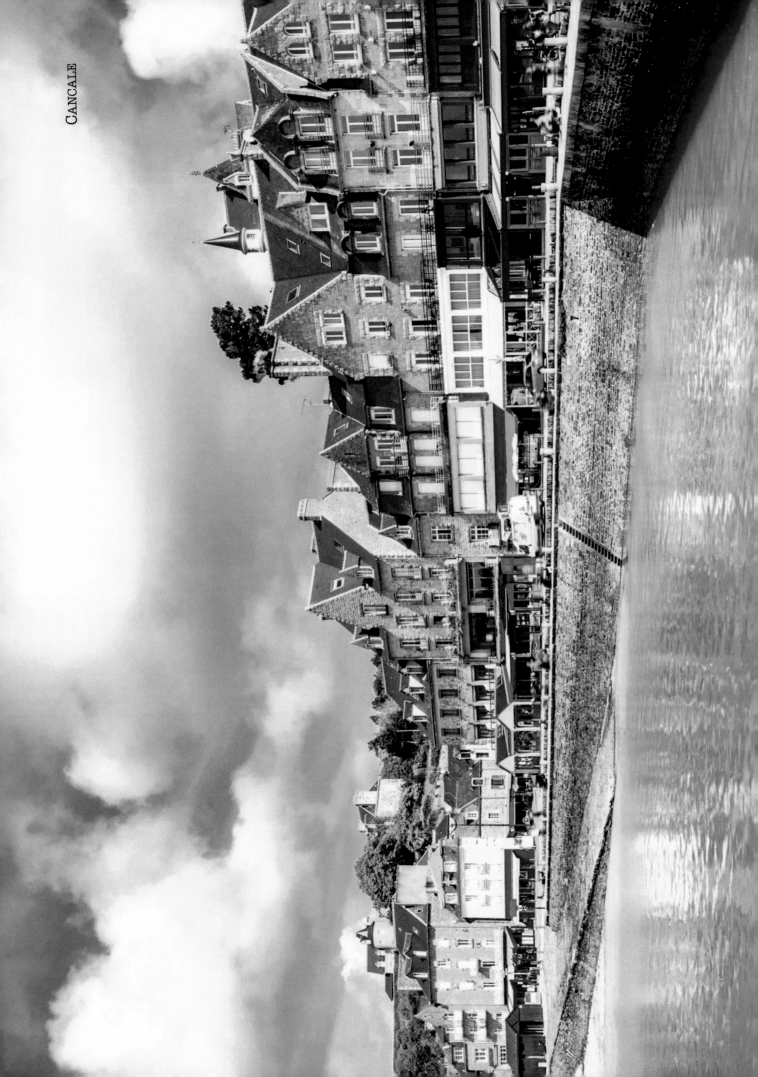
CANCALE

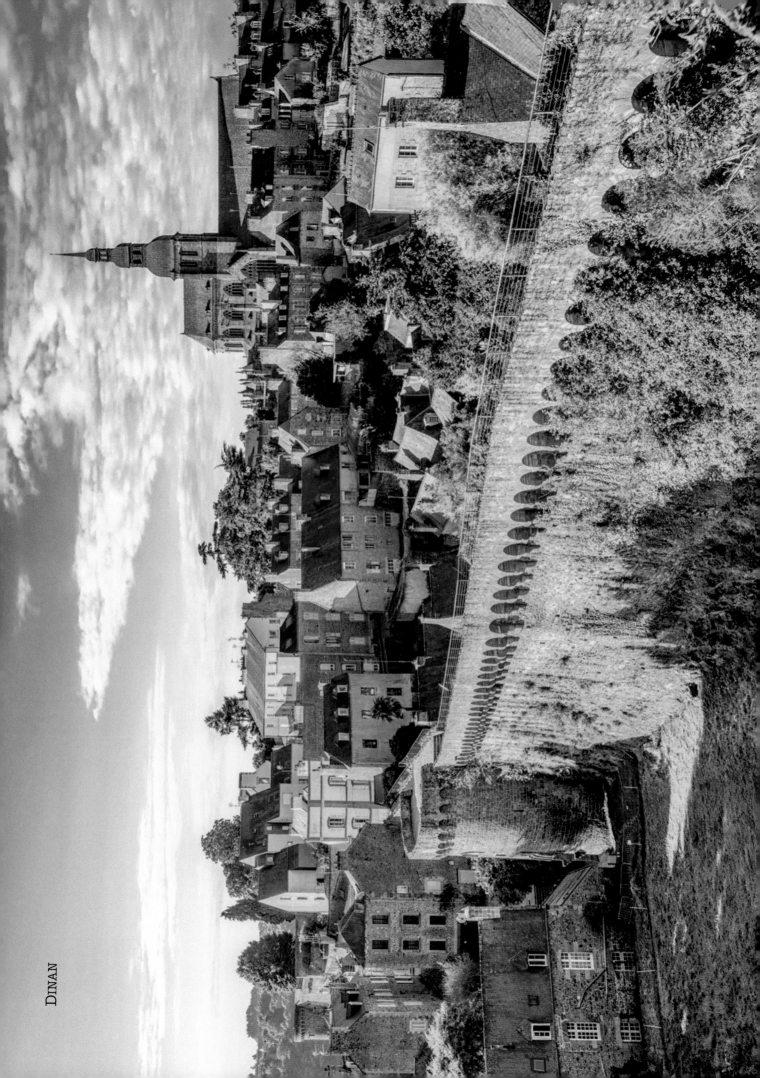

DINAN

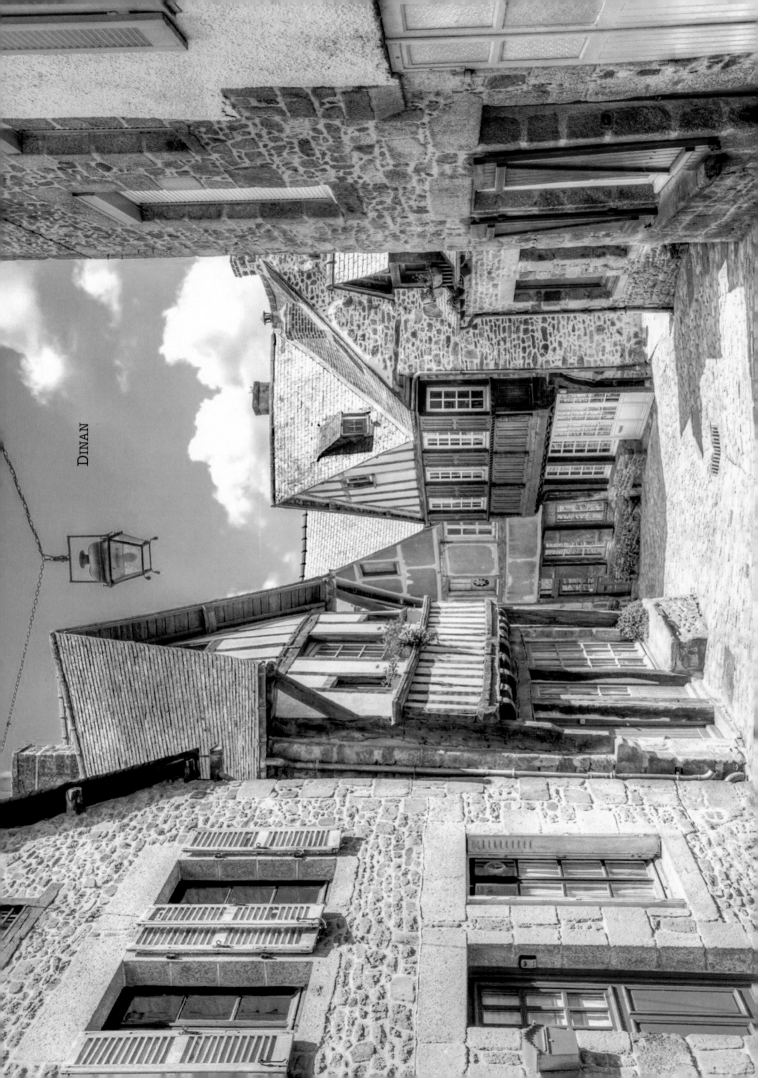

Dinan

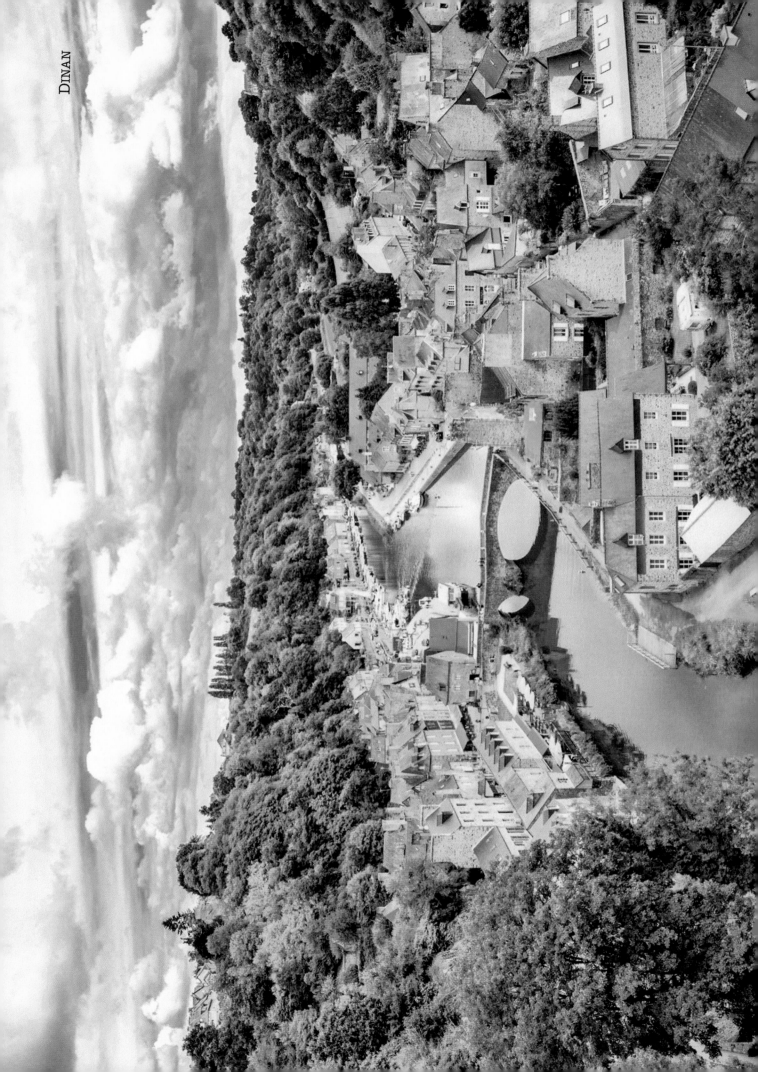

DINAN

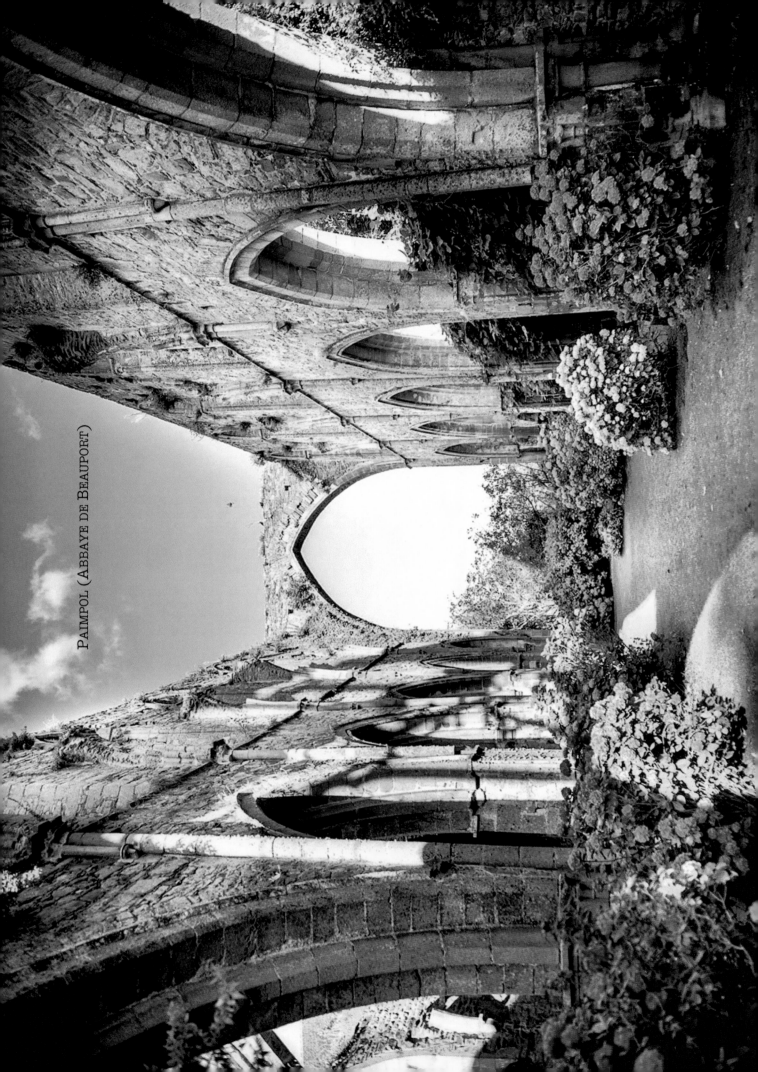

PAIMPOL (ABBAYE DE BEAUPORT)

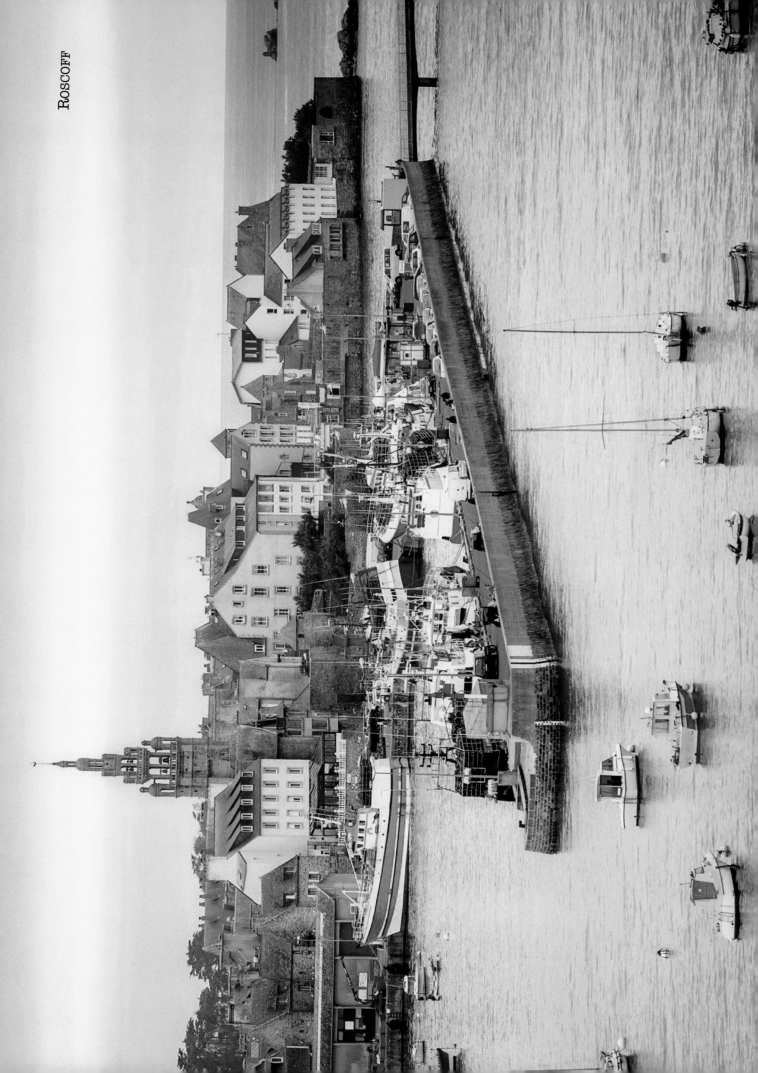

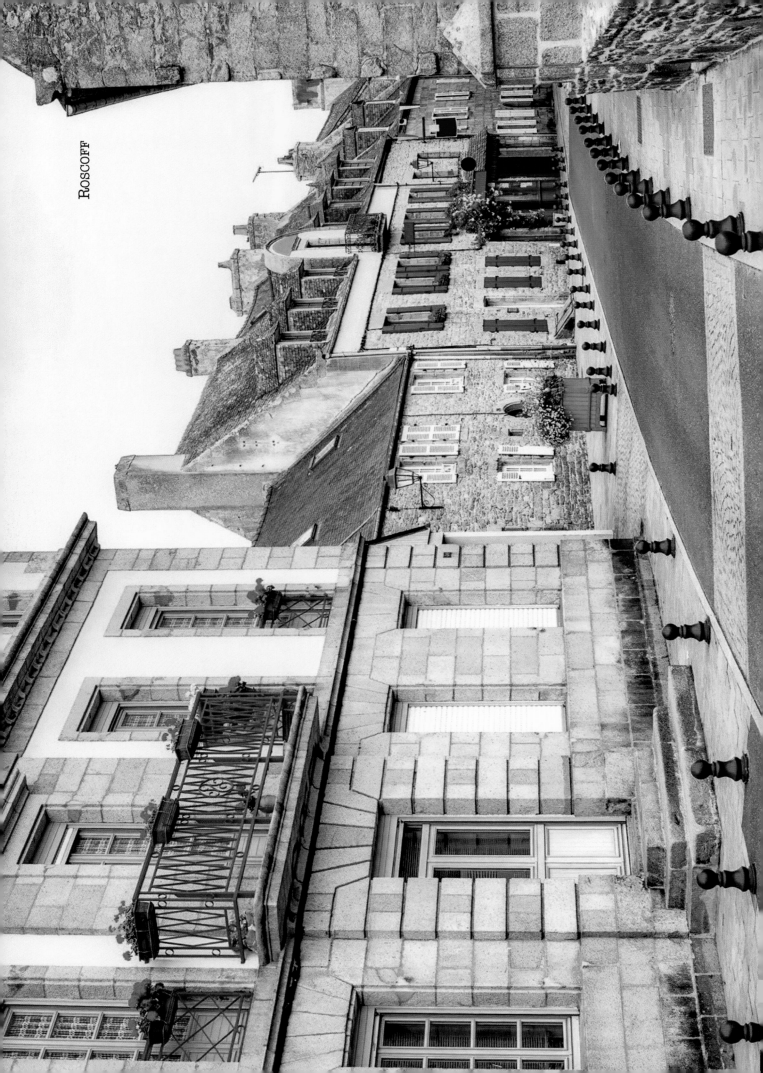

ROSCOFF

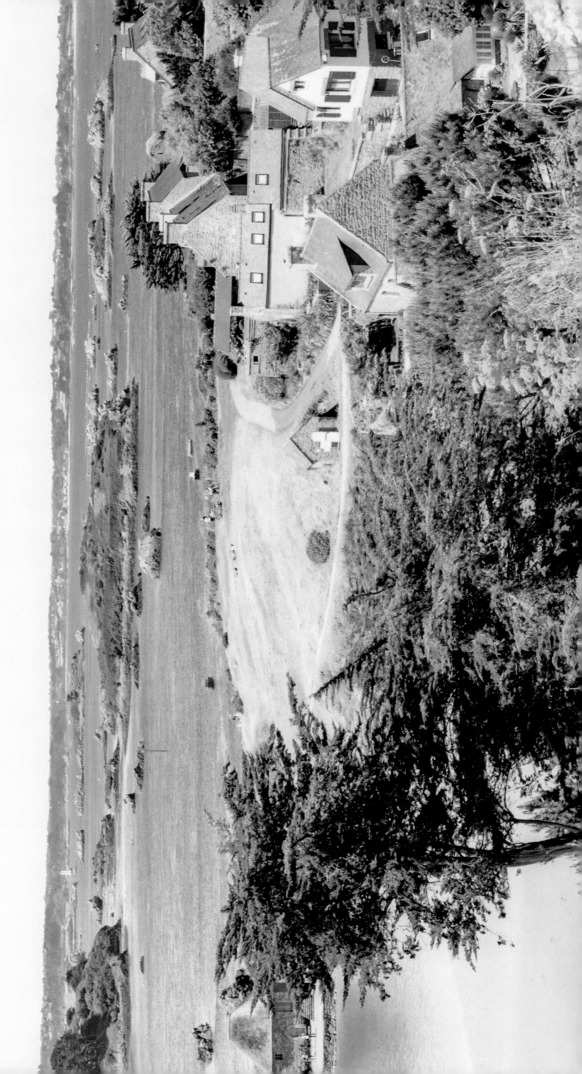

BRÉHAT

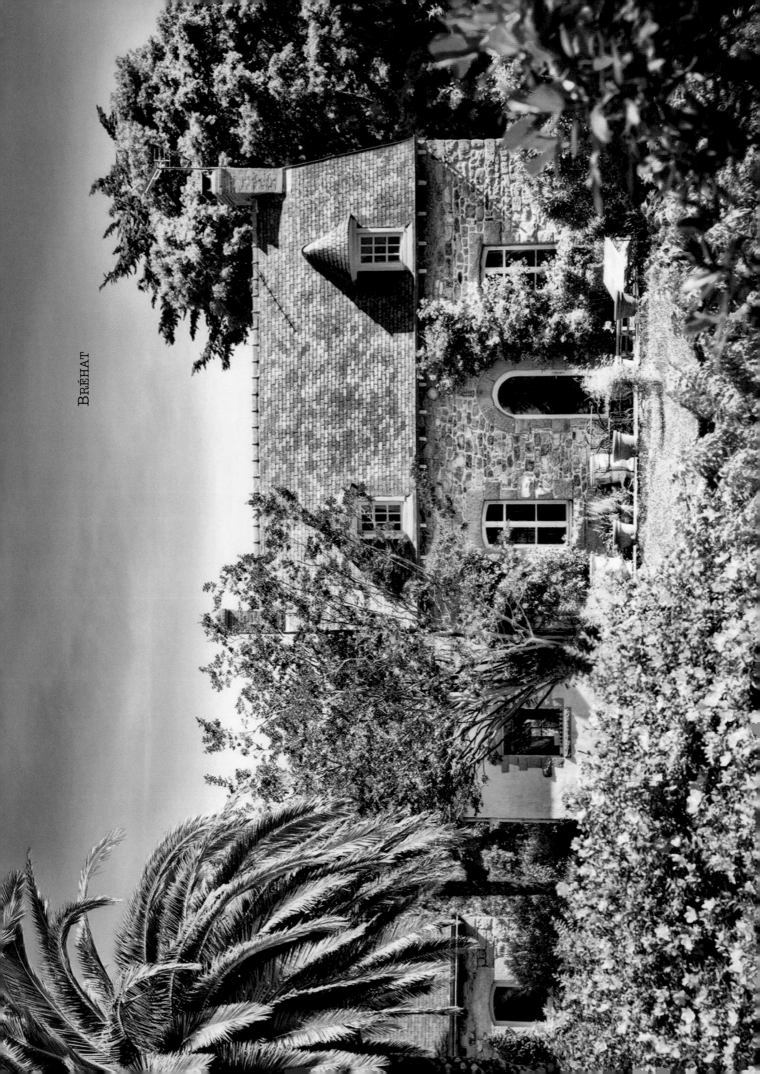

BRÉHAT

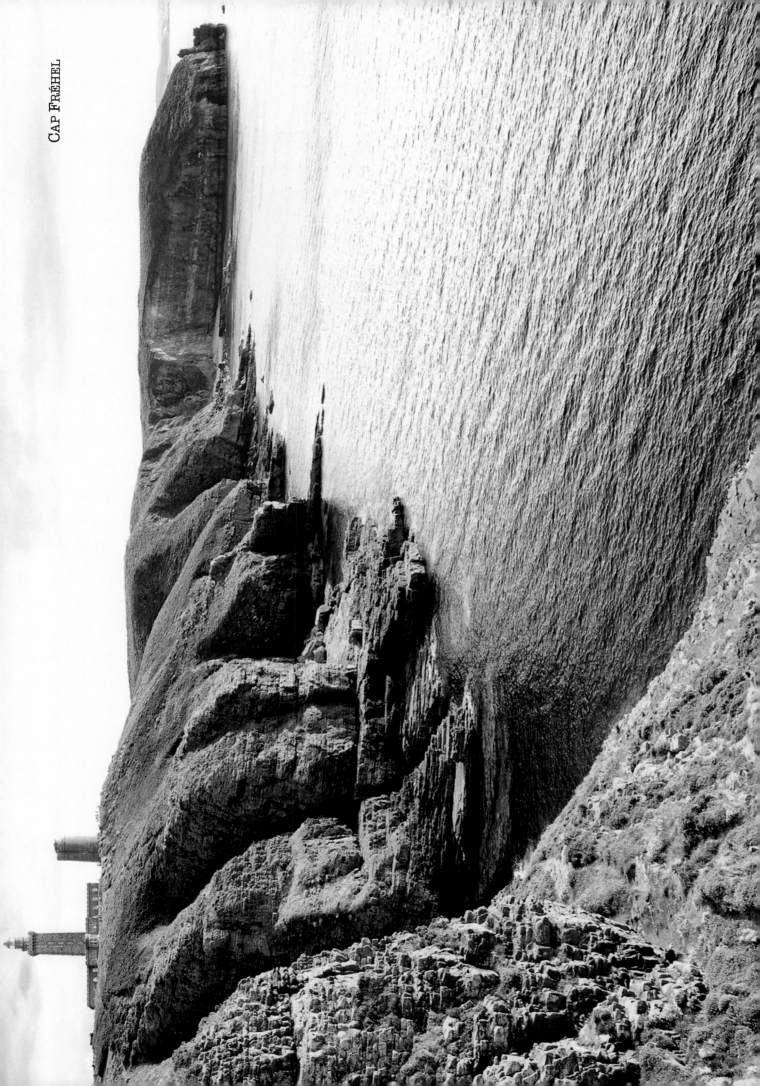

CAP FRÉHEL

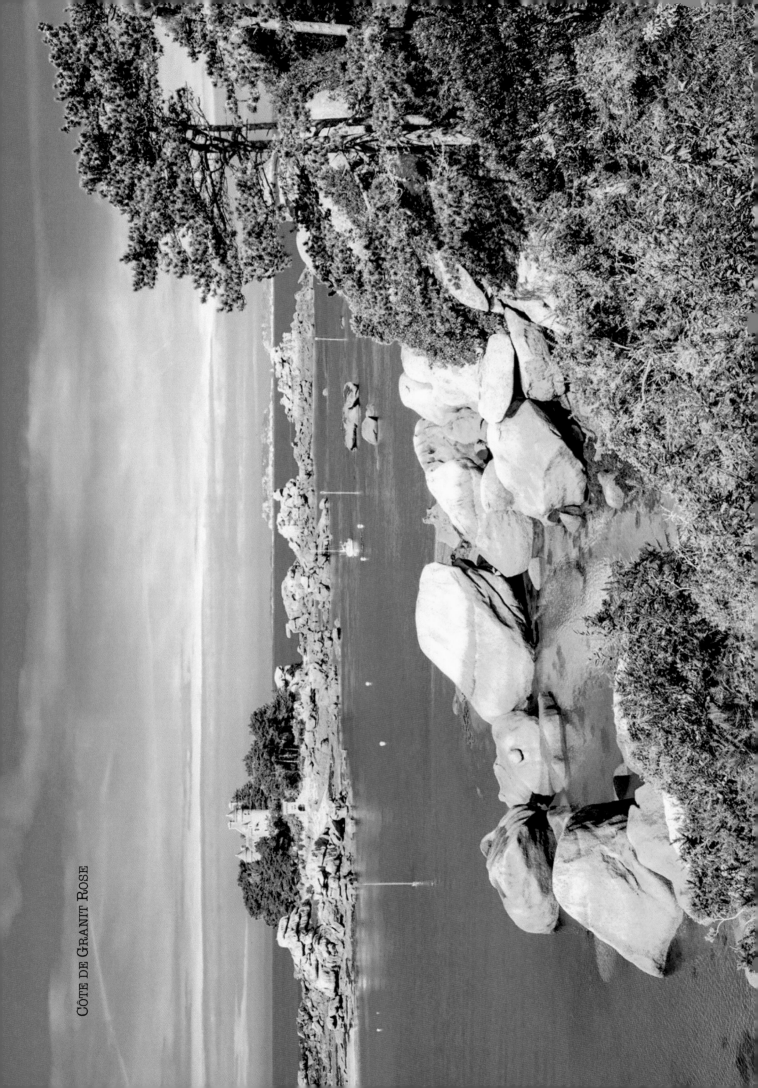

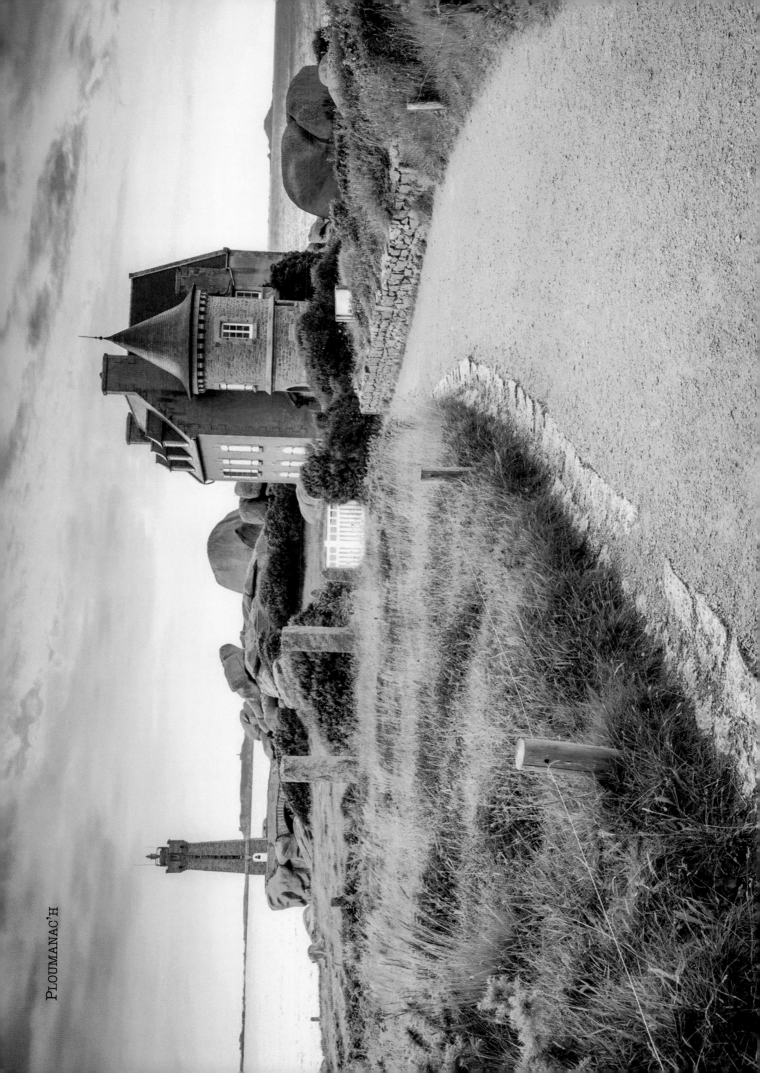

PLOUMANAC'H

PLOUMANAC'H

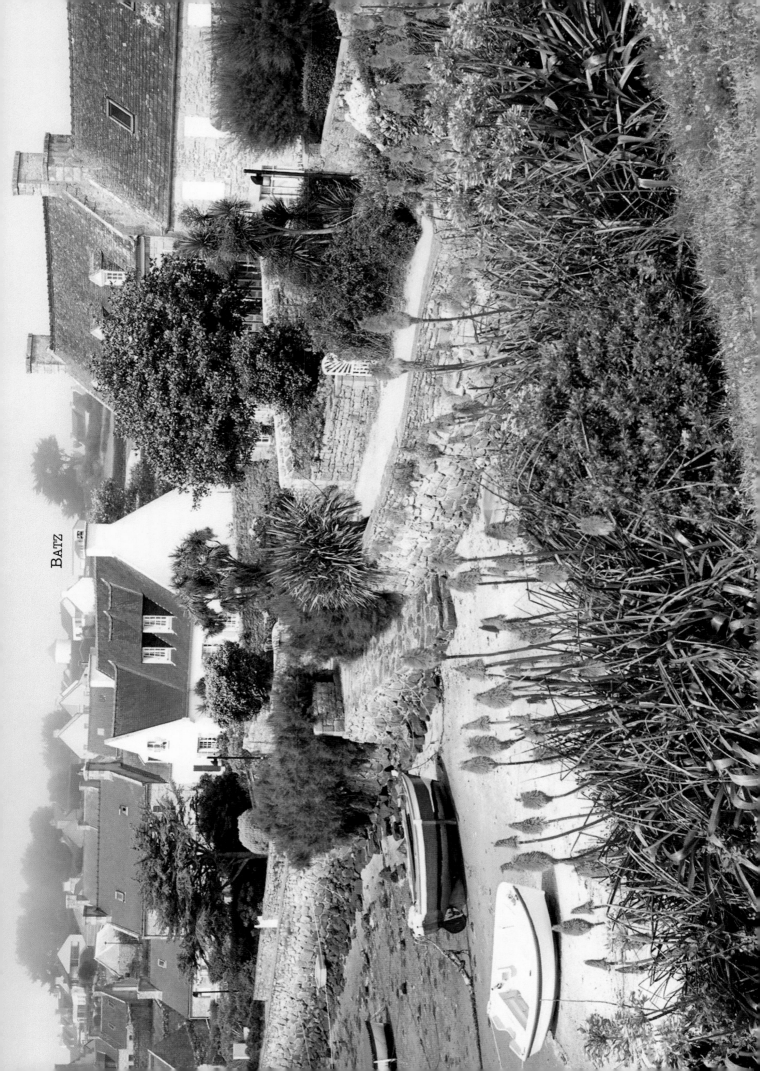

BATZ

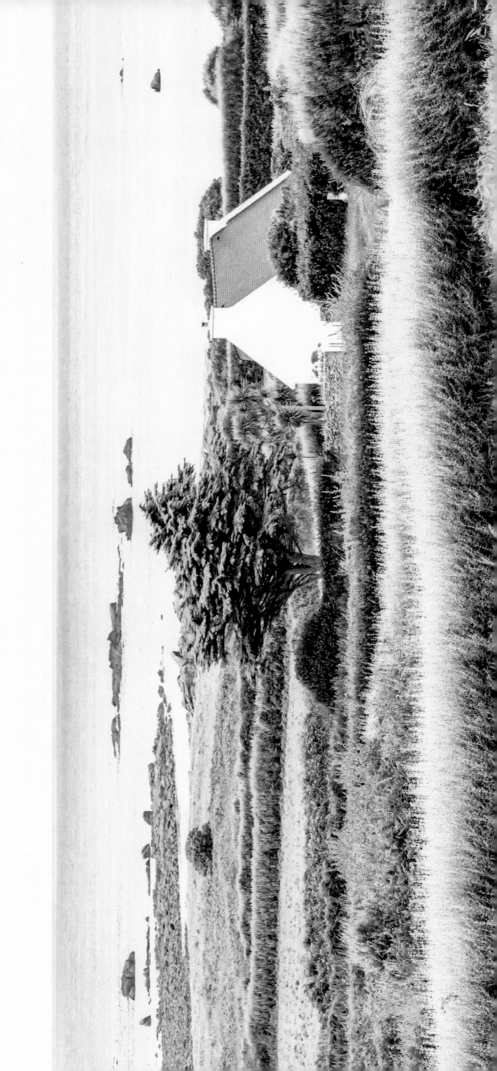

BATZ

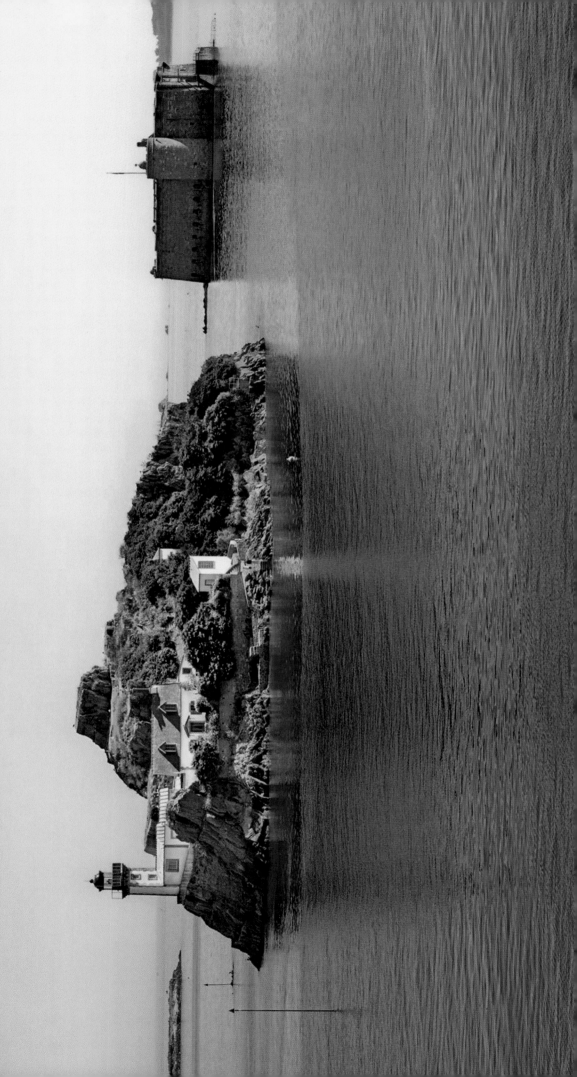

LOUËT

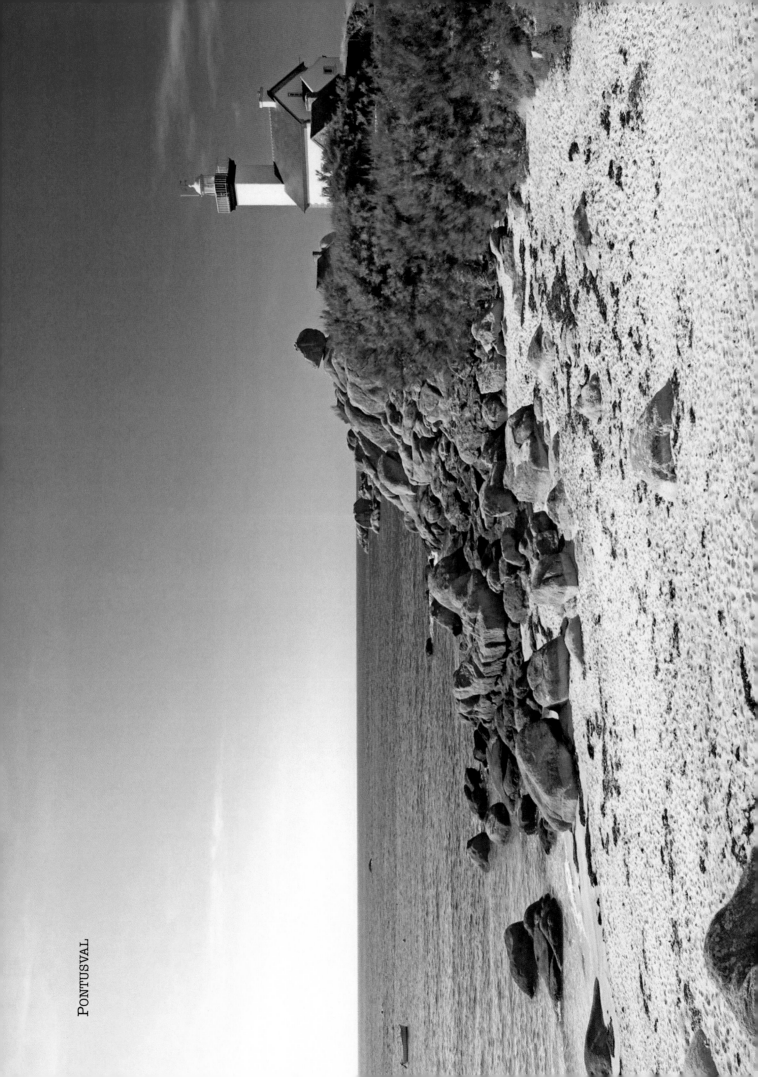

PONTUSVAL

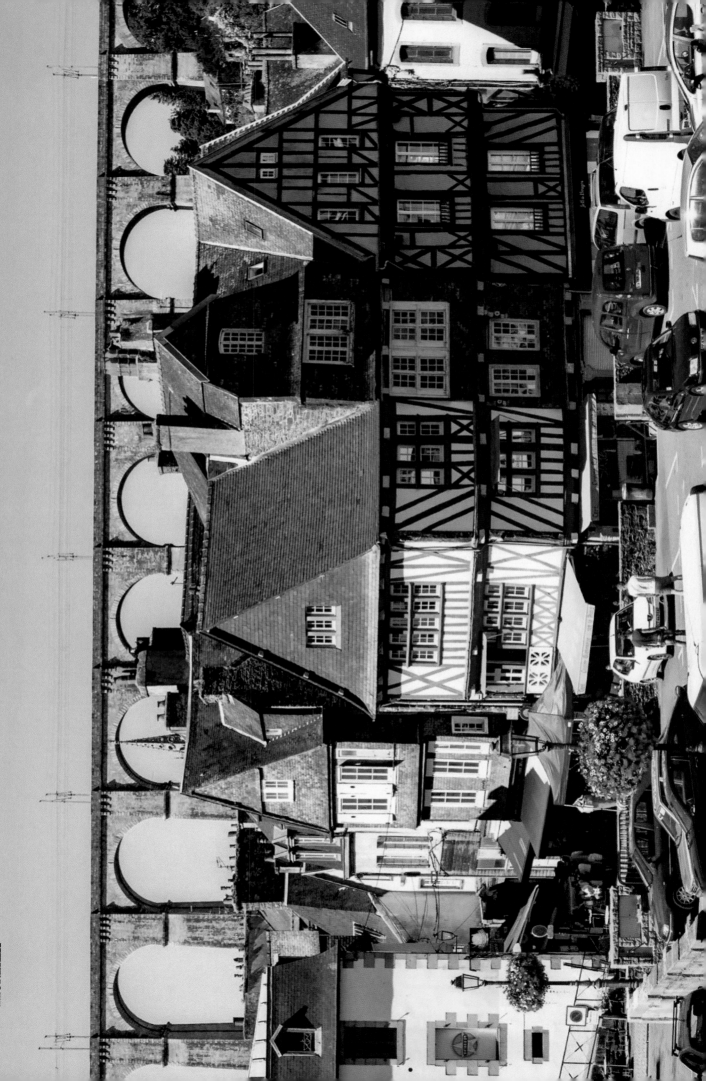

MORLAIX

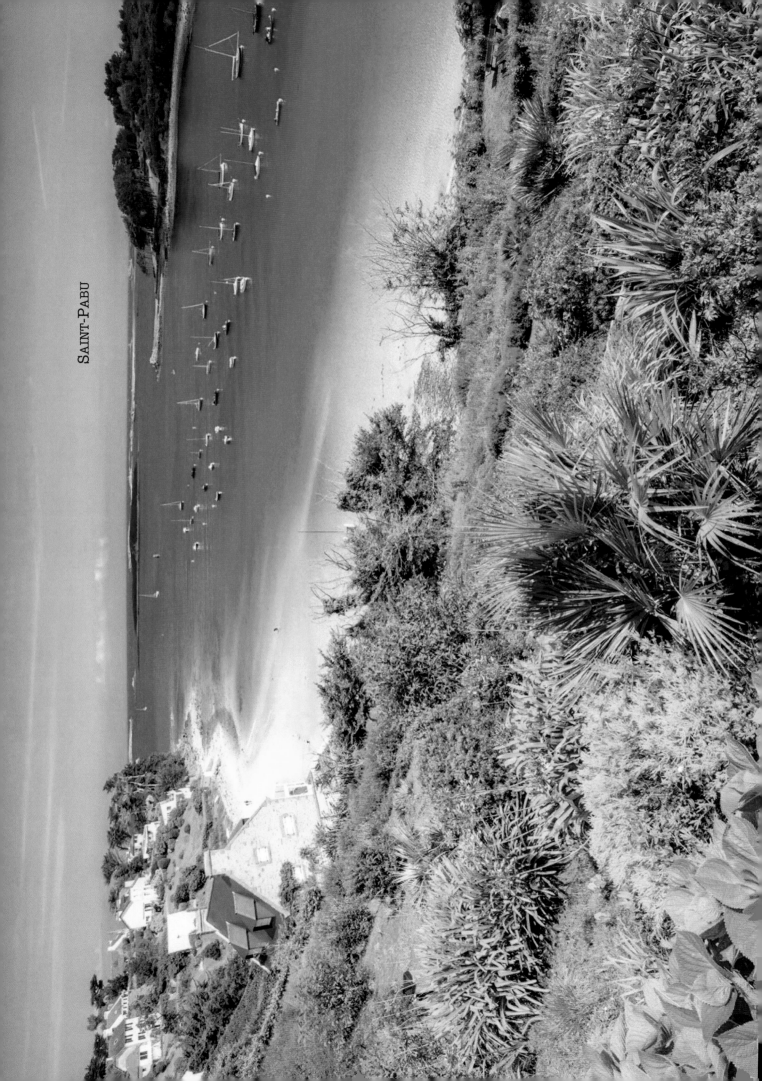

SAINT-PABU

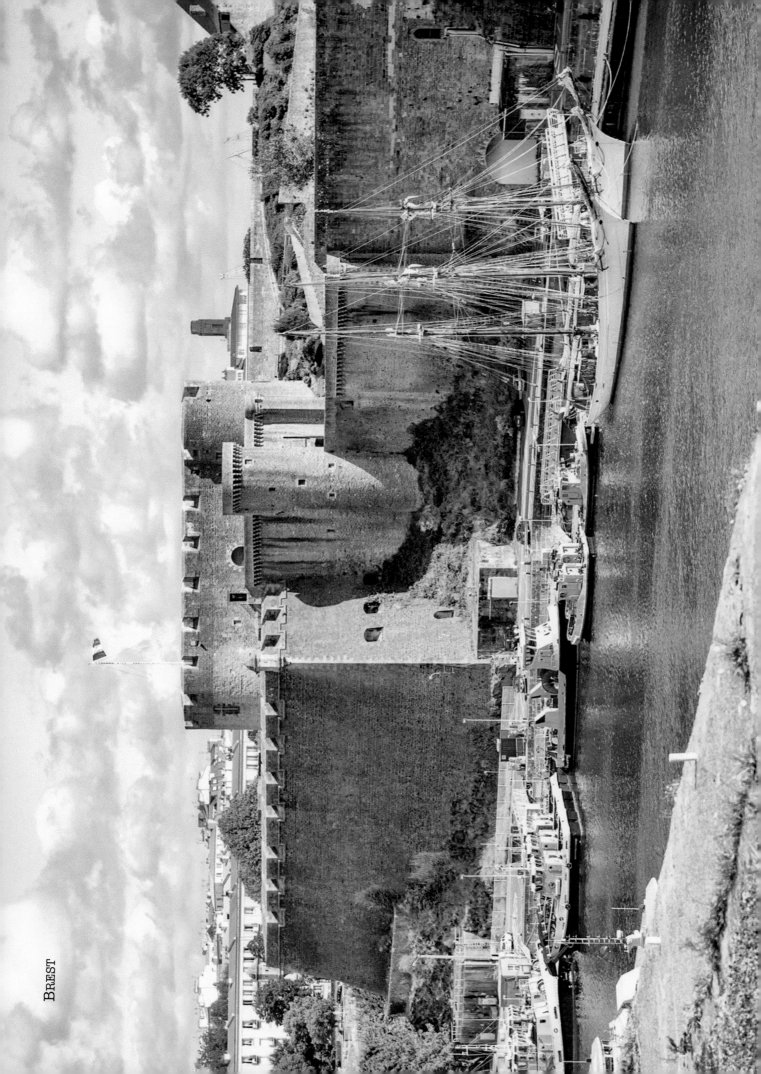

BREST

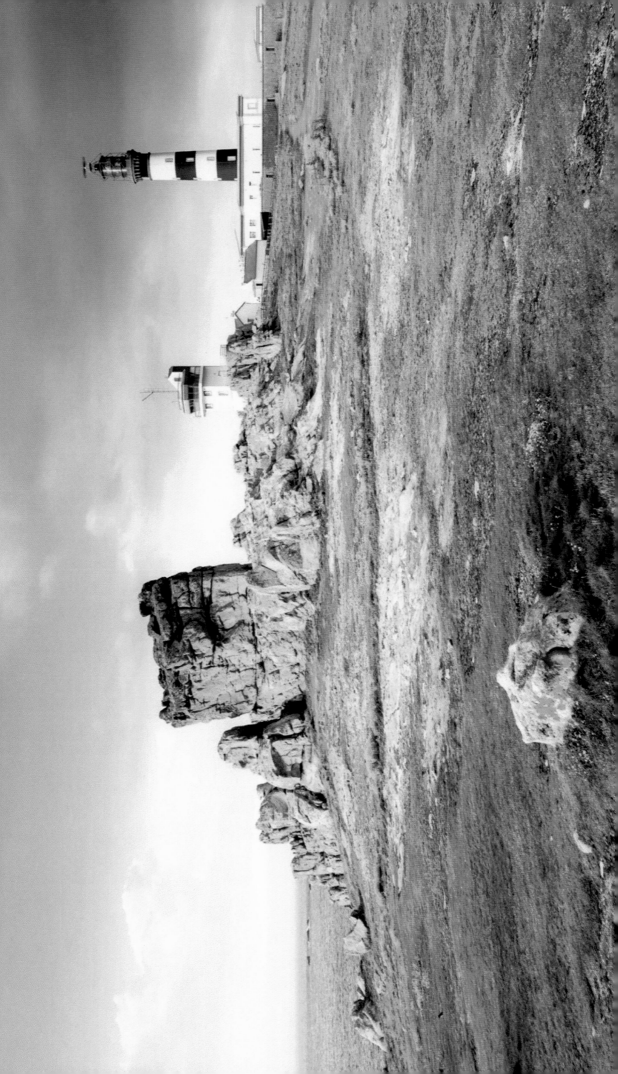

OUESSANT

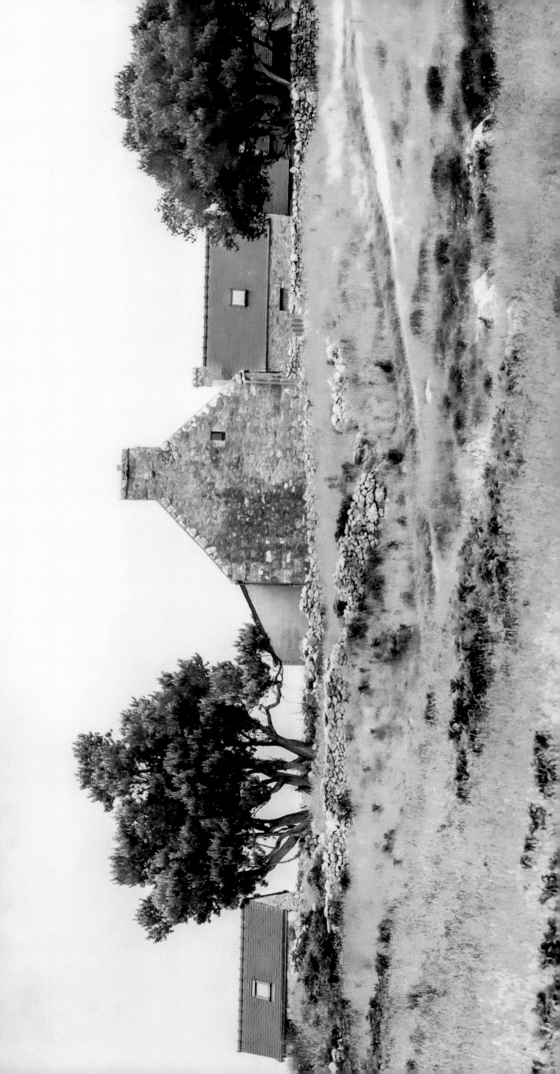

OUESSANT

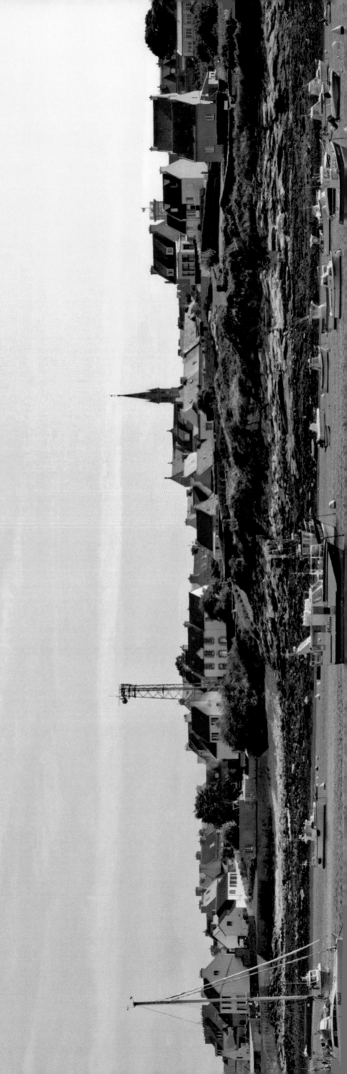

MOLÈNE

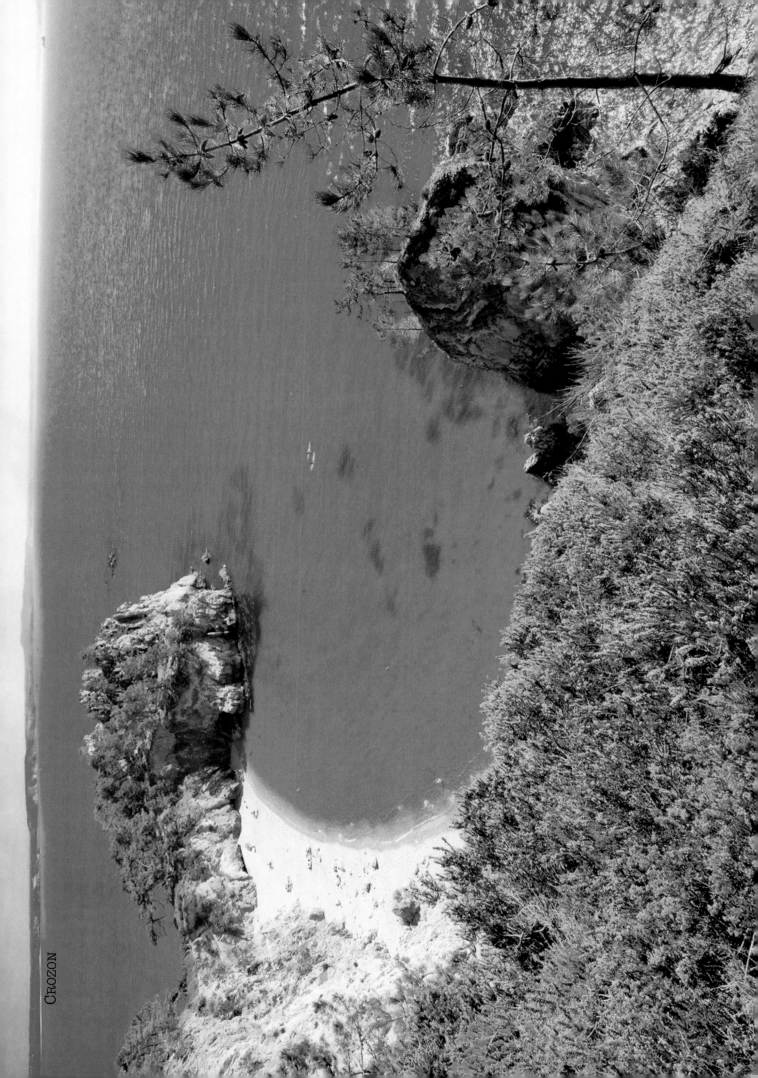

CROZON

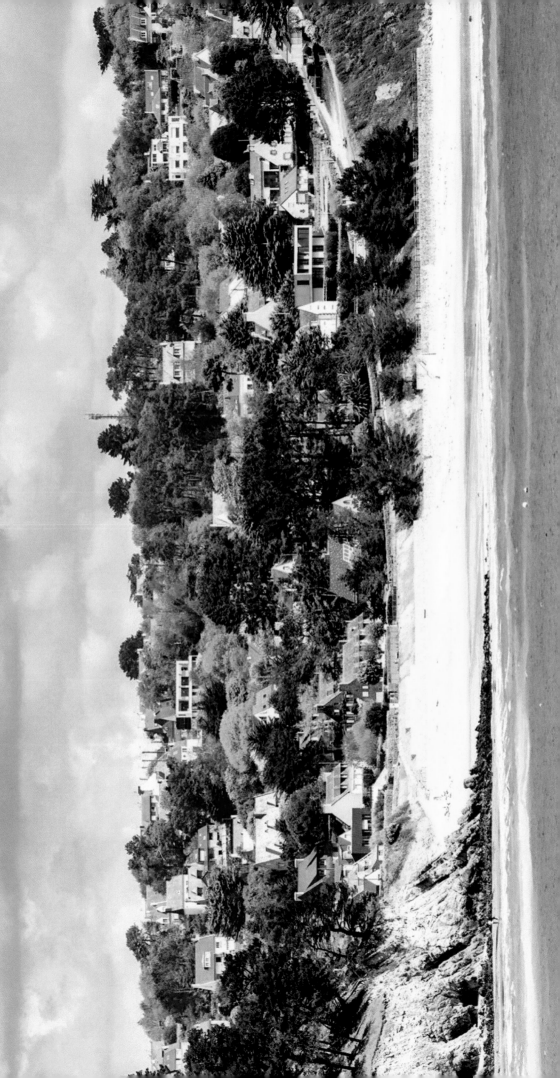

MORGAT

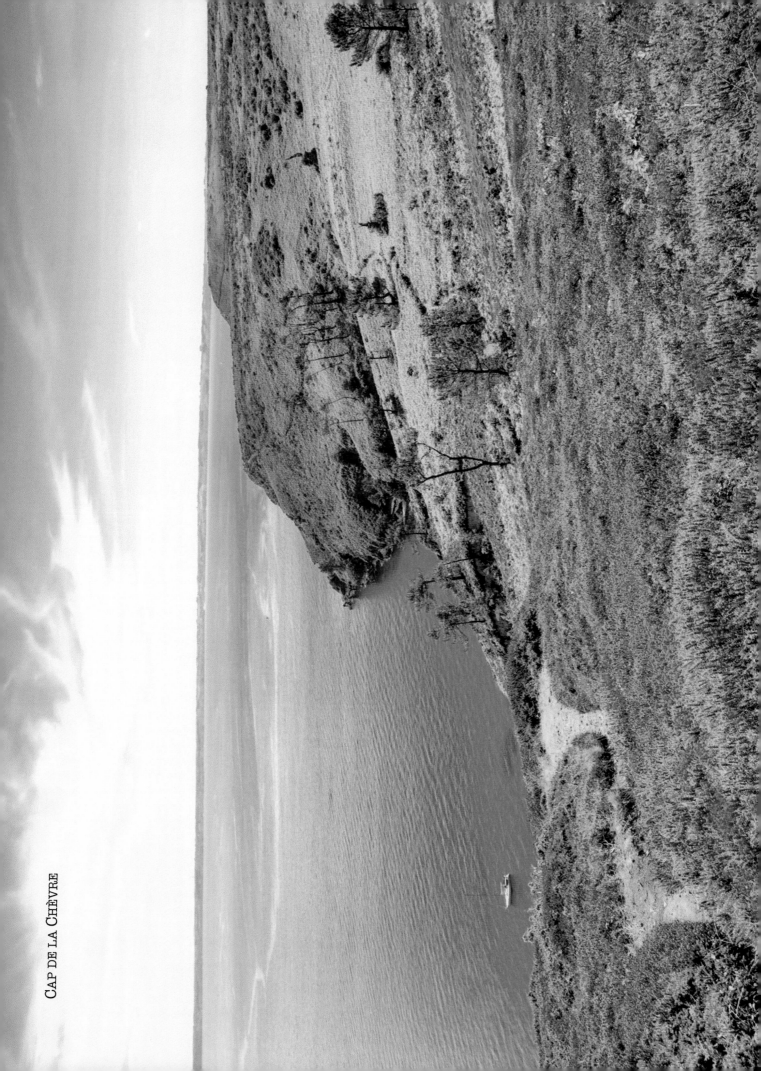

CAP DE LA CHÈVRE

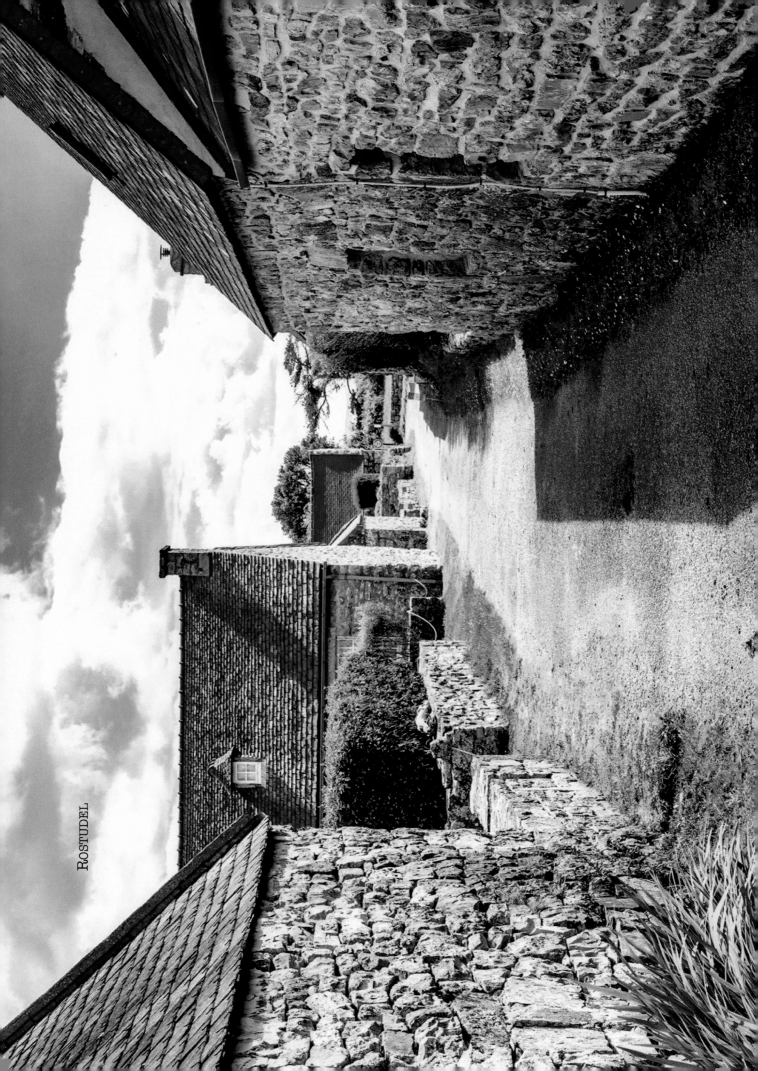

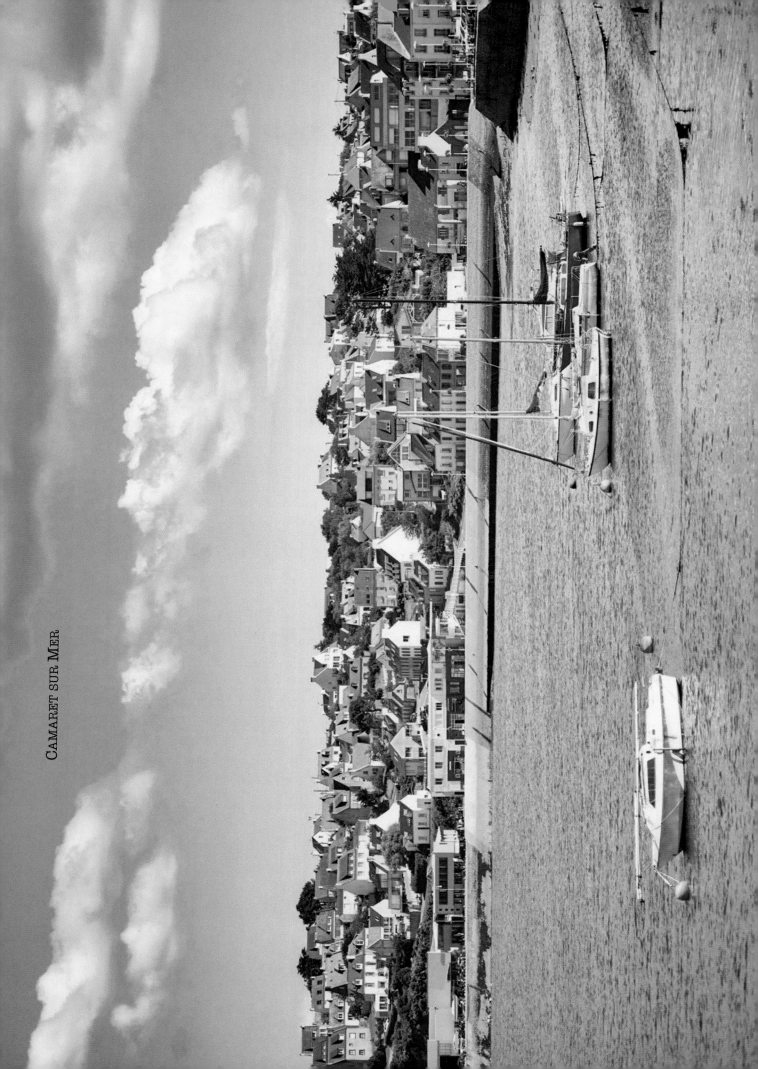

CAMARET SUR MER.

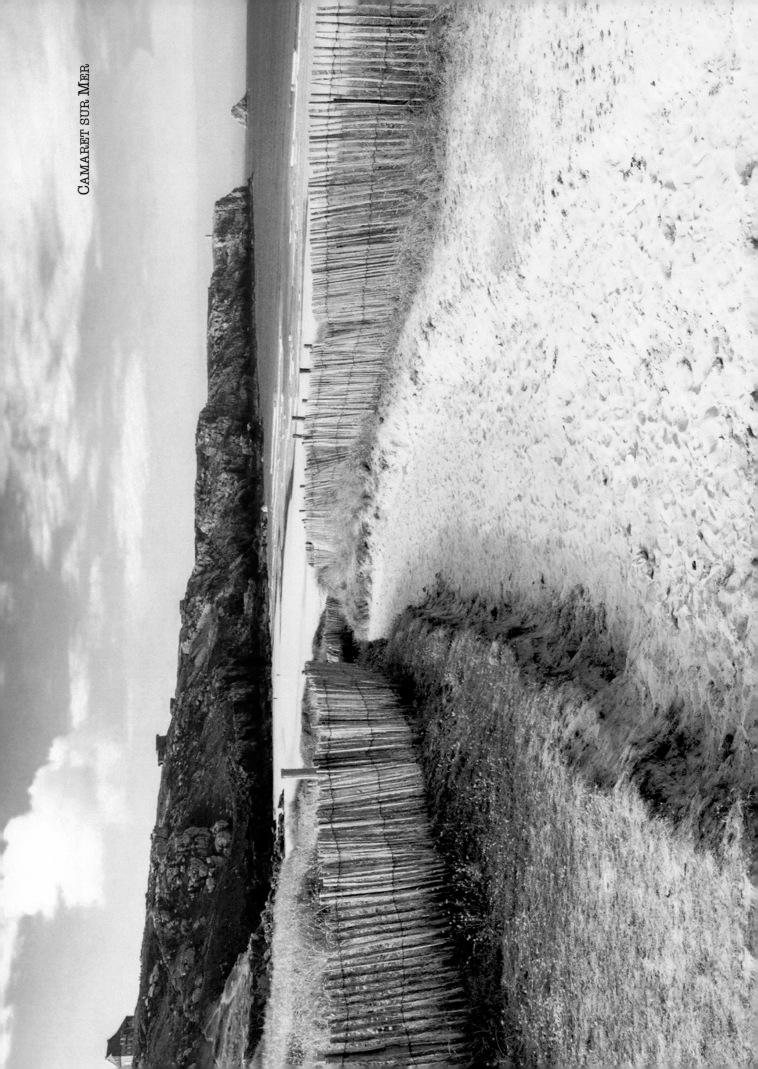

CAMARET SUR MER

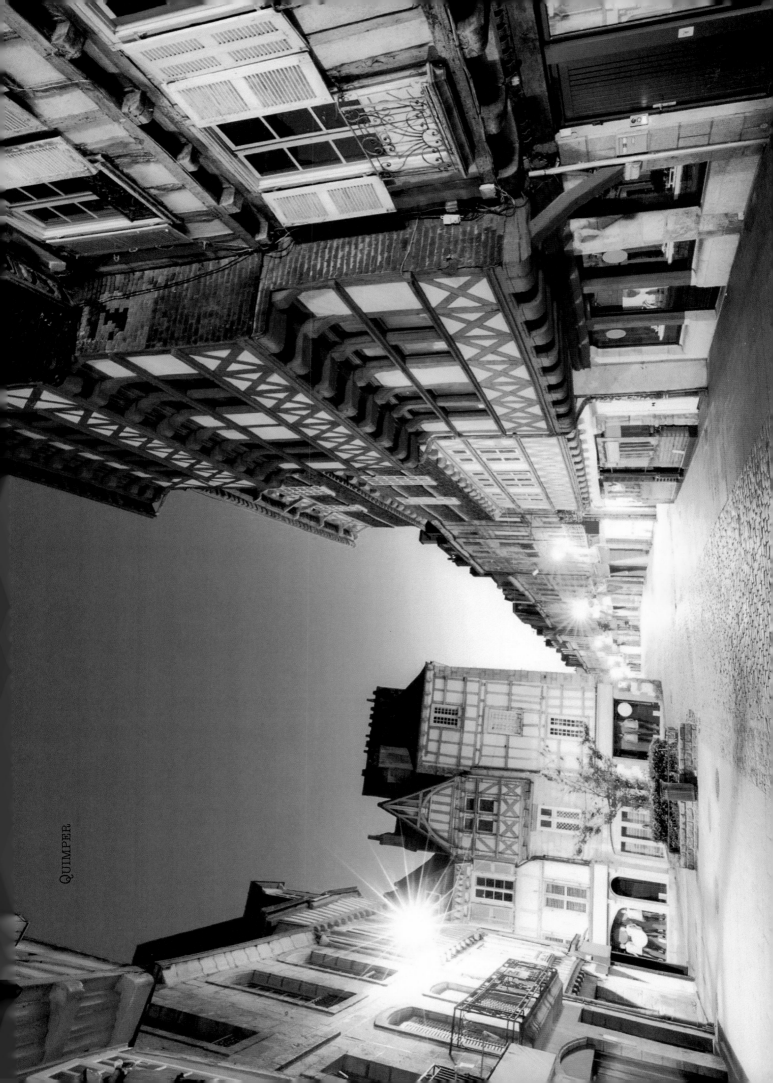

QUIMPER.

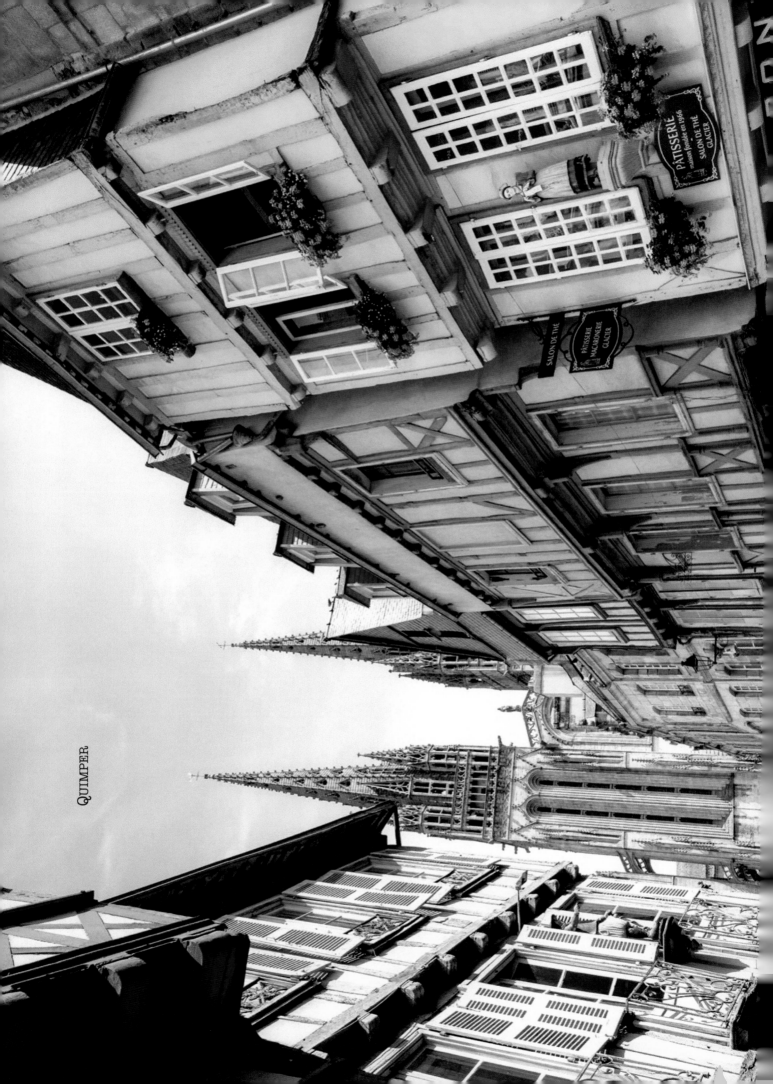

QUIMPER

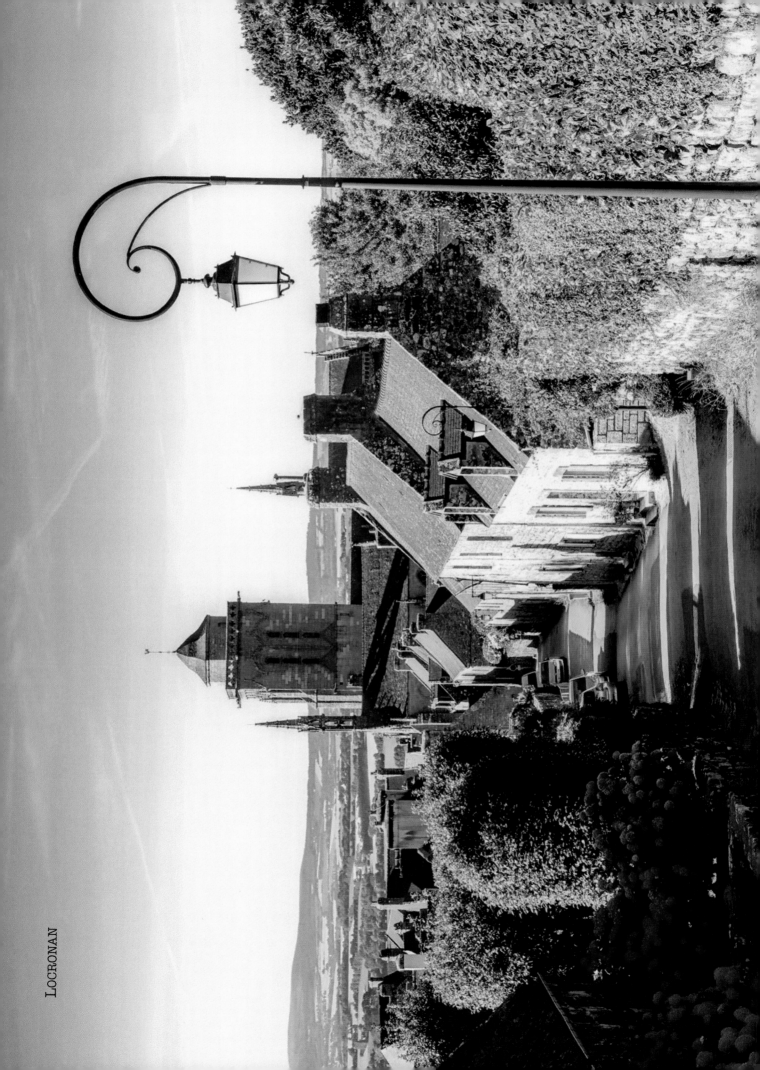

LOCRONAN

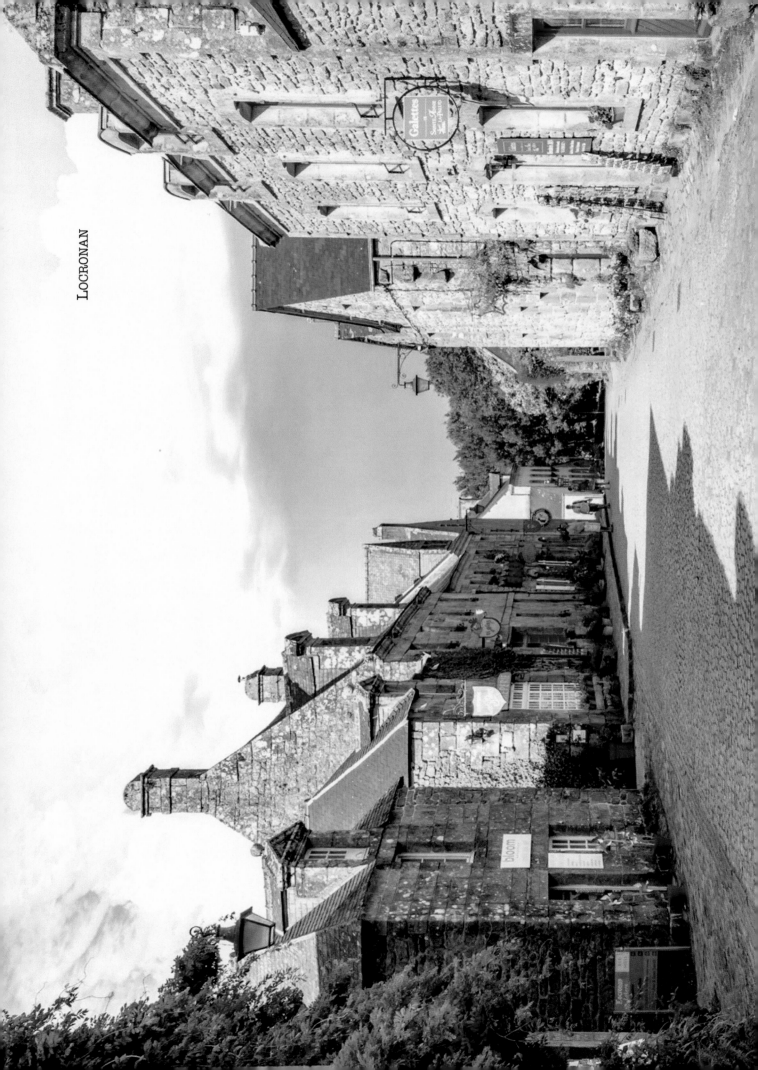

LOCRONAN

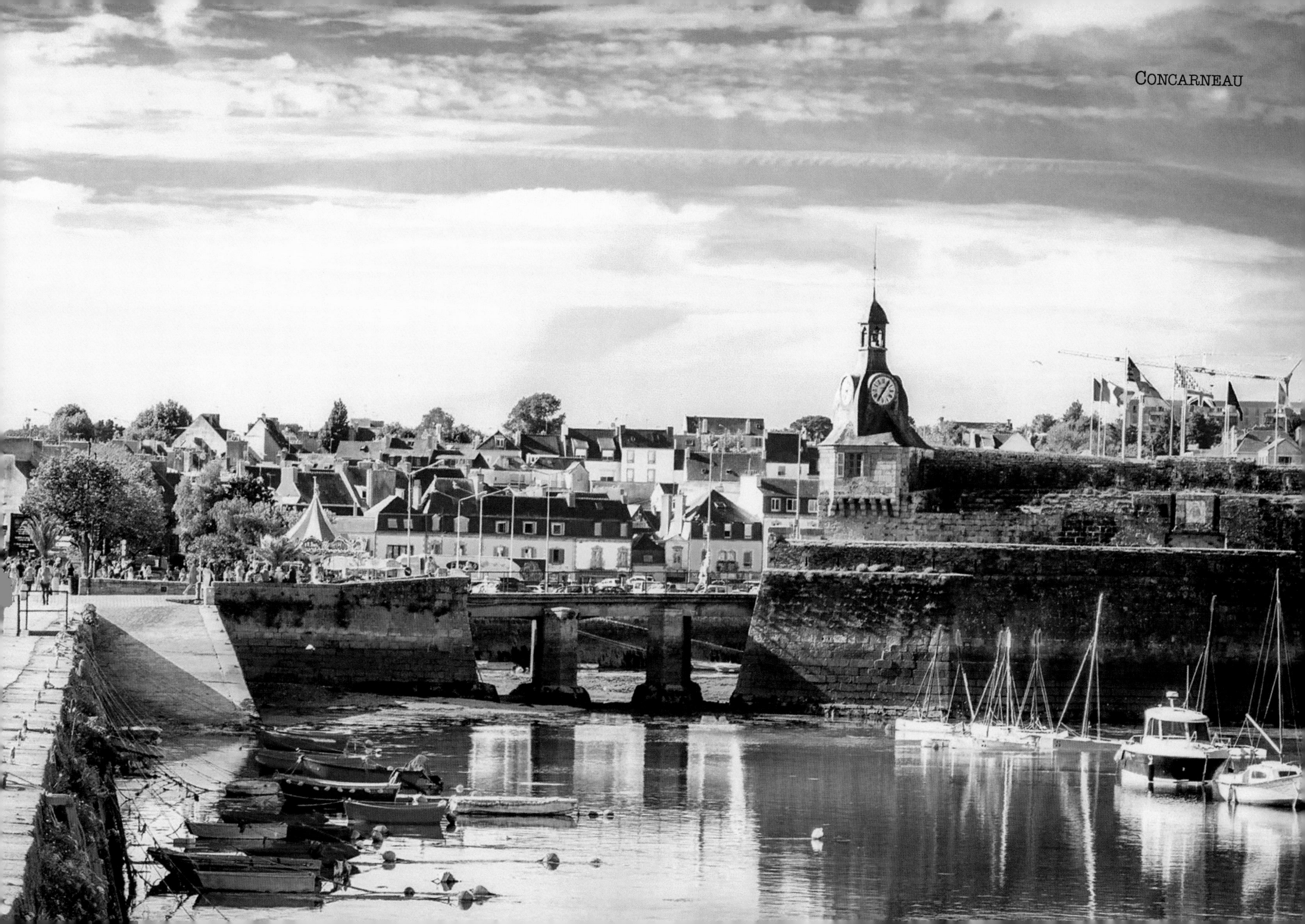
CONCARNEAU

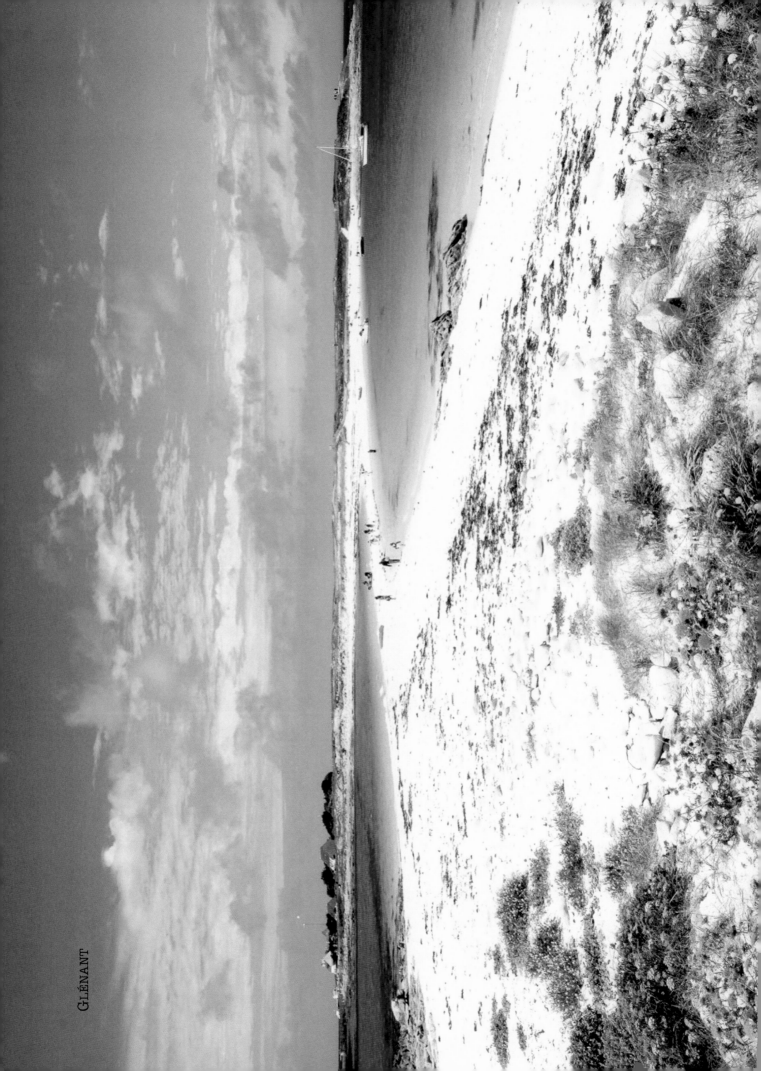

GLÉNANT

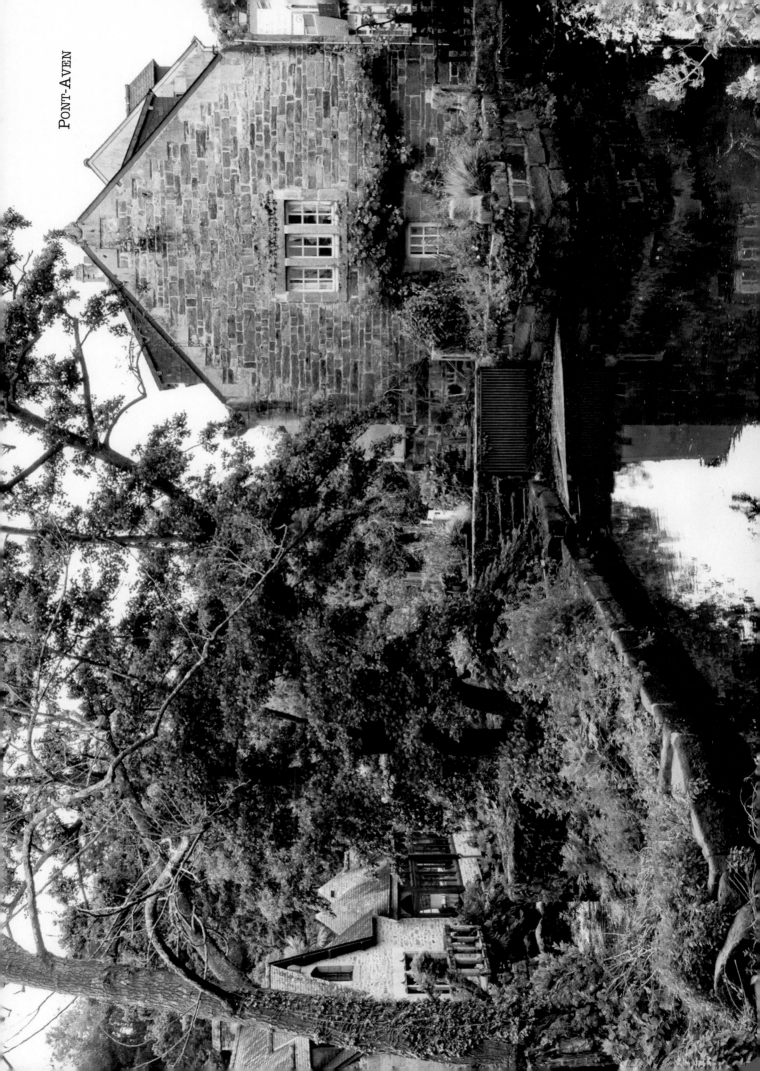

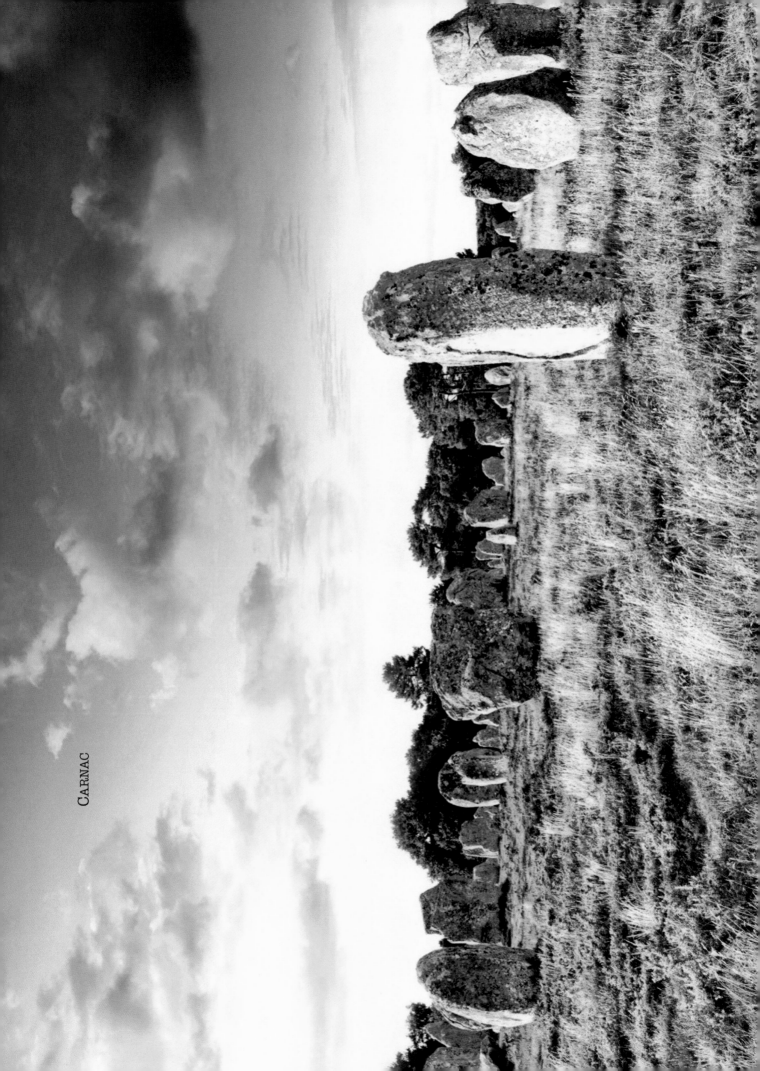

CARNAC

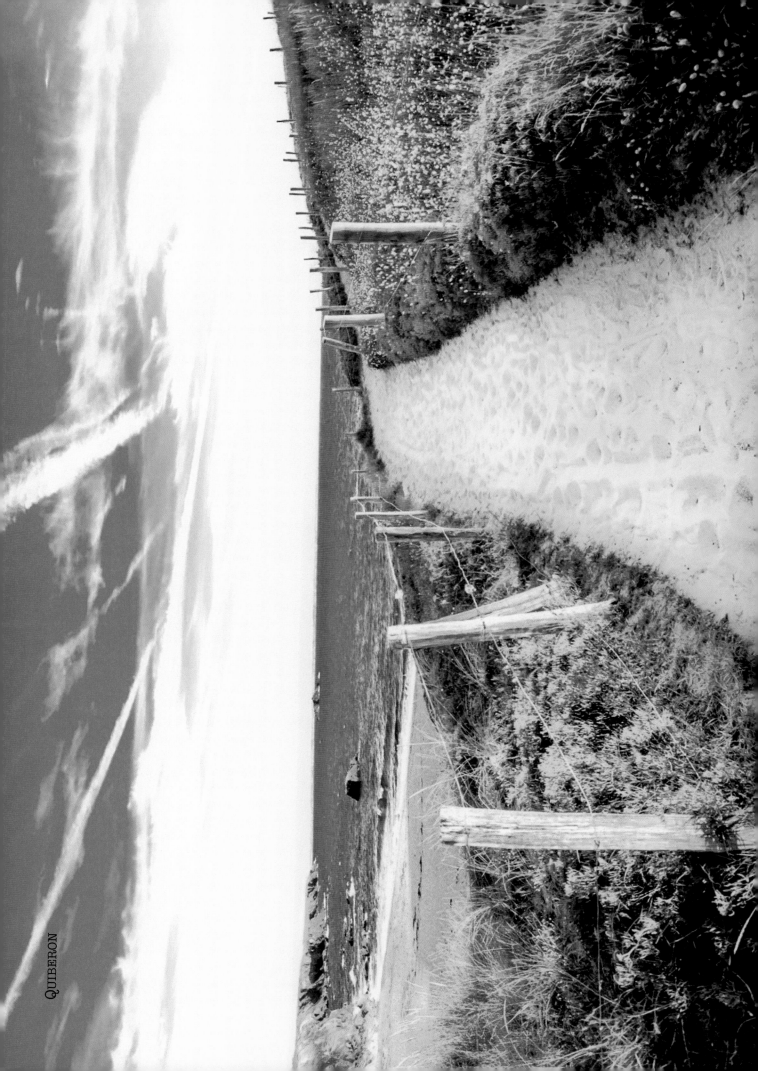

QUIBERON

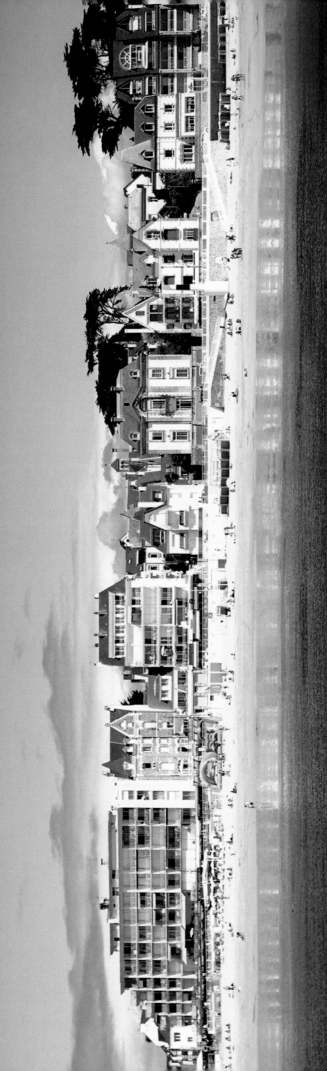

QUIBERON

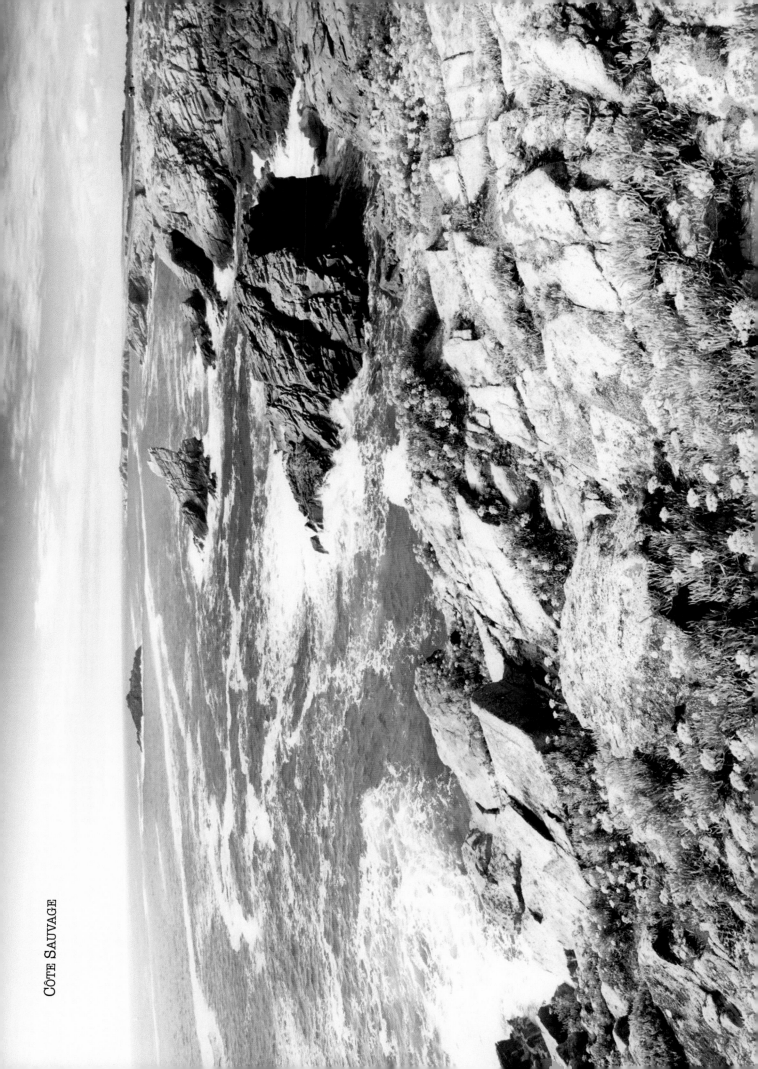

Côte Sauvage

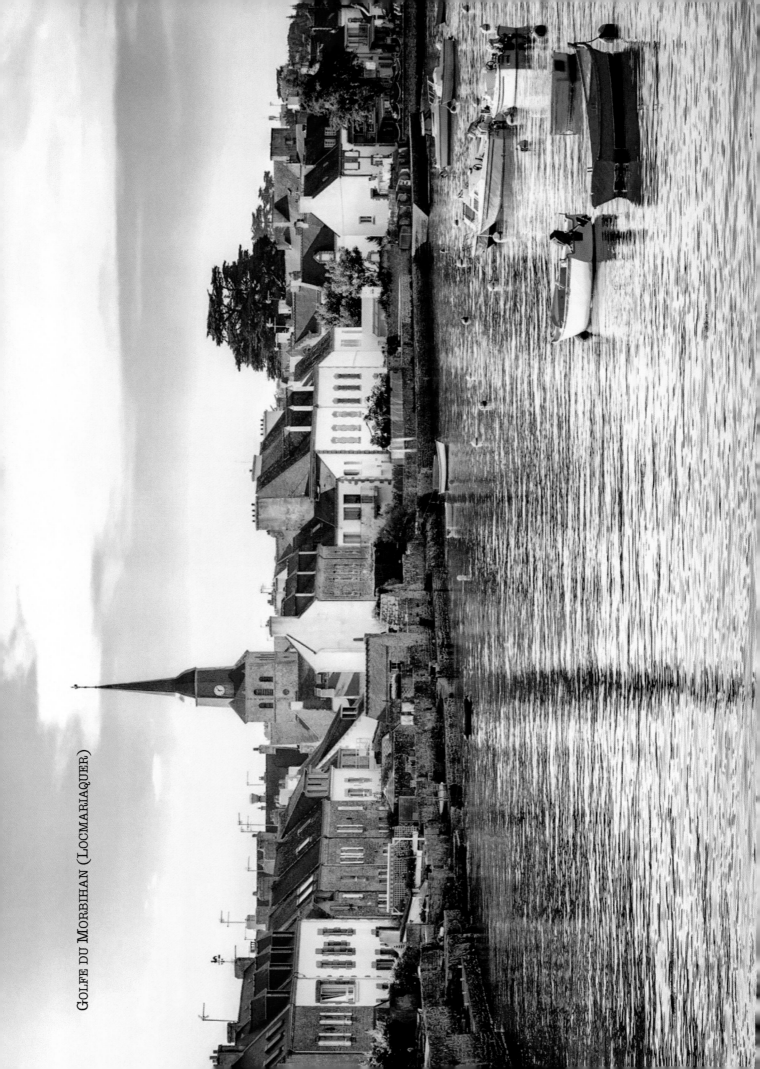

Golfe du Morbihan (Locmariaquer)

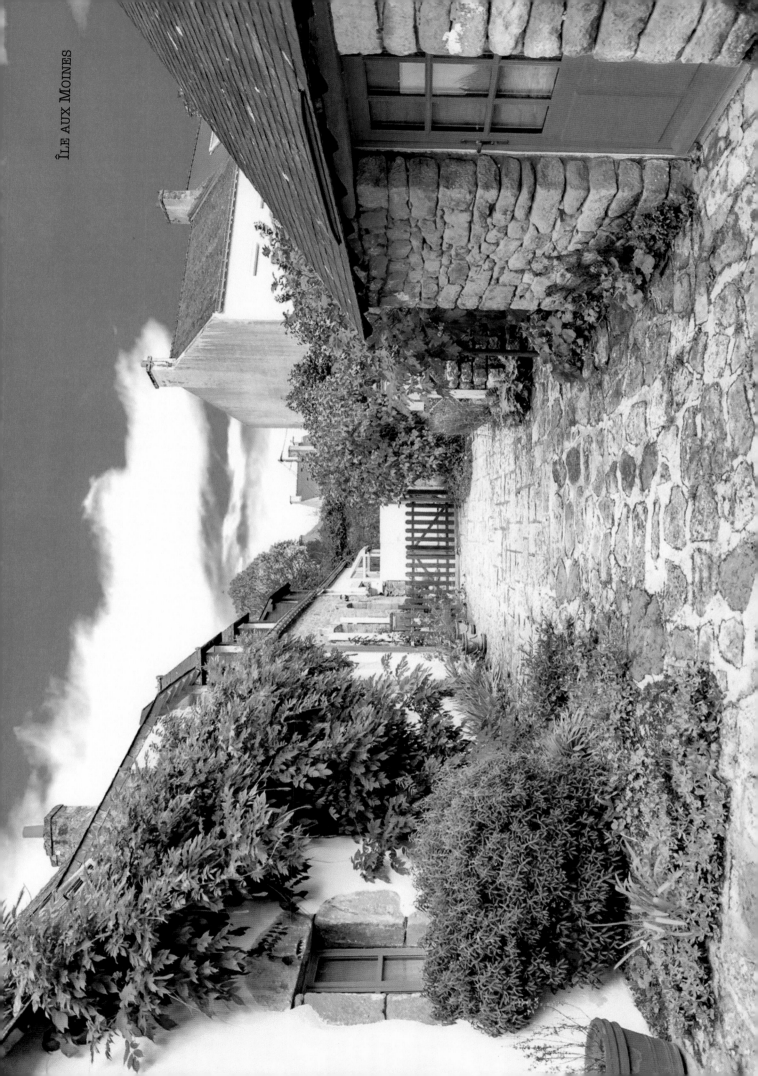

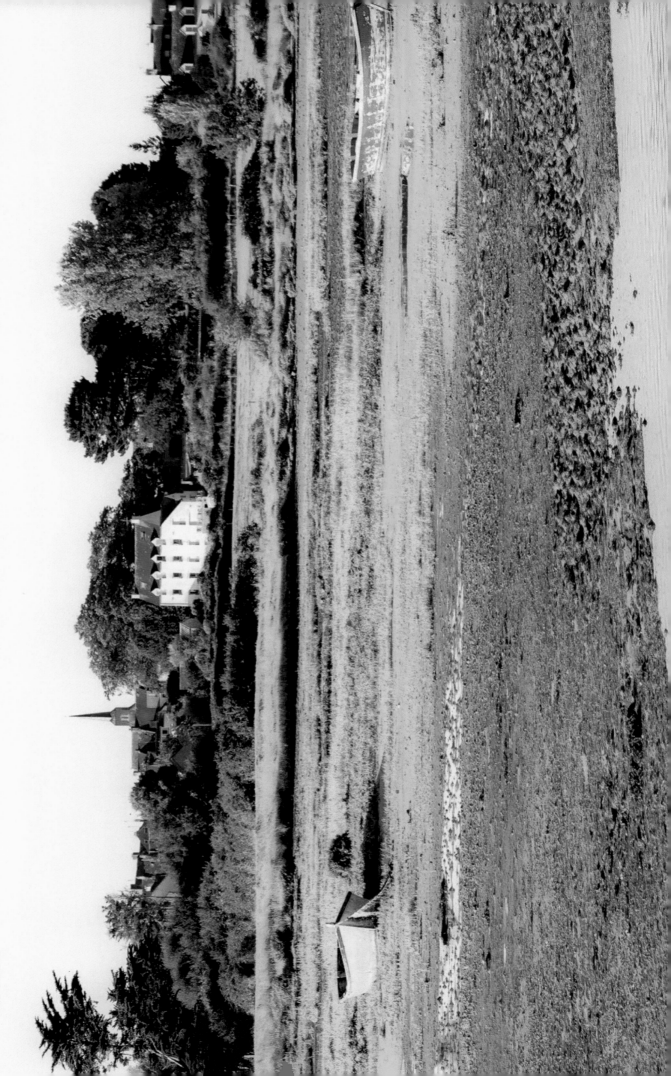

ÎLE D'ARZ

Belle Île en Mer (Sauzon)

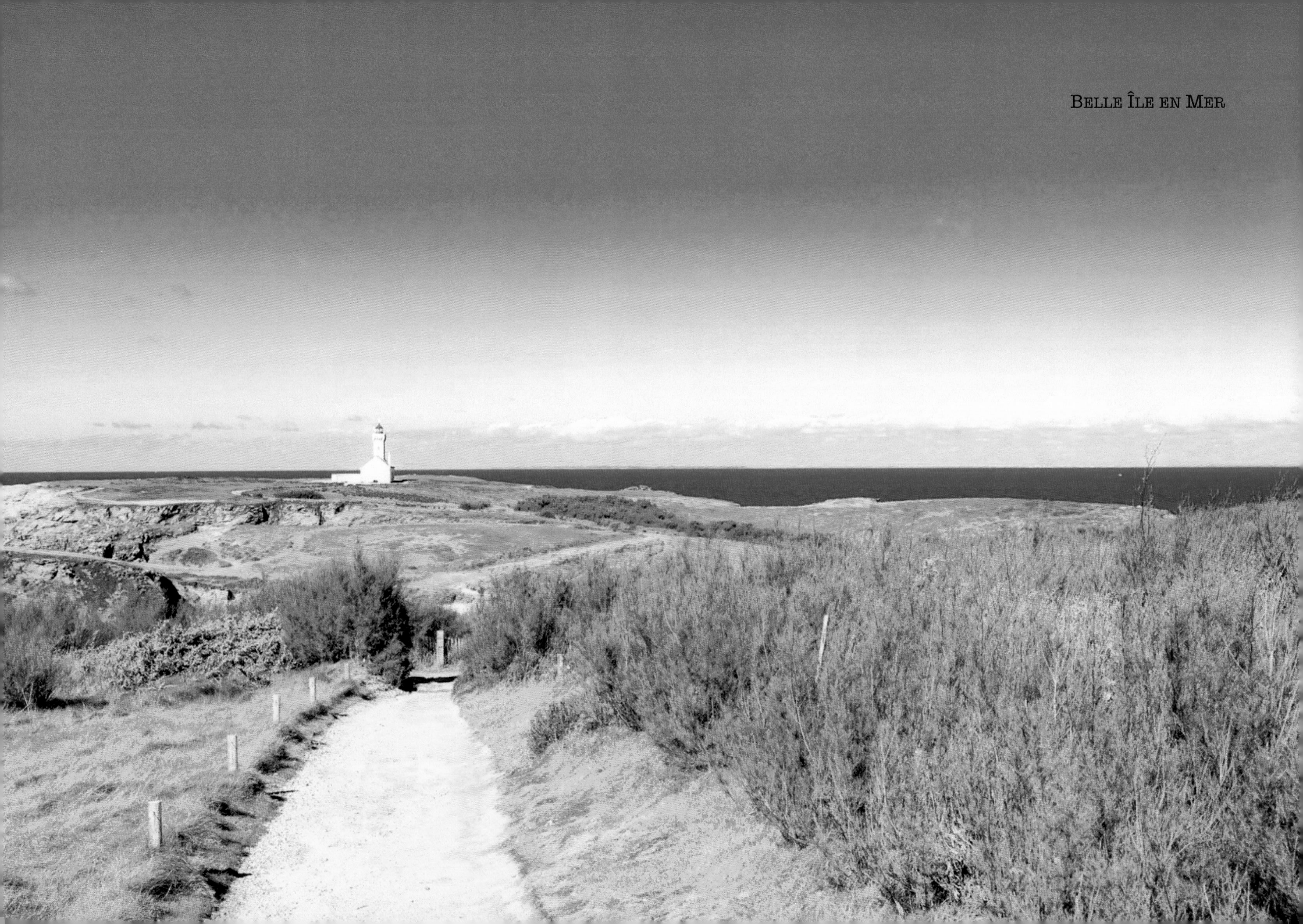

Belle Île en Mer

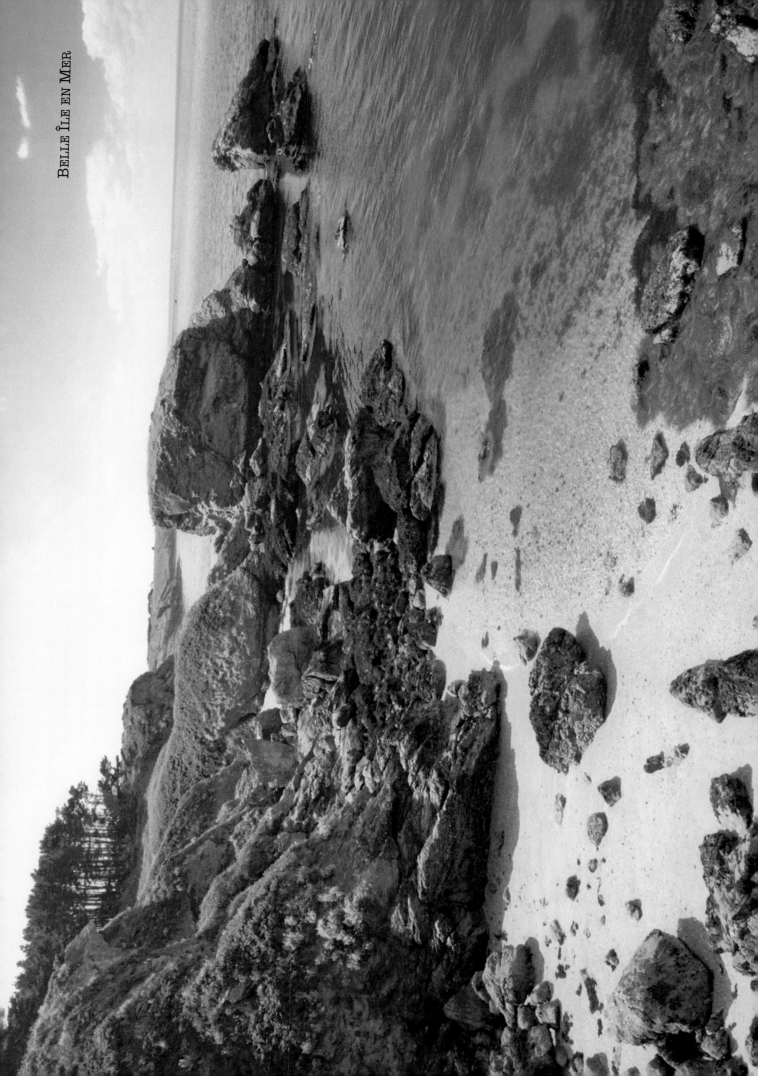

BELLE ÎLE EN MER

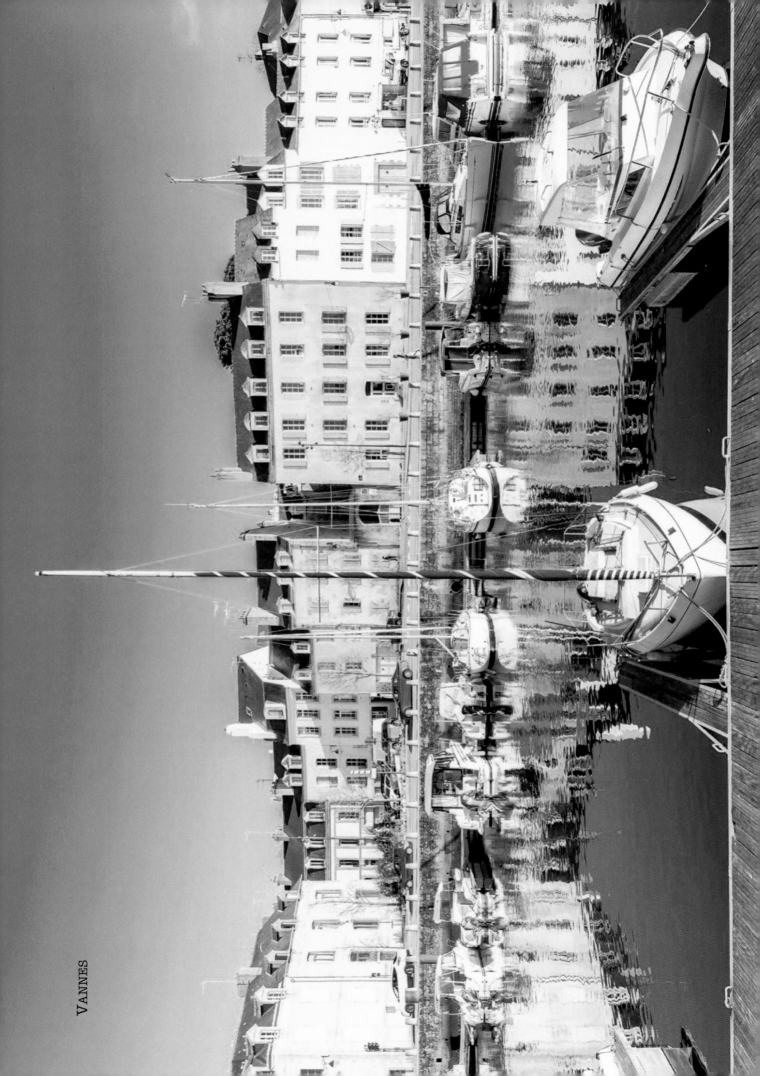

VANNES

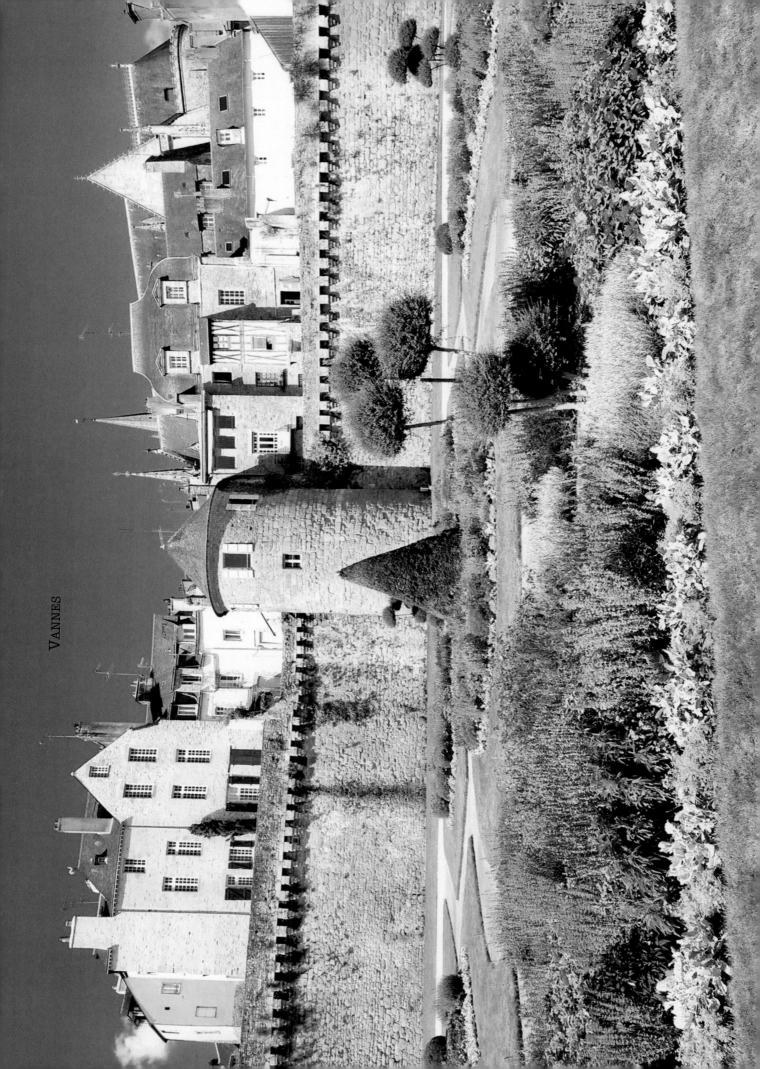

VANNES

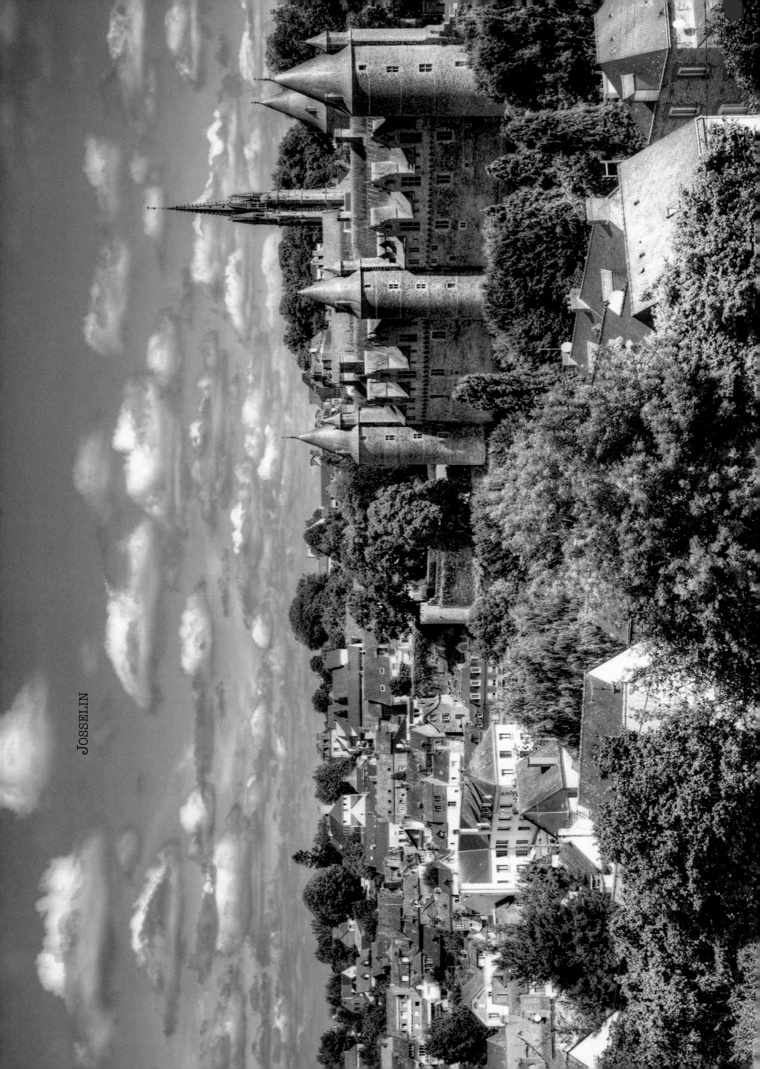

JOSSELIN

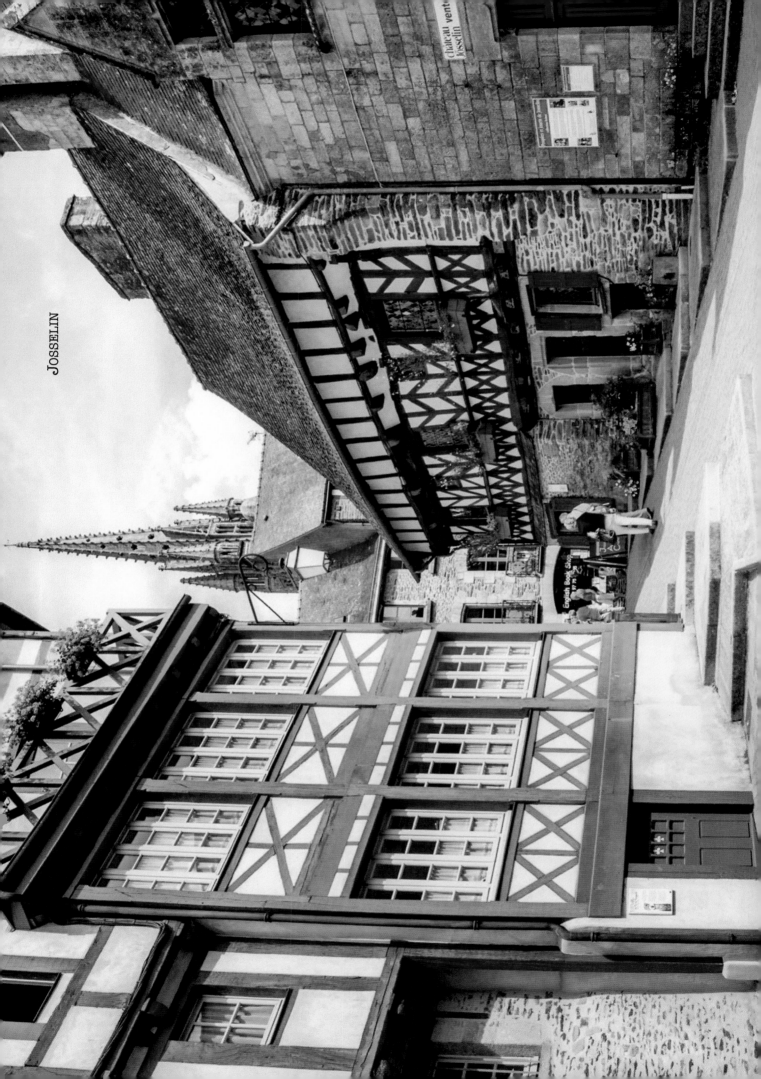

JOSSELIN

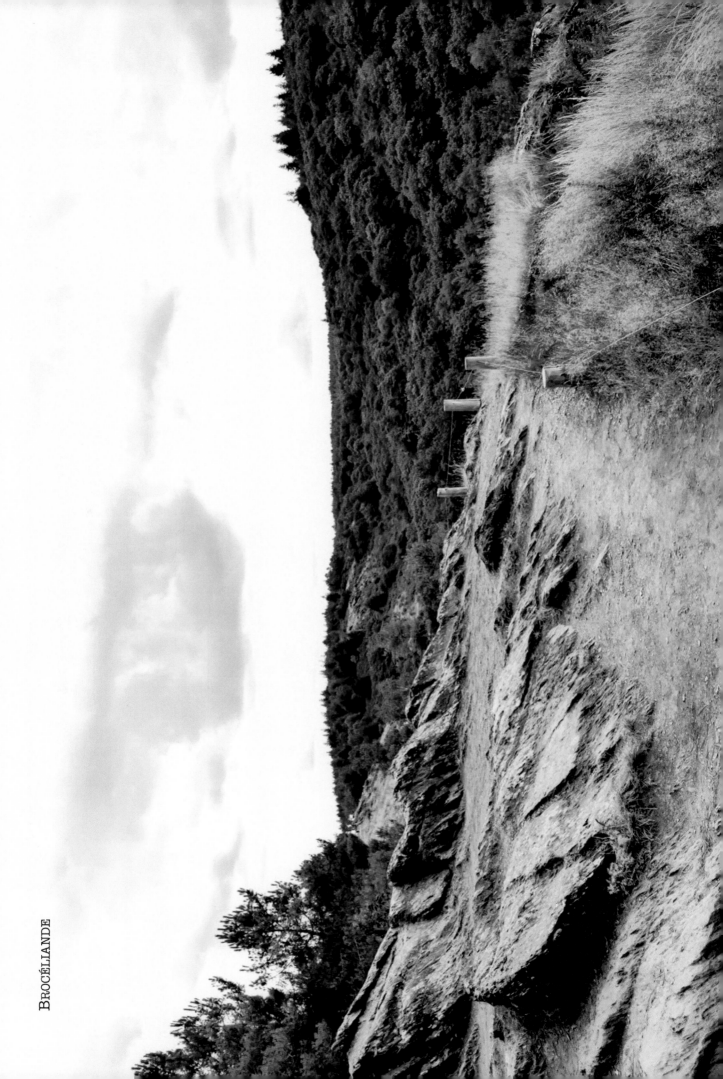

BROCÉLIANDE

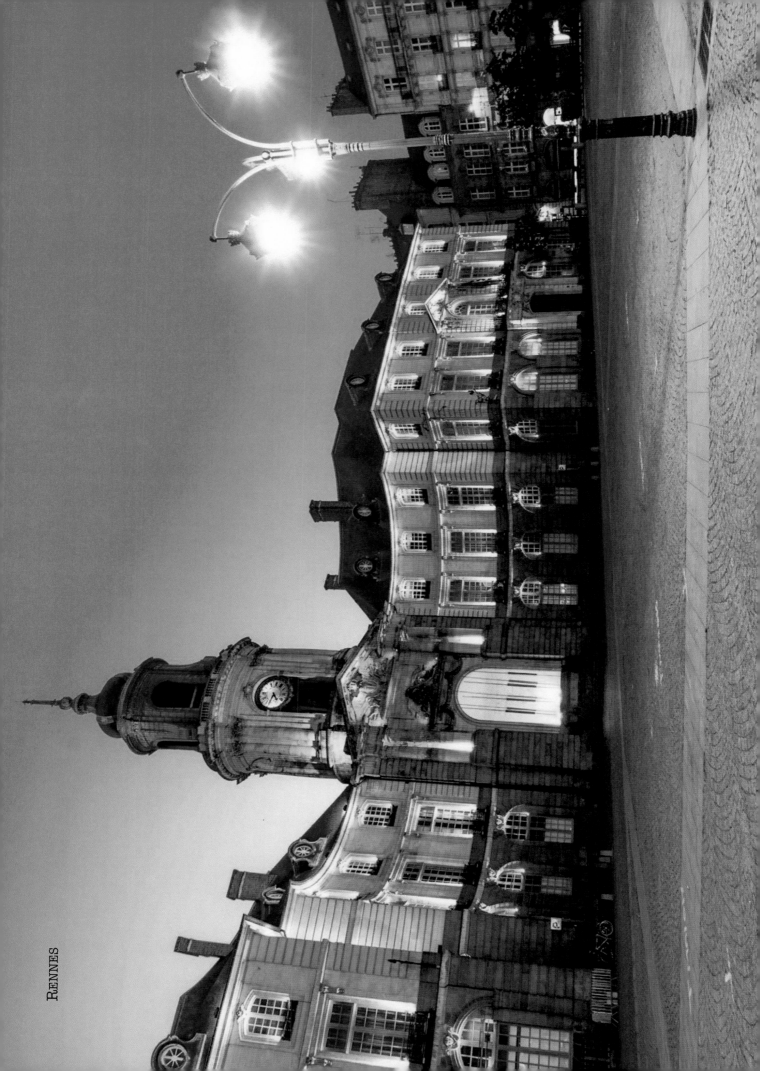

RENNES

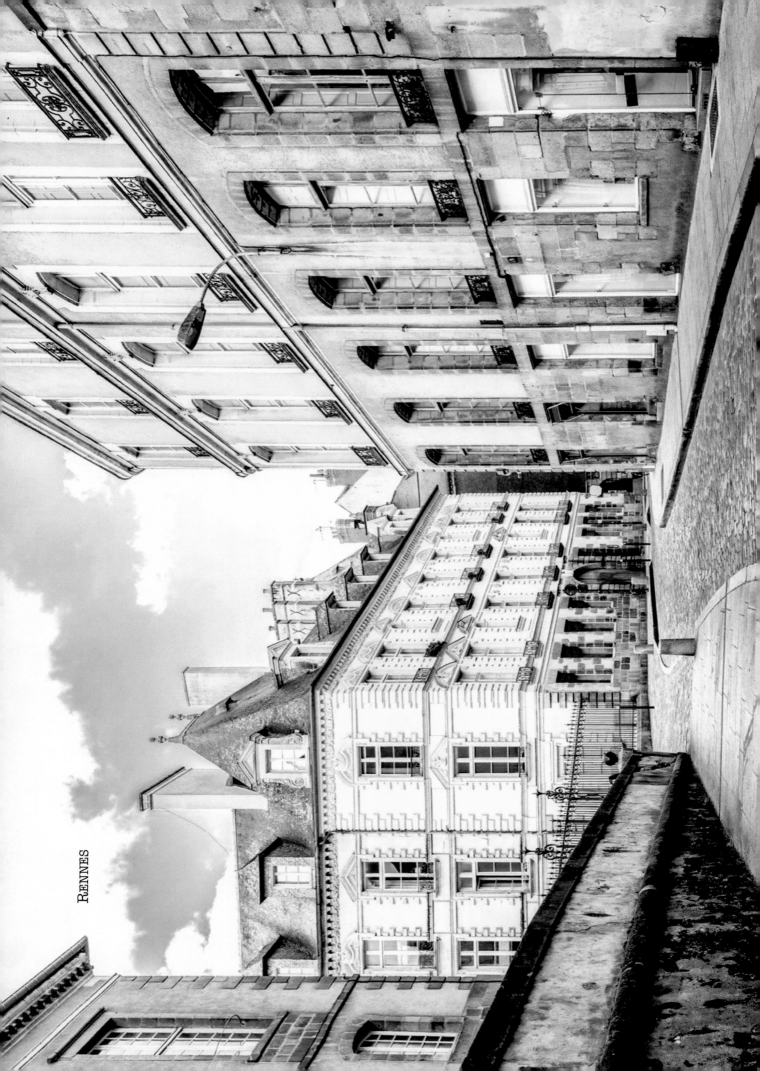

RENNES

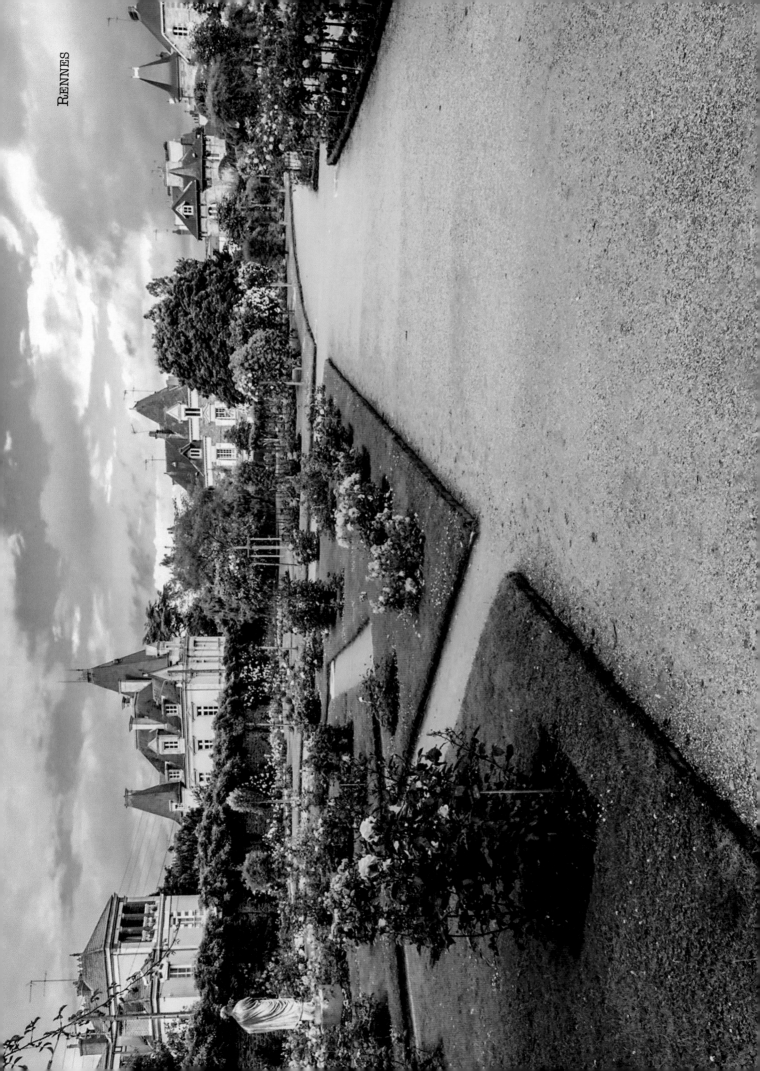

RENNES

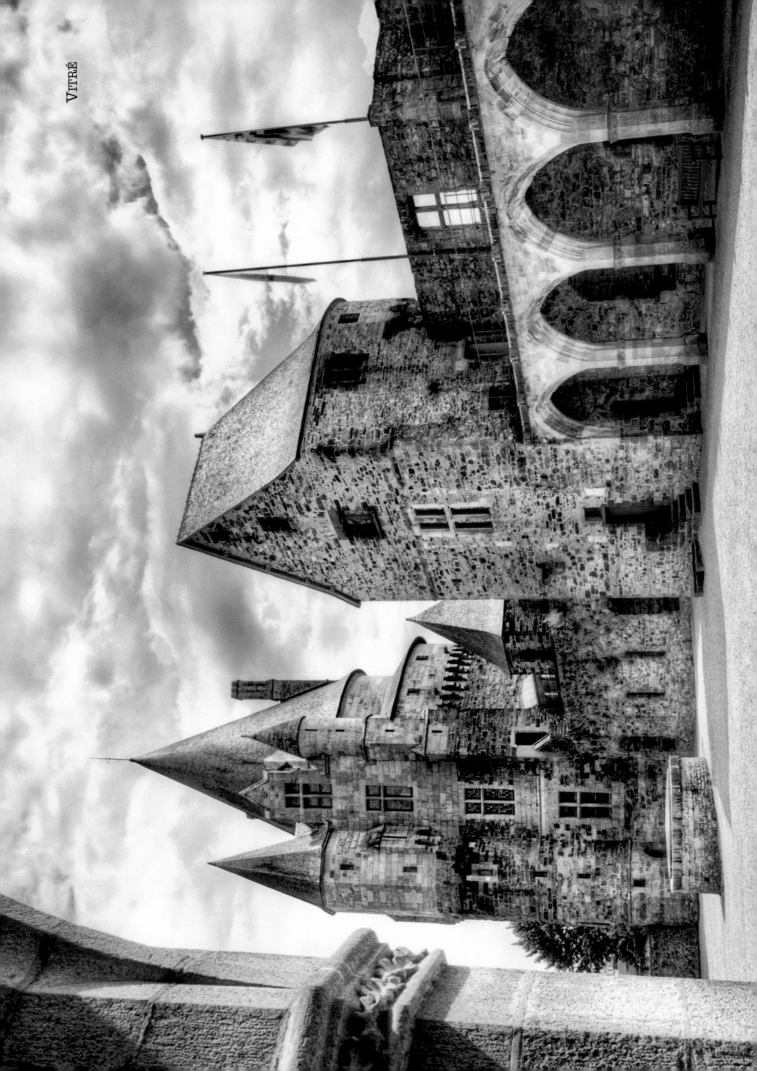

VITRÉ

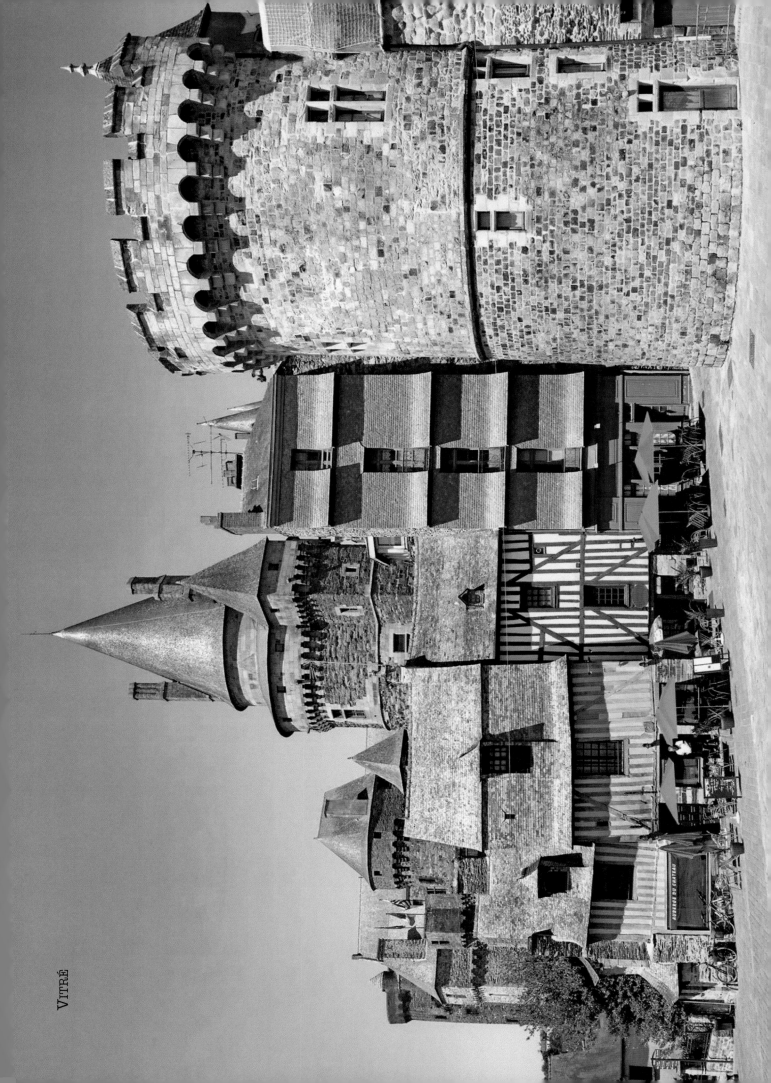

VITRÉ

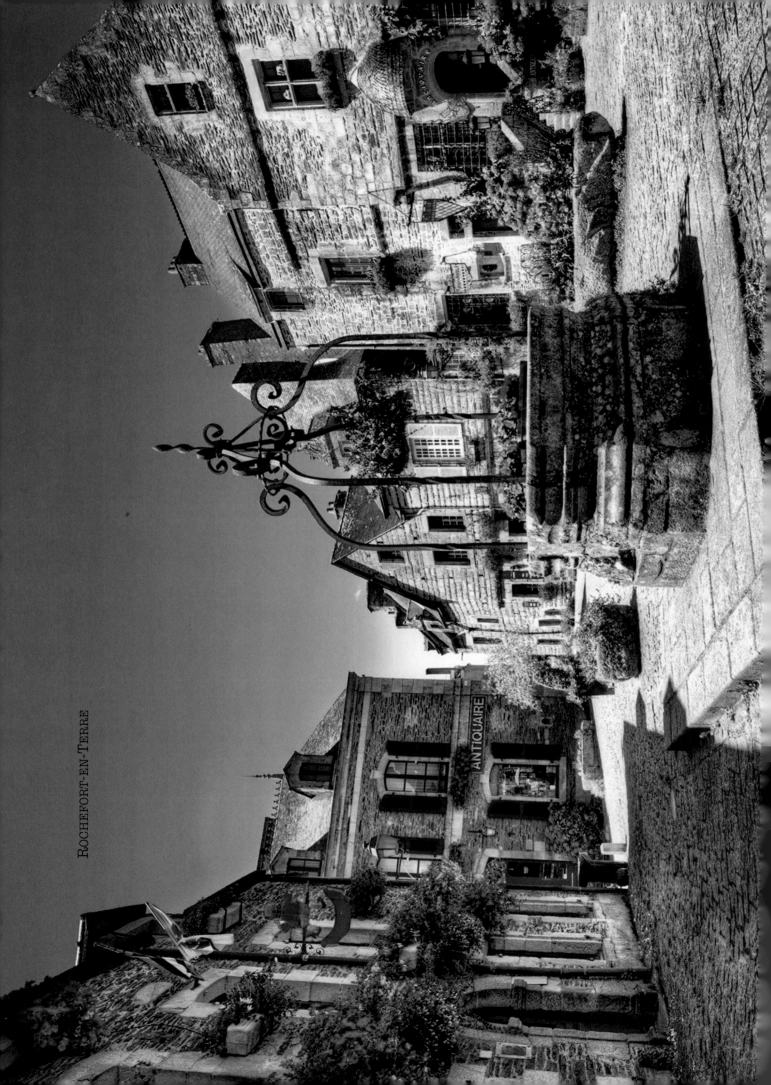

ROCHEFORT-EN-TERRE

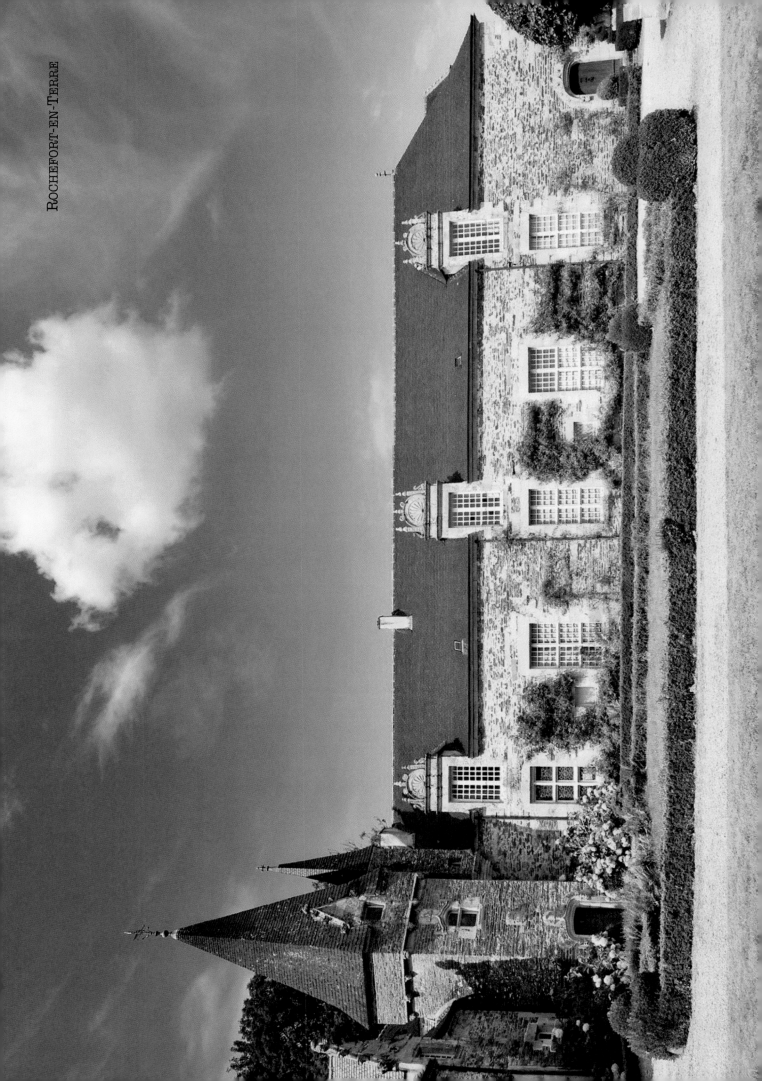

ROCHEFORT-EN-TERRE

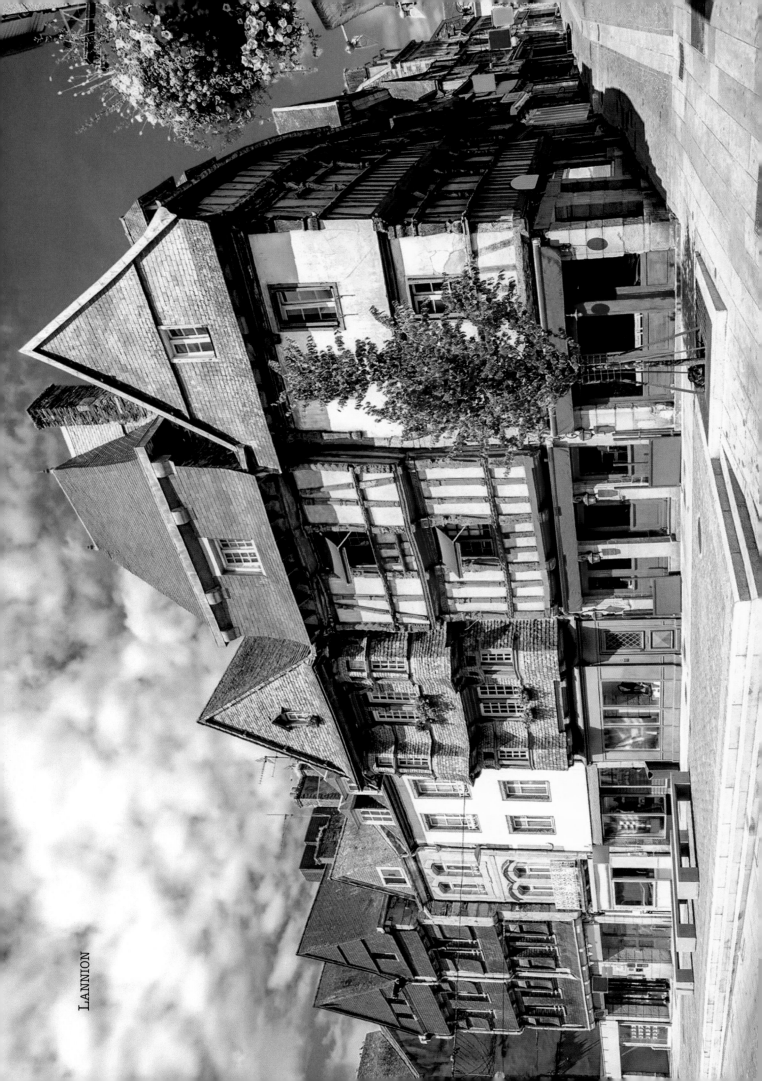

LANNION

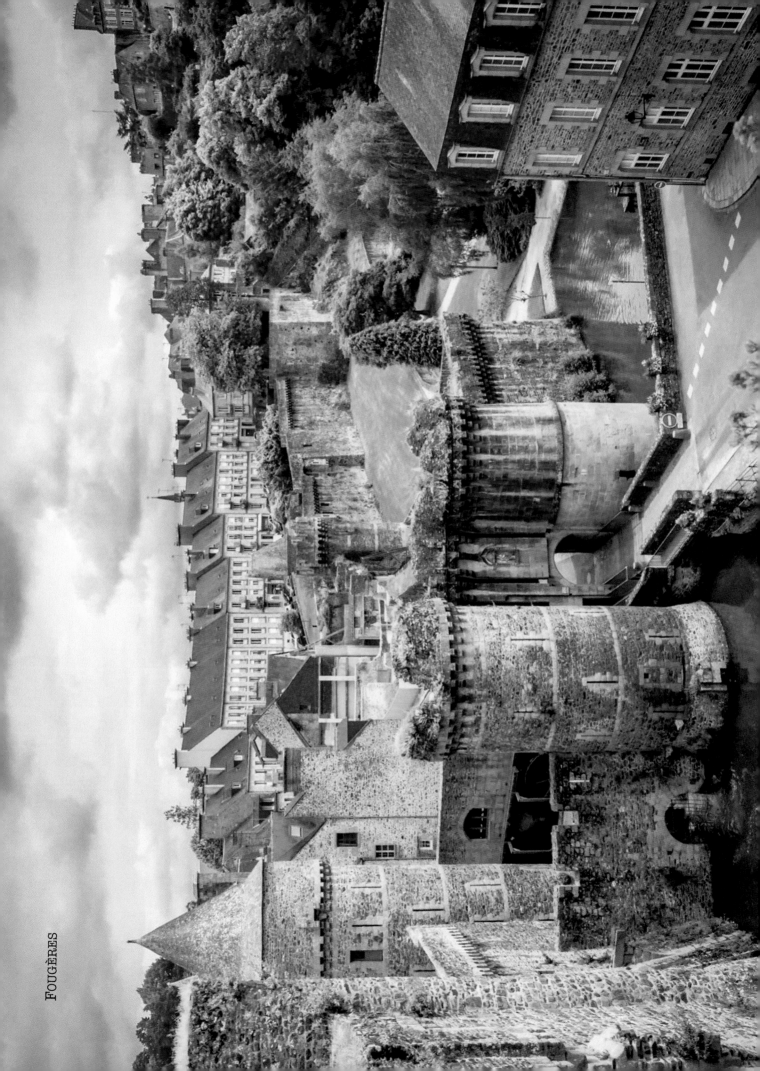

FOUGÈRES

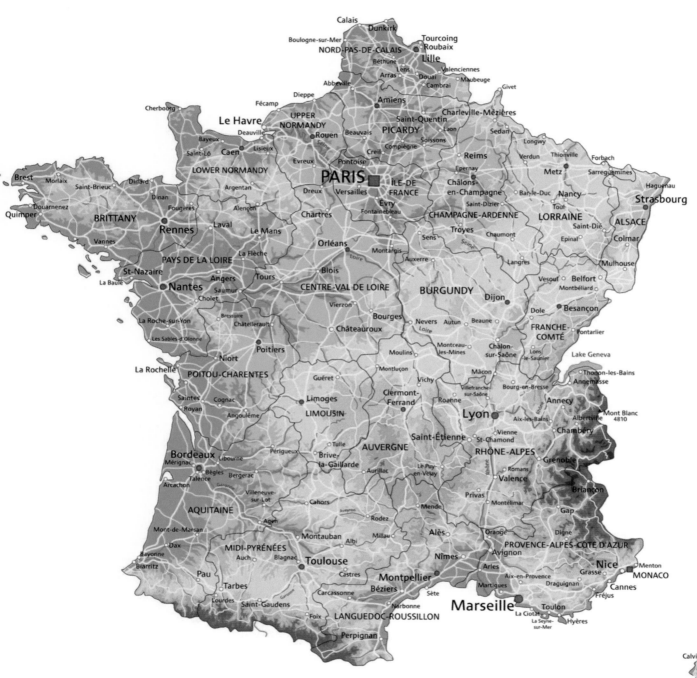

PHOTO CREDITS

Printed in Great Britain
by Amazon

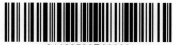